FORMS OF KNOWLEDGE

A Psychoanalytic Study of Human Communication

by

Anna Aragno, Ph.D.

PublishAmerica
Baltimore

First printing

ISBN: 1-60610-355-5
PUBLISHED BY PUBLISHAMERICA, LLLP
www.publishamerica.com
Baltimore

Printed in the United States of America

In dedication to Peter; beloved inspiration,
mentor, model, partner and guide.
Your patient listening and invaluable input
lives on in every page, as does
my undying love and passionate appreciation

"...we can know more than we can tell and we can tell nothing without relying on our awareness of things we may not be able to tell."

Polyanyi — 1964, p. X

TABLE OF CONTENTS

THE MORPHOGENESIS OF COMMUNICATIVE MODES AND REFERENTIAL FORMS

FOURTH MOVEMENT
PRINCIPLES OF APPLICATION

PREFACE

I was inspired to write this book while participating in a two-year supervisory training programme. One comes to this final step in psychoanalytic training as qualified practitioners, seasoned by years of personal, didactic, and clinical experience, only to find that what lies before, theoretically speaking, is still a vast expanse of uncharted terrain. This impressive new area of important phenomena, that recapitulates many clinical and group processes, provides a wealth of valuable data to be experienced, studied, observed and integrated into our metatheoretical framework.

The supervisory experience has been part of psychoanalytic training requirements since the founding of the Berlin Institute in the 1920's when the "Kontroll-Analyse" or "Analysen-Kontrolle," (so named in 1937) was still conducted by the candidate's own analyst. Many years later, considerable interest in the powers and pitfalls of this situation has focused discussions on its specific function in the overall scheme of training. These ongoing debates helped clarify the frame, contract and educative goals of this special psychoanalytic dialogue and a considerable body of literature has resulted. Yet, to date, only a few select supervisory training programs have been established specifically to study the supervisory process. I was fortunate to be part of a comprehensive program which, in addition to readings, lengthy supervisory case discussions and the supervised practice of supervision, also provided on-site observation opportunities. For two years, biweekly, we observed colleagues conducting supervisory sessions with a variety of supervisees through a one-way mirror in a room nicknamed the "fishbowl." These observed sessions were followed immediately by group discussions.

On these occasions, which lent themselves so beautifully for research purposes, I was struck by the vividness with which diverse unconscious transmissive processes and dynamic undercurrents became manifest. Amidst the heightened anxiety generated by the "fishbowl" experience, in the vital presence of tense process-narratives and tentative educative interchanges between novice supervisors and novice therapists, the rich dialogues that were engendered — replete with enactive, inductive, collusive, defensive, and parallel processes — provided an array of new experiential data. I adopted this situation for my observations since the conflicting goals of practice and research often render their simultaneous combination incompatible. And while the entire supervisory framework provides fertile conditions for the investigation of unconscious communications and collusive blind spots, nowhere was the interrelationship between these and diverse forms of affect-transmission and narrative forms more striking than during the observed sessions. My observations of the interactive phenomena within this triadic field, and how I understood their implications for teaching and learning the psychoanalytic attentional stance; understanding the processes of clinical and supervisory dialogues; examining semiotic progressions involved in making the unconscious conscious and, above all, adopting the psychoanalytic semantic as an epistemological window through which to identify the shifting morphology of human meanings, is the essence of this work.

The ideas that are developed in this book were crystallizing toward the end of the first year of the program as I began giving serious thought to the power and diversity of the multiple forms of unconscious communications that I was observing and discussing. These yielded a wealth of experiential information as unconscious interactive patterns from the clinical dyad and triadic supervisory dialogues permeated the group process, palpably impacting on the dynamics of the discussions that ensued immediately afterwards. My observations were guided and informed by principles of semiotic progression set forth in a previous revisionary effort (Aragno, 1997) in which was proposed a developmental model of mind based on the microgenetic steps of symbolization. These functional progressions can be traced phylogenetically, ontogenetically, and in microgenetic recapitulations of semiotic mediation in dialogues designed to make the unconscious conscious. More than merely an orienting backdrop, however, the conceptual framework in which this model is embedded proved encompassing enough to systematize a whole range of interactive phenomena, and had the explanatory power to illuminate and organize many more. The recasting of the topographical model into viable principles for how what is unconscious becomes conscious provides a unifying template for method and metatheory, gathering many conceptually disparate elements into one primary system of ideas.

Freud's prescience led him to uncover a method that is a "conversation." In this, and in his pluralistic metapsychology, he anticipated the philosophical *zeitgeist* and humanistic science to which we have access today by one hundred years. His expressed wish was that those who followed would continue to update and advance the science of psychoanalysis by daring to modify the conceptual underpinnings of a scientific paradigm that, he lamented, had not served him well enough. Today this is truer than ever. The old conceptual framework does not accommodate the full range of phenomena the method has illuminated. The proposed new model of the "mind's work"- or "symbolization"- rests in a paradigm of form and transformation, of pattern, design, and changing organizations of experience within the mutually impacting world of vital, interacting systems. This shift necessitates a radical reconsideration of the phenomena that are truly *relevant* to the science of psychoanalysis from a perspective which, as Freud intended, relates methodological stance to explanatory principles for how the method works.

As a point of entry, the study of psychoanalytic dialogue leads back to an examination of human communicative and interactive forms resulting in a more courageous integration of biology with the psychological findings of our method. This integration produces a genuine paradigm shift, a larger more fundamental metatheoretical reorientation, with significant epistemological implications. In turn, this allows psychoanalysis to include within its metatheoretical purview important phenomena that have been scrupulously excluded for their "unscientific" connotations, such as the reality of emotional-cognitions, the unspoken transmission of different kinds of information or telepathy, the transient dedifferentiation, or primal sharing, of the 'aesthetic' experience, the repetitive transfer of unconscious dynamisms — of forms, frequencies and patterns as *informing,* through different channels and in different ways. Readily recognized as the stuff of which psychoanalysis is made, these types of interaction—the underbelly of human experience and sentience—have yet to be integrated into a comprehensive framework that can demystify their regular occurrence in our semantic fields.

Consider the lacunae: to date, we have no integrated theory of affects despite their close connection to communication at the start of life, or of language and the therapeutic action of dialogue in our method of cure. Despite the outstanding benefits of a deeply transforming tripartite training approach we have no acknowledged theory of learning, tracing the confluence of soma and psyche as they interdigitate at all levels of human functioning. More seriously, despite the fact that we delve and dwell in a realm of "depth" phenomena, we lack a sufficiently comprehensive conceptual map for the simultaneity and interpenetrative frequencies of "the unconscious." Nor do we have an adequate vocabulary to identify its multiple dimensions or denote the fluid properties and qualities of the dynamically resonating fields of influence that are its phenomenological soil. We have remained curiously caught in the paradox of the practice of a transforming dialogical method that lacks a serviceable metatheory to encompass the ineffable quality of what we do daily.

But initial questions led only to further questioning: and as I searched for answers in ontogenetic roots I found instead that I was forced to face larger epistemological problems, to look at *how* we know what we know, at the sensory and semiotic sources of meaning-construction, and at the different channels of reception through which diverse forms of information are assimilated and understood. In short, I was forced to recognize that psychoanalytic methodology provides an epistemological lens to view the ways in which different kinds of knowledge are constructed, and the personal means by which we apprehend what we know

This line of thinking led to far reaching questions such as the nature of knowledge itself, the constitutive differences between unconscious and conscious communications and the diverse modes of responsiveness each engenders; the possible phylogenetic origins of these forms, how they can be traced ontogenetically, and how this relates to the mediation of consciousness and manifestations of change in our therapeutic method; the constitutive nature of empathy and insight; the impact of context purpose and discourse-referentiality on mind, and how these shape our accounts of experiences, influencing both channels of communication as well as narrative structures; the co-construction of meaning through contextual referents...all interrelated issues of enormous complexity and relevance to the psychoanalytic endeavor and to understanding of the art of interpretive dialogues

Needless to say, the more I observed and thought, the vaster did the topic appear. From an organismic perspective, human communication is always a reflection of the entire person; all the more so in semantic fields where *everything* is taken to be meaningful. A psychoanalytic study of communication, from an organismic/developmental perspective, would consider the underlying functional organization that is tied to each mode of interaction, beginning at the outset of life, and would then trace the mediational stages or steps that take place during language acquisition and socialization. This implies that communication and acculturation in development are closely connected, interwoven into psychic structure and that perhaps, via similar avenues, the power of dialogue continues to exert a quite formidable impact on inner organization. It also implies that the morphology of communicative forms reflects corresponding enduring modes of experience that are not necessarily lexically determined and that only psychoanalytic situations explicitly make conscious. Accordingly, this study is guided by semiotic principles that correlate with psychoanalytic discourse processes of therapeutic gain.

Given the obvious centrality of communication in psychological development, and in the psychoanalytic method, I wondered how such a conceptual schism as that between mind and communication could have come about since one emerges out of the other and, at some point, the two are one. Communication *is* the expression of mind and of personality; there had to be, I reasoned, a comprehensive system uniting the two. I also wondered why communication *per se* has received so little focused attention in psychoanalysis and why so many different kinds of unconscious meanings are still swept loosely under the broad rubric of non-verbal.

It has become customary in psychoanalysis to adopt terms for concepts that are loosely defined or multiple, unclear meanings: "intersubjectivity," "symbolized and un-symbolized transference," "projective identification," "countertransference," "empathy," even "insight" and "interpretation" are a few such words serving overly broad definitions, unattached to clearly articulated psychological principles. On occasion I have found it necessary to question their precise meanings and have tried to identify their referents in *operative* rather than *descriptive* term. Taking the liberties of a creative, revisionist approach, wherever needed I have devised differentiated terms for increasingly differentiated phenomena, some borrowed from music.

From the latter half of the past century leading figures from various disciplines have called for a unification of ideas underlying related areas of study as a way of bridging the unnatural discontinuity between biological, psychological and social processes. Psychoanalysis, in particular, requires this sort of synthesis and interdisciplinary foundation; the breadth of the bibliography reflects this. I am particularly indebted to my teachers and mentors for their encouragement and to the seminal works of Cassirer (1874-1953), Langer (1942, 1972), Werner and Kaplan (1963), Goodman (1984), Marshack (1972), Vygotsky (1934, 1978), Bakhtin (1981, 1984) and the father of sociobiology, E.O Wilson (1978); in psychoanalysis, to Freedman (1971, 1975, 1978) and T. Shapiro (1970, 1979, 1981, 1986, 1988, 1991) in addition to the Freudian opus, and to the research and ideas of the English evolutionary biologist, Rupert Sheldrake (1981, 1988, 1991), who has studied biological patterns of intraspecies information-transmission. Generalized ideas derived from an interdisciplinary foundation provide overarching concepts that are helpful to psychoanalysis. Communication is explored from a variety of psychosocial and cultural discourse domains, spanning multiple fields, in an overall developmental orientation that echoes the ideas of Werner and Vygotsky.

The developmental approach underlying this work, however, refers to a *general orientation*—a developmental paradigm—rather than ontogenetic study. In their opening remarks to the 14th Heinz Werner Lecture Series, Kaplan and Wapner (1981) illustrate this approach:

Convinced that developmental psychology is not merely a subject matter but is, rather, a manner of conceptualizing all psychological phenomena, Werner sought to encompass animal behavior, ontogenesis, pathological phenomena, products of collective activity, and behavior evoked in experimental situations, within a comprehensive system — a general psychology, grounded in the fundamental concept of development. (p.1)

Similarly, Vygotsky's (1978) methodological approach coincides quit remarkably with the psychoanalytic method:

> Our method may be called experimental-developmental in the sense that it artificially provokes or creates a process of psychological development. This approach is equally appropriate to the basic aim of dynamic analysis. If we replace object analysis by process analysis, then the basic task of research obviously becomes a reconstruction of each stage in the development of the process: the process must be turned back to its initial stages. (p. 61-62)

In recent years many symposia and publications have reflected increasing interest in the intimate and intense contact between therapist and patient beyond what is narrowly called *countertransference,* to paraphrase from a current brochure. Focus has moved to exploring moment to moment transient emotional experiences and intense states of mind in listening analysts, organized around making and losing contact, facilitating or impeding communication, feeling or being cut off, and the experience of attempting to engage someone with whom it is difficult to sustain contact. Awareness of this shift demands a reexamination not only of psychoanalytic technique but also of the range of interpretable referents: "communication" has undoubtedly come to the forefront. However, interactive and communicative phenomena are currently discussed primarily from a "relational" perspective in terms of the therapeutic *relationship* itself rather than in terms of the *forms of interactions* it lays bare. The point I will continue to stress throughout, is that it is not *relationship* per se that is of relevance to metatheory but the *nature of the interactive modes* and the *unconscious processes* highlighted in our semantic fields that constitute the "data" to be systematized by theoretical psychoanalysis. The predominant focus on clinical issues overshadows the need to integrate new phenomena into an updated conceptual framework—a metapsychology—sufficiently encompassing to accommodate them.

Accordingly, this study approaches psychoanalytic situations as specialized semantic fields, or discourse situations, that engender and highlight unconscious modes of interaction and transmission. From this approach derives a comprehensive model of forms of communication that reflects and corresponds with our current understanding of the psychical. In striving for theoretical synthesis and cohesion this work proposes principles of psychoanalytic thinking, teaching, and learning, which bring clinical and supervisory discourse-processes in line with the logical progressions of symbolic functioning in interpretive dialogues.

The seeds of this scientific and reflective endeavor are to be found at the source, in Freud's "auto-analysis." This well documented, halting and courageous introspective struggle, with its clearly marked phases of resistance, incubation and new insight, is the prototype for psychoanalytic inquiry; as the acorn to the oak tree, it is also a basic cognitive phenotype for the many genotypic branches that have stemmed from its singularly generative, interpretive epistemology — in training, practice, supervision, and research. What begins as a reflective process in the personal analysis, continuing privately via its own momentum, is the same analytic attitude and formulative effort that stimulates higher levels of symbolic thought, leading to verbalization and insight. I return to the many thematic leads thread through this introduction as ideas are developed and woven into the fabric of the book. This may be an apt place to add that I return again and again to Freud not because I wish to ignore all that has come since, but because Freud's goal was to devise a *general psychology* from psychoanalytic findings, a theory of mind, not only a *clinical* method.

Infact, one of Freud's major concerns regarding the future of psychoanalysis was that the 'therapy' not destroy the 'science'. Whatever his personal qualms about medicine, Freud explicitly laid out an ideal program of background studies for psychoanalysts, making it clear that neither the science nor practice of psychoanalysis are served by a medical degree. In his desire to see the scientific advancement of his methodology and metapsychology he specifically opened the terrain to broader intellectual discussion. At no time in its history has it become more pressing to place psychoanalytic phenomena within a compatible conceptual framework because at no other time has psychoanalysis been so widespread, so discredited, or at risk. Reformulations are not just desirable, they are *essential* for its continued credibility as an independent discipline, a valued treatment mode, and a science of mind.

I am keenly aware of Okham, wielding his razor of parsimony over my conceptual quandaries, yet the many complex issues raised in this Preface proved, in their development, to be anything but simple, or simple to unify. The fact that psychoanalysis is three things in one — a research method, a treatment mode and a general theory of mind — and when writing from a revisionist standpoint all three dimensions have to be encompassed more or less simultaneously, makes it all the more difficult. This may explain why despite the unanimous call for revisions, very few are attempted.

Since music and musical ideas inspire this work, the book is structured in the traditional four movements of classical symphonic form. Initially I wondered whether this was a devotional exercise, expressing my profound love and reverence for music or a deep seated need to shape my ideas into classical form. Only toward the end did I realize that it sprang from deeper source, and was a way of mapping out the formulation and exposition of a semantic of *significant* forms with meanings neither tied to, nor one with, language. A developmental model of human communication founded on principles of symbolization inevitably encompasses early pre-semiotic, sensory-affective forms of interaction, and even deeper transmissive pathways forming the enduring, ineffable underlay of human sentience. We have thereby ventured into the unexplored possibility of a "genuine semantic beyond the limits of discursive language," as Langer (1942, p.86) foresaw — a semantic, I would add, with which psychoanalysts are already familiar.

The musical form I had chosen to structure the book held up a mirror for me to identify the nature and substance of the problems of meaning I would be encountering in the development of its contents. Acutely aware of form Freud expressed similar ideas regarding the important interrelationship between form and content in dreams. His emphasizing the entire passage points to its importance; *"The form of a dream or the form in which it is dreamt is used with quite surprising frequency for representing its concealed subject-matter"* (1900, p. 332). Form may encapsulate and prefigure the essence of content in ways that are more immediate and succinct than the often laborious, linearizing processes of linguistic cogitation and exposition.

Turning to musical form and terminology for assistance in conveying new complex ideas, however, is an ancient and well worn habit. In medieval theology, Augustine(1973) sought melodic analogies to render the idea of God's will and design, and Kepler, similarly, invoked celestial choirs to describe the harmonious precision he observed in the moving firmament. The anthropologist Levi-Strauss (1964) made copious use of musical structure to illustrate his ideas on myth; the philosophers Langer and Goodman, and psychoanalysts such as Reik (1948), Kubie (1953) and Edelson(1075) all refer to music, some (like Edelson) even providing in-depth musical analyses to illustrate their points. My reliance on orchestral, instrumental and musical analogies has been a way of anchoring complex processes and concepts ill defined by words, fashioning a sustained metaphor for those ineffable sources of sentience and signification with which music is suffused.

And it is fitting, I believe, that such ideas should come from psychoanalytic thought. Psychoanalysis is the first interpretive method to formally operationalize a semantic inclusive of unconscious, sensory-emotive and directly transmitted meanings, the first epistemology to enable inference of their broad significance through phylogenetic reconstruction and neurophysiological mappings of the mind. This book confronts the fact that the field of semantics and the range of human meanings is broader, deeper, wider, by far, than that currently defined by words, and that language is not the only, or even the best, symbolism by which to understand all human meanings. A psychoanalytic developmental model of communication founded on logical principles of symbolization opens the door to a comprehensive theory of knowledge encompassing forms of *understanding* prior to and different from those designated by words. As far as I can see, it points to essential sources; to primal emotive patterns, the base metal out of which human meanings, perception, and experience—felt and expressed – issue; to the morphology of expressive form, of which music and dreams are the purest reflection. And it does so considering both the aesthetics and therapeutics of interpretative dialogues. Already in 1942, Langer wrote:

> Discursive thought gives rise to science, and a theory of knowledge restricted to its products culminates in the critique of science; but the recognition of non-discursive

> thought makes it possible to construct a theory of *understanding* that naturally culminates in a critique of art. The parent stock of both conceptual types, of verbal and non-verbal formulation, is the basic human act of symbolic transformation. The root is the same, only the flower is different. (p. 148)

She claimed such questions for her own field, declaring them to be *philosophical* in nature, "requiring logical study, and involving music:"(1942, p. 219) for she believed that to be able to "define 'musical meaning' adequately, precisely, but *for an artistic, not a positivistic context and purpose,*. . . is the touchstone of a really powerful philosophy of symbolism" (Langer, 1942, p. 219). But the conditions for discovering a "language of music" or of 'significant form' of any other sort than language" (Langer, 1942, p. 219), given the work here undertaken, lies squarely in the province of psychoanalytic investigation, whereby the study of human expressive formulations and the communication of unconscious meanings may be articulated in the logical terms of symbolization, through which interrelationships between form and content are most clearly exhibited. My desire to write a symphonic book then proves to be a compromise between an impetus to formulate my understanding and another to express my formulation.

More importantly, it is a way of honoring the conceptual centrality of interrelationships between form and content, a metatheoretical leitmotif that pervades the thinking underlying this work. Like symphonic music, the instrumentation of human communication is a polyphony of sounds, feelings, thoughts and expressions, multitoned, multistratal, multidetermined. The whole emerges out of condensations of many diverse strains and timbres. We who listen and observe must remain open to the entire spectrum of contributing moods, sounds and instruments, regardless of how dissonant or discordant they may appear. And we must ourselves learn how to keep such channels of resonance and attunement open to the entire orchestration — from the slimmest sliver of a sound to the loudest, most strident — to be sensitive to the slightest modulation or transposition, all of which contribute to the sonorous outcome of a meaningful whole.

FIRST MOVEMENT

PRESENTING PROBLEMS, ORIENTING PROPOSITIONS

We require a single method of approach which avoids the partly verbal problem of the relations of "matter" and "mind," and deals with the changing structure of experienced and observed relationships. It will therefore be assumed that a unified theory is possible,...in which "material" and "mental," "conscious" and "unconscious" aspects will be derivable as related components of one primary system of ideas.
Whyte, 1960, p. 19

In this metatheoretical study, communication is examined in process, from both sides, observing an interplay of diverse forms and modes of interaction, as unconscious meanings are brought to consciousness through linguistic interpretation in semantic fields that bring these shifts into sharp relief. Psychoanalytic situations are used here as research venues to observe and systematize various forms of interaction and to isolate the specific semiotic, referential and dialogical mediations by which the unconscious is made conscious.

This is therefore a multidimensional, analytic study, filtered through the unifying template of a modern, semiotic developmental model of mind (Aragno 1997) leading us into the immensely complex domain of meanings, forms of reference, and sources of knowledge. In the physical sciences function follows form: in the science of mind functional-form expresses or denotes *how* something is experienced. This *functional* role of form in the psyche only becomes apparent when one considers the interaction of many unconscious elements in relation to the whole. For purposes of understanding and interpretation the examination of interrelationships between function, form and content provides a theoretical basis for the grammar, or architecture of human meanings. Accordingly a preoccupation with feelings, meanings and form begins early and threads through this entire work, anchoring psychological manifestations firmly in their biological roots.

The advantage of a broadly inclusive, metatheoretical approach is that it brings together many different dimensions of communicative phenomena under one system of ideas. The disadvantage is its inherent difficulty: it makes for immense complexity of organization and exposition while revealing many conceptual lacunae that have to be filled without the benefits of an existing terminological common ground. Transdisciplinarity of scholarship becomes a necessity in a work that will move in liminal regions of knowledge, synthesizing and integrating at points of juncture and overlap with related disciplines that span from philosophy to semiotics, neuroscience to narratology, biology to dialogicality. The purpose of this exhaustive interdisciplinarity is to find concepts at the cutting edge of contemporary knowledge that can adequately articulate the interactional phenomena of psychoanalytic semantic fields. Yet this amalgam of cultural cogitation has always been the underlying intellectual stretch of psychoanalytic theoretical discourse.

From the beginning I encountered three broadly grouped sets of problems – terminological, organizational, epistemological. The first have to do with the inadequacy, or non- existence, of differentiated, experience-near terms or, in fact, a comprehensive enough conceptual vocabulary to speak about the plethora of process-phenomena that unfold in psychoanalytic dialogues. New distinctions are now being made, but without a cohesive conceptual framework and fitting terms to name the phenomena, these observations remain undefined and ungrounded. For instance, differentiations have to be made between i) *countertransference*-proper, ii) reactions stimulated by projective mechanisms, and, iii) responses to unconscious transmissions engendered by resonance to *form*. Each is quite distinct, signifies something very different in psychodynamic terms, and must be used quite differently. Yet their differences are subtle and very difficult to detect on the spur of the moment. Also, in effect, the 'primary' and 'secondary' processes, Freud's dichotomized principles of mental functioning, are, at this point, too conceptually broad and impressionistic to accommodate the many gradations and formal shifts that are encountered along the continuum from unconscious to conscious. What is needed is a willingness to enter into a whole new way of thinking about the kinds of phenomena that are scientifically systematizable, remembering Freud's (1917) statement that "What characterizes psycho-analysis as a science is not the material which it handles but the technique with which it works....What it aims at and achieves is nothing other than the uncovering of what is unconscious in mental life."(p. 389).

As part of a larger conceptual reorientation, I propose introducing morphological principles into our thinking or incorporating the morphological dimension into our metapsychology. Morphology subsumes many organic functions involving normal and abnormal biological growth and change. It accounts for the pathological permutations brought about by aberrant development, trauma and disintegrative breakdown as well as those of regeneration, healing and growth. Associated with natural, organic processes within and between vital systems, it creates a conceptual link between biology, psychology and the social sciences, making the possibility of finding concordant principles between them more likely. Morphological ideas accord with a cybernetic paradigm of pattern, organization and design, a paradigm for understanding the recursive embeddedness of synergistic systems that are dynamically interactional, open-ended, responsive to and affecting their environments. Inter-systemically, morphological principles refer to the reciprocal impact of organisms meeting at the interface with other dynamic systems; intra-systemically they accommodate qualities and kinds of shifts in the interrelationship between parts or elements of a whole. This cybernetic paradigm lends itself to the study of communication, to an understanding of dialogue as root human condition, and to an appreciation of its immense power to impress, mold, mend and impact upon the human psyche, in both destructive and constructive ways.

The second problem is posed by the enormous complexity condensed in the simultaneity and immediacy of all psychical manifestations. This compounds the difficulties of an analytic presentation that has to contend with identifying, ordering and sequentializing a linear account of what actually happens all at the same time. When studied from the perspective of depth-psychology, the fluctuating confluence of projective transmissions, enactments and speech, produces cross-referenced meanings along the vertical axis as well as semiotic and referential progressions toward awareness over time, along the horizontal line. A process-analysis of our dialogues encompassing polysemic, polyvocal and psychodynamic dimensions of unconscious communications becomes an enormous organizational feat.

The architecture of this complexity corresponds to the complexity of music. As already mentioned, my solution has been to conjure this organizing metaphor and to hold in my mind's eye the analogue of an orchestral score as a visual display from which to draw conceptual parallels between the two systems. The most important of these parallels has to do with the functional fabric, the constitution, they share resulting, in both, from compositional interrelationships between multilayered parts of a whole that is constantly moving forward in time. Even referring to chapters as "movements," in addition to adhering to musical form, is designed to convey the idea of dynamic progressions propelled forward in self-modifying, self-qualifying modulations. In the book, the gradual accretion of ideas builds upon itself; it is in this sense that I wanted the relationship between its form and content to mirror the compositional qualities that music and communication share. In effect, we are talking about process-phenomena; a musical and a communicational, process. Both systems are generated by combinatorial elements, composed and sequenced by phrases and developmental progressions that, in great part, impact in subliminal ways.

When analogizing from music to communication I assume some familiarity with both, enough to make comprehensible the comparison between patterns of sound-combination (for which there *is* a comprehensive notational system of signs) and modes of information transmission-and-reception that still lack terminology. The assumption also presupposes the reader's recognition of deeper differences in experience when listening to a melodic development versus a tune, a symphonic poem versus a quartet, a march versus a minuet, the sound of an oboe versus a clarinet, not only in terms of their distinct tone and timbre, but especially for the *qualitative* difference in evoked emotional response that each engender. For how and in what ways these deeper sense-registrations induce the listener's response represents a very central point of our study, and belongs to that innominate realm of experience to which the musical analogy most applies. Because emotional-cognitions are more congruent with musical than with linguistic process, music expresses and can evoke forms of sentience that are not easily put into words.

Common roots in a semantic that encompasses emotional sensibilities, given the organismic orientation of this work, makes the analog of a musical score as template for human communication quite powerful. Both rely on a receptive interpreter in order to be grasped, and every translation is also a transposition in form. In order to better understand and interpret the unconscious, there has to be fluency in the transposition of its manifest forms into common every-day speech. We need to become more conversant with the vocabulary and grammar of 'the psychical'. From a theoretical standpoint, we have to identify discrete facets of the unconscious, their diverse modes of transmission, and our responses to them. To name and systematize their differential forms, as observable referents of the human psyche, is the task of theoretical psychoanalysis. One of the goals of this work is to begin to devise just such a conceptual and terminological vocabulary.

But the implications of what it uncovers are wider still. For the fact that diverse communicative forms evoke different types of response and, indeed, carry and transmit different kinds of information, suggests that we are endowed with different sense-frequencies or modes of registration to receive different forms of knowledge, and that once identified, we may be capable of tuning-in to these diverse epistemological perspectives in order to resonate with, register and identify, a whole new range of different types of facts. What this implies for a general theory of knowledge is for another work. But what this implies for a study of communication, from within psychoanalytic semantic fields, is that through our specialized attentional stance we can isolate discrete modes of resonance and attunement that orient toward registering different types of unconscious meanings – and that their inherent forms will dictate how we are to understand them.

This leads logically to my next proposition, namely, that the locus of our inquiry must be what transpires *between* people, the forms of the interactions themselves, examined from both sides, all metapsychological dimensions, *in process,* and in terms of how interpretive transactions impact on psychical organization. Our paradigm of in-forming transformation enables us to divorce completely from reifications of any kind, including the fateful Cartesian split between experiencing subject and observed object, by means of a reflexive methodology in which both subjects must themselves collaborate in becoming their own objects of analytic inquiry and introspective interchange. Methodological use of the entire spectrum of human interactive-channels obliges us to recognize sensory-emotive registrations as important and valid sources of in-formation in psychoanalytic research. The splitting of the 'ego' in the service of analytic observation is a key methodological tool in the instrumentation of this 'method' of investigation. Cartesian divisions are explicitly undermined where full integration of the mind/body unity and the ability to *enter into*, while observing the interactive field, are not merely desirable, but essential. This adjustment of methodological stance in relation to the *kinds* of phenomena under investigation is the clearest indication of a shift from a paradigm of causal explanation to one of compositional elements in mutually transforming interactions.

A book that begins to examine the functional role of form in the dynamics of human interaction is part of a paradigm revolution in communication sciences of which the most recent and exciting advance is the study of the operative properties and interconnectedness of complex networks (Barabasi, 2003). In representing a psychoanalytic contribution to this new cutting-edge scientific paradigm, this work may also be fulfilling a prediction made by D.D.Olds that "the underpinnings of the theory of mind that we will find most useful for a new psychoanalytic model will include, as conceptual contexts for our research, semiotic theories and the theories of complexity (non-linear dynamics, chaos theories, connectionist paradigms) (2000, p. 526).

All at once we find that we have been embedded in a methodology that is also an *interpenetrative epistemology*, a dialectical means for uncovering *how* we come to know what we know. The yields of its inquiries bifurcate into two branches each expanding human consciousness in different ways: the one, via the analysis of the personal unconscious, leads to therapeutic insight and personal change; the other displays the mediational progressions in dialogical processes involved in the transformation of experience into higher more abstract levels of verbal symbolization.

For what Freud uncovered in the different formal organizations of the primary (Ucs) and secondary (Cs) processes, his two *principles* of mental functioning, and what this expanded semantic implied, was originally the province of philosophy, as Langer (1942) pointed out, "traditional theory of mind is epistemology — theory of *knowledge*" (p. 51). Had Freud's metapsychology been constructed on fluid principles of transforming organizations of experience (to which he frequently alluded), rather than on borrowed metaphors from physics (to which he took recourse), it would have been evident long ago that psychoanalysis is a methodological epistemology for the interpretive study and theoretical understanding of human, bio-semiotic processes bridging unconscious and conscious dimensions of meaning and knowledge.

The organismic, bio-semiotic foundations of this study, I believe, provide the correct underpinnings and logical principles for understanding how communicative behaviors intersect with referential and interpretive activities to create semantic fields that can transform the range of human awareness and knowledge. Grounded in this conceptual framework our analytic study yields principles of discourse that have universal applicability. It opens the door to an objective theory of the subjective and to empirical foundations with communicative modes as observable referents. This approach evaporates residual dichotomies silently implied, still present, of a Cartesian-rationalist frame dividing body and mind, sense and cognition, emotion and reason, art and science, even psychology and philosophy, polarizations long with us that have obfuscated and obscured rather than clarified and enlightened our understanding of human nature.

The book is structured so as to build toward the developmental model of communication that is its centerpiece, in Chapter 3. Beginning with a series of brief essays that examine and reformulate key conceptual underpinnings so that human communication becomes an empirical window for the study of the psychical, the nature of the phenomena that are of relevance to the science of psychoanalysis are redefined and their systematic study begun. Through a three-part examination and rearticulation of epistemological, methodological and phylogenetic foundations in Chapter 1, rendering communication a prime referent for the study of mind; and a reorientation of our five metapsychological dimensions toward ' human-interactions' in Chapter 2, the groundwork is laid and the reader prepared, step by step, to a full understanding of the revisionary implications of the hierarchic model presented in Chapter 3, and its practical applicability in Chapter 4. Laborious and multidimensional as this may appear, psychoanalysts of all persuasions will recognize it is as being essential for a radical recasting of the conceptual language of theoretical psychoanalysis, if the study of its method and practice is to yield universal principles.

Because an overarching reconsideration and comprehensive synthesis is long overdue, the book works hard to subsume the contributions of major critical thinkers in psychoanalysis, spanning our 100 years in existence, on a number of crucial issues that, to date, have gone unresolved. However, my goal is not so much to encompass the literature as to chronicle the historical trajectory of psychoanalytic thought on the subject, from select early contributors to the subject, to current shifts in technique. Psychoanalysis brings together scientific and humanistic pursuits in a methodology that unifies rigorous empiricism with the intellectual practices and aesthetic values of the traditions of ancient Greece. The tributaries of these two strains and traditions, which jointly stream from Freud's own thinking, enable us today to observe and classify new psychological facts.

It follows that a psychoanalytic study of communication will not approach its subject matter as an abstraction, but will enter into the pragmatic and dynamic speech activities that constitute its dialogical interactions and processes. The usefulness and applicability of a developmental model of human communication that begins with affects, or natural, biological form, and moves along a semiotic continuum culminating in a discourse analysis of the psychoanalytic clinical and supervisory situations, is exemplified in the last three sections of the book where the yields of the study provide principles for bio-psychological models of empathic listening and learning, as well as an exploration of what exactly is artistic in the interpretive art of our dialogues. This entire work recasts the conceptual underpinnings of theoretical psychoanalysis into the language of communication and discourse, offering new and different unifying propositions based on semiotic, dialogical and referential processes.

I join those philosophers, philologists, psychologists and anthropologists whose vision encompassed the possibility of an authentic, unified science of humankind, in appealing to my psychoanalytic colleagues to adopt "the humanistic skills" that would enable us to "live more comfortably in those territories where the masters of human thought and art have long been dwelling…"(Turner, 1974, p.17). By applying our methodology to the study of an "innovative, liminal creature, to a species whose individual members have included Homer, Dante and Shakespeare, as well as Galileo, Newton and Einstein" (Turner, 1974, p.18) it may be possible to cultivate more intensely the relationship between the sciences and the humanities. We have in the Freudian legacy an optimal method for the study of mind — a way of listening, observing and understanding — crafted by a prescient genius, combining science and an interpretive art. As a scientist, Freud sought explanatory hypotheses for unconscious mental functioning; as a literary artist he discerned meaningful form wherever form presented itself. It would be foolish to miss the full breadth of opportunities afforded by a method that accommodates scientific insight as well as artistic expression, and the forms of knowledge igniting both.

MATTERS OF MIND

> Common sense is accustomed to the division of the world into mind and matter. It is supposed by all who have never studied philosophy that the distinction between mind and matter is perfectly clear and easy, that the two do not at any point overlap, and that only a fool or a philosopher could be in doubt as to whether any given entity is mental or material.
>
> B. Russell, 1915, p. 120

> The hypothesis we have adopted of a psychical apparatus extended in space, expediently put together, developed by the exigencies of life, which gives rise to the phenomena of consciousness only at one particular point and under certain conditions — this hypothesis has put us in a position to establish psychology on foundations similar to those of any other science, such for instance, as physics.
>
> S. Freud, 1940, p. 196

> Aristotle conceived 'matter'...as being pure potentiality awaiting the incoming of form in order to become actual.
>
> A. L. Whitehead, 1927, p. 36

This little exploration of large matters is designed to accentuate the unique value of viewing human communication as prime manifestation of the human psyche, and to trace the philosophical roots of this pre-Descartian approach to the Hellenic unity of body and mind, as articulated by Aristotle. Building on his great predecessors Socrates and Plato, while anchoring his ideas in organic and teleological principles, Aristotle's conceptual fusion of form and matter, makes utterly comprehensible the pervasive presence and expression of psyche in all human acts.

In Aristotle's philosophy, living organisms are composed of matter and form; the body, or material substrate, and its vital essence, psyche, the soul. These two components are inseparable, except in thought, and organismic functioning cannot be understood outside of this unity. 'Form' actualizes the potential functioning of the material substrate, so that a "full possession of form is equivalent to the proper performance of function" (Guthrie, 1960, p. 134). By introducing the idea of potentiality and actualization as inherent in the directional dynamisms of development and growth, Aristotle provides conceptual foundations for both change and continuity in the transformations that take place over time and that characterize of organic processes of maturation. Being entirely immanent, form is not independent of its material manifestations. Rather, it is that which bestows upon a substance its unique shape and structure as well as what impels its developmental dynamisms (Tarnas, 1991).

So fluid in Aristotle's doctrine is the fusion of form and matter that the basic principles it yields can be applied to understand the recursive, mutually transforming, effects of all vital, dynamic phenomena; "the actualization of a form can in turn lead to its being the matter out of which a higher form can grow" (Tarnas,1991 p.58). Form becomes a potentiating principle of matter, like the human mind, expressing its own distinctive nature only through actualized, observable manifestations.

Through the ages we have witnessed an irrepressible urge toward splitting this inherent unity culminating in Descartes' incisive division of matter and mind, the physical and the 'spiritual' worlds. The division between body and mind, and inner and outer worlds, resulted in a sharp epistemological bifurcation in our search for knowledge, deepening the chasm between the sciences and the humanities, with advances in our grasp of the operative laws of the natural world rapidly outpacing our grasp of the formulative, compositional laws that govern the nature of mind.

Stated succinctly: the mind makes 'matter' out of the same formulative processes from which it has itself been made. What the eye sees and the ear hears is carved out and chiseled selectively from the great sea of stimuli that meet the senses. And the mind further picks and chooses what to retain and what to reject, what merits attention and what's best to forget, by its own intensely personal criteria of value and judgment (and even these are often set by biological or psychological needs). Everything our senses record and process is filtered through the linguistic and conceptual categories that our symbol systems provide, and through the cognitive and communicative capabilities that serve our purpose at any given time. Most of what is registered is shaped by what is already known and by our arranging our perception of experiences in such a way as to match the 'patterns' with which we are already familiar. Much cognition is re-cognition, and everything depends on our current perspective. The versions of reality we create are limited by the functional organization through which we construct them, and constrained by our semiotic means.

Philosophically, and particularly psychologically, the division between the object of perception and the eye that sees, the subject of understanding and the mind that understands, between what we know and how we know it, is untenable.

Knowledge is formulative, and rests on systems of perception that are interpretive constructions; "the forms and the laws in our worlds do not lie there ready-made to be discerned but are imposed by world-versions we create — in the sciences, the arts, perception, and everyday practice." writes Goodman (1984, p. 21) emphasizing that "The arts and sciences are no more mirrors held up to nature than nature is a mirror held up to the arts and sciences" (p. 21). Timidly we point to the fatal flaw in the empiricist's fallacy that facts are found and not made, for they too result from the selection for registration of certain categories of experience, or certain features and aspects of material or of a series of events that are then sequentialized and interpretively understood to mean something in a particular context, according to its purpose and rhetorical form.

Not only do our interpretive systems and referential perspectives themselves determine which kind of sense-data we will register and include in our cognizing, but our contextual objectives and current communicative intent will further slant what we perceive and the significance we attribute to it. Quite literally we note what we denote. The mind makes its own matter by what matters to it, by means of signs and symbols, the only instrumentation it has. Our perception and what is knowable to us is always a fusion of sense-registrations and the mediated thought modes through which we currently formulate or pattern significance, so that the "problem of observation is all but eclipsed by the problem of *meaning*" writes Langer (1942, p. 21) and the "triumph of empiricism in science is jeopardized by the surprising truth that our *sense-data are primarily symbols*" (p. 21).

Having harnessed to such flagrant advantage the operative laws of the physical world, rather, the idea is handed down that the oculocentric empiricist approach is *the* way of science itself and that the whole paraphernalia of the empiricists protocol — controlled experimentation, observation, induction, validation, replication, quantification, etc. — the only means of obtaining it. While the outcome of the empiricists scheme, paired with mathematical logic, has led to all the stunning technological feats that pepper our modern world, the forced application of these same principles to matters of mind leads only to the manipulation of brain chemistry and titration of ratios of neurotransmitters, not to any remarkable insights or advances in our understanding of the multidetermined, synergistic and dynamic principles of mental functioning. No one has fared well or forged forward our grasp of the constitutive features of the "psychical" by imposing onto its shifting, compositional condensations the causal principles and static structures of matter, and Freud's mental "apparatus," an hydraulic mind-machine, was no exception. To his great credit he never intended that this temporary hypothesis be taken for anything more than what it was, a "fictive" metaphor through which to *describe* not explain his extraordinary observations. And to his great merit he left us a methodology, discredited because its yields have been misrepresented, through which we could continue what he had begun.

More and more, as we grow accustomed to the idea of multiple versions of truths and the provisional, partial nature of all knowledge — ideas that have been our rudders in this age of perspectivalism — some, involved in matters of mind, have become keenly aware that there are different ways of knowing different things and that by purposefully employing expanded modes of attention we can identify different types of facts. This implies, indeed necessitates, that we neither favor nor discredit any cognizable source of sensory or emotive impression as potentially informative but rather that we tailor our apperceptual modes and fit our referential perspectives to the kinds of forms that the phenomena dictate — once we have identified what the significant phenomena are.

Having now, ourselves, become multiperspectival observers we can attest to the veracity of Lord Russell's (1914) prescient pronouncement that "What is feasible is the understanding of general forms" (p.109). The "scientific philosophy" (p.109) that he envisioned for accomplishing such a task would concern itself with the "analysis and enumeration of logical forms, i.e., with the kinds of propositions that may occur, with the various types of facts, and with the classification of the constituents of facts" (p.108). Were we to have such a general theory of knowledge in place today we would already have factored in to all understanding the pivotal role of human responsiveness *in its totality* as participatory in the investigative scheme. Since all knowledge is guided by systems of interpretation and we, ourselves, are the formulative agents, it is for us to hone our sensibilities while adopting the most propitious methodologies for the subjects and purposes at hand; and in this exercise the forms and phenomena *themselves must determine how we are to understand them.* .

Clearly there are different ways of perceiving and understanding things of substance that can be seen, touched, weighed and counted, from apperceiving and understanding things insubstantial that must be inferred, sensed, felt, and interpretively surmised through their manifest attributes. There are different ways of approaching organic from inorganic substance, different stances for understanding operative functioning from interpreting personal meanings. Where quantity matters in things 'material,' *quality* matters in things of meaning. Facts like phenomena are fluid, their relative weight and value varying from context to context; their informative sources shifting from observation, causal cognition and calculation in one, to observation, feeling and emotional-recognition in another.

A participatory epistemology such as the one I am advocating would approach all "things" according to their particular function and nature, depending on the purpose of the context or investigation. It would require that we "sensitize our cognition" as Goodman (1984, p. 8) puts its, to recruit and include emotion and feeling as important, primary registers for discriminating various forms and patterns of information, and that we observe the investigative process itself as a means of understanding how better to understand. In this sense, it is not so easy to disentangle epistemology from psychology, science from art.

From the supraordinate standpoint of such a grammar of logical forms, we would enter each investigative context equipped with a current dictionary for the vocabulary of the language in which the forms of those phenomena speak and we would make it our business to try to amplify and enrich our fluency in that vocabulary as our familiarity with those forms increases. But we will understand little or nothing at all if we impose on our phenomena the categories and grammars of another language, if we confuse 'matter' that is constructed out of bricks and mortar with 'matters' that are composed of meanings and memories. Mind — or the concept of mind — materializes through formulation; and whether it is first a signal that cries, a sign that denotes, or a symbol that represents, the mind can make a 'thing' out of process, pattern or structure alike: "We make a star as we make a constellation, by putting its part together and marking off its boundaries" (Goodman, 1984, p. 42). A word makes a 'thing' of anything.

But 'psyche' or mind, does not exist outside of its manifestations. Because the *concept* of mind, or psyche, is, similarly, a linguistic abstraction that enables us to talk about phenomena that we infer as being 'mental'. And therefore it is for us to select the most apposite point of entry and organizing framework through which to identify, differentiate and understand the broadest possible range of 'psychical' phenomena. I have chosen to look at human communication though a psychoanalytic lens, first because it is the very soul of our method, and second because it is the clearest, most immediate, direct and accessible dynamic condensation of our symbolizing cognition and social disposition; simultaneously it exhibits what is on our mind, in our mind, what it means to us, in what ways we are willing or able to share it, and, of course, everything else that we express or transmit via unconscious channels, outside of our awareness.

The formulative processes and functional organizations of mind are governed by logical principles of symbolization; signals, signs and symbols each creating and capable of conveying different types of meaning, different forms of reference, different modes of thought. The mind's instruments are semiotic forms filtered through symbol systems, coded, dressed, and patterned in different ways; and each mind orchestrates its instrumentation according to its current capacities, goals and dynamic intent. "We are the music" writes the poet: and the philosopher echoes "...the edifice of human knowledge stands before us...as a structure of *facts that are symbols and laws that are their meanings*." (Langer, 1942, p. 21). And a symbol, as Goodman (1984) reminds, "may inform in as many different ways as there are contexts and systems of interpretation" (p.12).

In psychoanalysis we investigate unconscious processes and meanings: for therapeutic purposes we interpret the personal unconscious, for metatheoretical purposes we try to identify and systematize psychological principles. Our investigations take place in discourse situations and our metatheoretical insights are immensely increased if we observe our "data" through the logical principles of semiotic forms. And because our method is designed to make what is unconscious conscious, the nature of the phenomena through which our "data" are manifest will be pre-semiotic (biological or somatic), enacted, as well as symbolically organized communications. We are particularly interested in understanding the transformative factors and transmutative principles that bring about intrapsychical shifts resulting from our interpretive activities. The mind makes matter by 'signification', but the *meanings* thereby construed by that mind and their transitional phases are *contingent on the person's current, overall functional organization and state,* and this *key* interpretive factor for psychological understanding, can only be articulated through a developmental paradigm.

Given the psychological processes that are aroused by the particular conditions and analytic perspectives set by our method, we are given a unique vantage point from which to observe the rekindling of certain processes of development and maturation. We are also put in a position to note those formulative moments of semiotic progression in which ineffable, unconscious experiences and emotions are becoming accessible to words and, potentially, available to working-through consciously. But since we, the interpreters and observers of unconscious phenomena, have at our disposal only the same mind whose unconscious forms we are trying to detect, a crucial aspect of our methodological mandate will be to continuously monitor and reflect upon our own modes of apprehension. A methodological analysis in this sense becomes indispensable; a brief reflection on which now follows.

METHODOLOGICAL REFLECTIONS

> The human being has the peculiar quality of being able to observe himself and then bend back upon his observations and make a theory. He can explore observations, explore observations of observations, etc., and make theories about that. There is no end to it. It is most peculiar, most frightening, most enchanting.
>
> ...But the coin has another side; it has to do with methodology. The bending back of science upon itself to see scientific interrelationships between its own constructs and theories — that is methodology.
>
> D. Rapaport, 1944, p.172

The consequence of not having already subjected psychoanalysis to a methodological analysis is a field in theoretical disarray; without a clear conceptual understanding of what the relevant phenomena of our science really are, or a unifying vocabulary through which to speak about its many aspects and dimensions.

The reason that such an analysis has not been undertaken is, first, because we have been looking the other way, and second; because it's hard to swim upstream. The field has bypassed the painstaking labor of an analysis of method and the search for underlying principles, in favor of fragmentation and specialization. This has culminated in the externalization of the multidimensionality that is inherent in psychical phenomena, into ideologically splintering clinical 'schools' that lack a comprehensive, unifying metatheory. Each of these practices a 'version' of the conversational 'method,' but given the wide discrepancy in stance and predominant interpretive perspectives, it is doubtful whether they can all be considered truly 'psychoanalytic' in the methodological sense of the term. This makes a methodological analysis all the more imperative; because an examination of the unique features of the method, within the framework of a cohesive, unified system of ideas, will identify the kinds of 'phenomena' and 'data' that can be systematized and understood.

We know, because Freud left ample documentation, that the investigative 'method 'he called 'psychoanalysis' sprung from his own observational/ listening stance and growing interest in the 'unconscious'. Freud arrived at his hypotheses through the integration of clinical observations, his own auto-analysis, and the 'interpretation' of various unconsciously determined universal phenomena such as dreams, jokes, and slips of the tongue. At the genesis of this new science, everywhere we look, we see Freud authoring works at an astounding rate of output, confiding his new insights to Fliess in their correspondence, and dialoguing with those who began forming a movement that gathered around him. Freud's psycho-analytic observations and ideas began creating a pool of 'referents' for a growing body of experiential-research and theoretical hypotheses that rapidly generated a 'discourse' through which further articulation of new findings could take place. The objectification of psycho-analytic 'data', furnishing new kinds of psychological facts unveiled by this nascent science, occurred by means of this threefold process. And the inherent three-pronged span of his investigative method greatly expanded Freud's meta-theoretical goals: hence psychoanalysis evolved into a method of empirical investigation, a therapeutic modality, and a general theory of mind.

The consequence of an investigative method with diverse objectives is a context with different interpretive aims; i) to isolate unconscious processes and phenomena; ii) to interpret the personal unconscious for therapeutic insight; and iii) to understand the transformational principles of mental functioning along an unconscious/conscious continuum.

"It is very difficult to treat the methodology of something which is three things," wrote Rapaport (1944, p. 68), who believed a methodological analysis to be indispensable for the scientific advancement of our field; "It will have to be done before we get very far into a really systematic psychoanalytic psychology. That I am sure of." he emphasized (p.166). Understanding what many have not, that the mark of a science is a cohesive system of ideas correlating the process/phenomena identified by its method with the theoretical constructs that attempt to explain them, Rapaport realized that first and foremost we would have to distinguish between those psychoanalytic phenomena that are systematizable (and relevant to theory) and those that are not: "Methodological treatment of something means that you investigate what consequences adopting this method has for the material to be obtained and what kind of consequences it has for the theory that must be built to encompass, to make understandable, to unify these observations" (Rapaport, 1944, p.171). His questions wavered between the epistemological and methodological because psychoanalysis implicates both. If we ask, then, simply: How does it inform? (an epistemological question), answers point to methodological features; an expanded, multidimensional interpretive semantic, purposeful discourse situations guided by the mutual fit between a free-associative speech form, an attuned attentional stance, and a superordinate investigative goal, "...nothing other than the uncovering of what is unconscious in mental life (Freud, 1917, p.389).

But herein lie some of the key problems: we are dealing with three entirely different categories of phenomena, *psychological, epistemological* and *logical,* each operating according to different sets of principles while converging in the events of one methodological dialogue. Psychological principles are probably best understood along various developmental dimensions; epistemological principles have to do with how we 'know'; but, even when articulated along developmental lines (Aragno, 1997), principles of symbolization are logical — and logic is of the mind. These principles are not *directly* observable, yet they underlie how the method works. What transpires in psychoanalytic contexts reflects the practical application of the operative *principles* underlying these three above mentioned classes of phenomena.

We have, then, in one method, three primary investigative orientations, each guided by different aims, operating with different sets of referents, addressing different aspects of the phenomena, at different levels of abstraction. Because psychoanalysis is three things in one, each of its investigative pursuits requires adjustment of the interpretive and referential orientation in accordance with the specific focus of inquiry. Insofar as our primary methodological goal and interpretive pursuit is to make knowable what is unconscious, an important, albeit little appreciated, additional attribute of the method is its ability to uncover our modes of apperception, or ways of knowing, themselves. Rapaport (1944) understood the broader implication of this potential window into epistemology when he wrote; "The claims of psychoanalysis are so enormous that they include scrutiny of any kind of methodology, because any person who thinks about methodology does so with his psyche, and psychological functions can be scrutinized by psychoanalytic methods...." adding "You are dealing with a science which claims that it can bend back upon any kind of science or thought product. It is like being in an elevator with mirrors on two opposite sides. You look into one and see yourself looking at yourself in the other, and so on into infinity" (p.179).

This brief analytic reflection on psychoanalytic methodology is undertaken in the belief that an examination of its unique features and characteristics will point to the kinds of phenomena that are of relevance to our science. Psychoanalytic phenomena are pluralistic, multidimensional, hence Freud's multiperspectival '*meta*psychology' with its five dimensions, each contributing its own facet of inquiry, generating its own developmental lines and investigative yields. And psychoanalytic phenomena are interactional, uncovered through the dialectical interchange of a reflexive dialogue. As a research methodology, psychoanalysis anticipated the protocols of contemporary Naturalistic Research by a hundred years: as a therapeutic technique it expands our ability to 'know' ourselves; and as a theory of mind, psychoanalysis lays bare the operative progressions and logical principles of semiotic mediation (Symbolization, Aragno, 1997).

First, among the unique features of psychoanalytic methodology is its highly particularized, **participant-observer attentional disposition**, a stance that is markedly different from the traditional empirical approach. The listening/observer is required to *enter into* the field of observation, engaging the whole sensorium, becoming a resonant, interpretive 'instrument' of its unconscious currents. In addition to an internal splitting between the experiencing and the observing self, this details a requisite 'referential distance' from both, designed to safeguard an *interpretive* rather than an *entangled* position that can look inward and outward at the same time, while simultaneously monitoring processes arising in the dialogue. In psychoanalytic situations sensory-emotive modes of attunement not only *participate in cognizing* unconscious transmissions, they are central to their detection and understanding.

The injunction to the practicing analyst is to "turn his own unconscious like a receptive organ toward the transmitting unconscious of the patient" (Freud, 1912, p.115); interpretation, for Freud (1917), meant "finding a hidden sense in something" (p. 87). Freud left notoriously few, loose "recommendations" regarding when and even *what* to interpret (other than transference and resistance) but he did leave detailed instructions on *how* to listen, because in psychoanalytic semantic fields both the stance and the experience of the listening/observer are central to the receptive understanding unconscious forms of communication. One of the key features of this pliant, evenly suspended attentional disposition is a methodological insistence on *finding* rather than making sense of something: of allowing the phenomena to speak for themselves. This basic "hands off" interpretive stance is fundamental to psychoanalytic understanding, in its therapeutic aims as well its scientific investigations

A second prominent feature of psychoanalytic methodology is its **reflective/reflexive referentiality**. This results from a participant-observer stance that must monitor various internal, interactional and process events simultaneously. It was this extraordinary ability to register subjective experience, while identifying various contextually-arising unconscious patterns, that enabled Freud to detect the regular appearance of transference and resistance, even in their subtlest forms, to identify the repetition compulsion, to decipher the grammar and vocabulary of dreams, trace neurotic guilt to childhood passion, and pull all these disparate unconscious manifestations together into a comprehensive, multiperspectival interpretive approach encompassing five supeordinate meta-psychological dimensions.

Psychoanalytic contexts are **dialogical** situations; hence they are intrinsically **interactional,** methodologically. The human psyche/mind germinates and develops through and within the dialectics of social interchange: its developmental history and structural characteristics, likewise, emerge through a specialized dialectical discourse-method that revives its most salient patterns. The analysis of transference and resistance became the defining cornerstones of a psychoanalytic treatment because Freud realized that the contextual process provided a far more immediate and direct experiential avenue to achieve the intended therapeutic goals. He harnessed these contextually vital interactive process-phenomena, making them vehicles rather than impediments to the treatment. By deriving *from* the emergent process, advocating a *contextual* rather than a retrospective approach, he set the stage for the scrupulous, uncontaminating use of the self as a methodological necessity. This newly devised interpenetrative epistemology utilizes human responsiveness, *in its totality*, as its instrument; and we are the players *and* the music. Therefore how the method works is intimately tied to how it informs.

In addition to the dynamic, structural, and topographical dimensions, psychoanalysis is defined by its *genetic* orientation: and genetic understanding, as Rapaport (1941) wrote, is "the discovery of the laws of development" (p.78). To study something developmentally or historically, to use Vygotsky's words (1978), "*means to study it in the process of change:* that is the dialectical methods basic demand." he stressed, "To encompass in research the process of a given things development in all its phases and changes." (p.65). The "*search for method*," therefore, as Vygotsky (1978, p.15) emphasized, is one of the most crucial problems of the whole enterprise. Psychoanalytic contexts, in this Vygotskian sense, could be considered 'developmental/experimental' insofar as they foster conditions that engender a concentrated recapitulation and emotional resolution of childhood experience in a dialogue that, through personal insight and integration, promotes psychological maturation at higher more articulate levels of symbolic reorganization. The situation, and its referential processes of working-through and verbalization, put us in a position to observe these transformations taking place *before our very eyes*, so that "the past and present are fused and the present is seen in the light of history" and "we find ourselves simultaneously on two planes: that which is and that which was." (Vygotsky, 1978, p. 64) We observe this not only in terms of the history of the *personal* unconscious, but most especially, in terms of the transforming *processes* themselves. The study of these processes belongs to psychology, wrote Langer (1967) "but the basis of that study is the conception of living form and function, which takes one from biology into psychology, and further into the strictly human part of that discipline, the investigation of mind and all its reaches and expressions" (p. 444).

Whereas secondary repression and the dynamic unconscious are the referential cornerstones of the interpretive framework for the classical model of clinical psychoanalysis, now pre-semiotic experience (pre-oedipal and primary repressions) have entered our interpretable spheres of interaction accessing more primitive states and earlier, more pervasive etiologies. In recent years psychoanalytic practitioners have learned to become attuned to deeper more amorphous types of transference organization originating from different points along a developmental continuum some of which require resonance to very early sensory-affective reenactments in order to be identified at all. Non-verbal signal-patterns and behavioral signs now serve indexical functions in an interpretive discourse in which everything is to be funneled through words. The nature of the phenomena that are to be included as informative 'data,' and the range of stimuli from which we infer meanings, today, now reaches to the minute gesture, transitory sense-impression, the fleeting expression or image evoked, the transmitted affect-state, degrees of connectedness or withdrawal, all experienced beneath the limen of everyday awareness.

The success of the method can be measured in part by this increasingly widening scope of interpretable, unconscious referents now sinking practically to biological levels of expression. Yet this is precisely what psychoanalysis has always asserted in its second, fundamental hypothesis, "It explains the supposedly somatic concomitant phenomena as being what is truly psychical, and thus, in the first instance disregards the quality of consciousness" (Freud, 1940, p.158). Freud's "method" harnesses for apperceptual and formulative purposes virtually all sense-modalities, in a methodological fusion of intent that creates a synthesis of feeling and intellect, observation and introspection, emotional resonance and discursive articulation, all funneled through the interpretive focus dictated by the situational purpose. Identifying unconscious forms and interpreting unconscious meanings, however, also requires a multipaletted repertoire of referential perspectives coupled with an especially receptive mode of attunement that orients, at will, toward different forms of transmission and organizations of meaning.

What is handed down, more valuable still than the talking 'cure,' is Freud's own way of coming-to-know, his 'methodological' stance. What is of immeasurable value is the *method* itself, of which it can truly be said that, "...it is simultaneously prerequisite and product, the tool and the result of the study" (Vygotsky, 1978, p. 65). Insight into 'psychical' reality is the new dimension of understanding gained by this methodology. Psychoanalysis provides an instrumental situation that is an observational lens for gaining access to a whole range of experiential processes and phenomena of 'mental functioning,' and for interpreting unconscious meanings, that are not accessible by any other means.

One cannot but marvel at Freud's modernity in uncovering and crafting a curative "conversation" that adopts only language as its instrument; or but be impressed by the prescience with which he essentially anticipated the whole sway of relativism and perspectivalism that was to sweep over twentieth century thought. His radical alteration of the relationship between 'observer' and the 'object' of observation anticipated, and had already implemented, what Heisenberg (in physics) was to introduce as a *principle* of uncertainty, on the heels of Freud's death.

Striking, in particular, are; a) Freud's willingness to become part of the investigative field, making participant-observation and the technical instrumentation of human responsiveness, central features of the interpretive task; b) his multidimensionality of viewpoints, both metatheoretically and interpretively, aiming at identifying unconscious patterns and enactions arising from within the dynamisms of the contextual process, from numerous perspectives, simultaneously c) Freud's adoption of multiple modes of apprehension—introspection, empathy, listening, observing and feeling—in an integration of symbolic objectification of subjective observations and experiences; d) his implicit instrumentation of the dialectical dimension, emphasized by Dilthey (1883/1911), as fundamental to human understanding, by adopting the bi-directional reflexivity of reference upon which the therapeutic dialogue depends; e) Freud's incorporating all of the above features of his investigative style and molding them into a comprehensive, interpretive methodology for studying the human mind; and finally, f) Freud's steadfast conviction of the *scientific* value and potential of this new methodology with respect to its generativity and universal applicability.

The provenance of such perspicacious insights can be traced to the talents, temperament and interests, of the mind that had them; one cannot readily separate methodology from the traits of the man, its founder. Chief among Freud's natural gifts was his verbal dexterity, a lifelong drive to translate observations, impressions, experiences and ideas into discursive thought, to formulate, order, author. We are greatly indebted for the extensive record of this progressive, searching mind, to the discursive stream that flowed fluidly from his pen—twenty-three volumes strong, as well as a staggering correspondence. A man of genius with a twofold talent, Freud combined the mentality and investigative eye of the scientist with the formulative, interpretive flair of an author. It comes as no surprise that he would devise a method encompassing both these traits and apparently divergent aims—the uncovering of the operative principles of mind and the interpretation of the personal unconscious, two interweaving streams that run through his entire opus. We are indebted as much to his observational acuity as to his discursive drive for the breadth of his legacy. For in Freud the requisite, rare amalgam of natural gifts and creative rigor, scientific insight and literary artistry, moral courage and humanistic integrity, were present in equal parts. Psychoanalysis is the first scientific psychology the methodology of which combines science and art. And while the idea that science and art are not as antithetical as they might once have appeared, does not strike us today as so very strange, in Freud's day they were still sharply divided.

Were it not for his empirical optic, neurological background and physicianly intent, Freud might not have detected the many dynamic configurations that he did, or isolated the distinctive clinical patterns of experience and enactment that were to become the shibboleths of the method. Without its 'therapeutic' bent to shape the context, Freud might not have devised the "procedural" processes, or discerned the healing properties of a "talking" cure. For without the therapeutic motive—tied to etiological belief—to slant the interpretive code, procedure and intent might never have converged in a dialogue.

Freud could also not have deciphered the structure and vocabulary of dreams, the dynamic fuel of jokes and verbal slips, the diverse grammars of the primary and secondary processes, or identified the replay of past in current enactment, grasping the intensely recapitulative nature of the clinical encounter, were he not exquisitely sensitive to form. And lastly, Freud would not have sought out the origins of neurotic misery in infantile passion, or come face-to-face—from both sides of the mirror—with the tenaciousness of resistances and discomforting tensions of suspended closure, were he not willing to turn his investigative eye back upon himself in an auto-analysis that used the clinical dialectic to arrive at insights ricocheting between his understanding of 'others' and of himself. Were he to have been any less reflective or less compelled to observe and 'understand,' he would not have *experienced* his way to the method, or brought his experiential understanding to bear on how he utilized the emergent processes as he encountered them; "Such is the *personal participation* of the knower in all acts of understanding" (Polanyi, 1964, xii).

Polanyi's (1964) "Personal Knowledge," however, was only to confirm what Freud's method had already amply demonstrated, namely, "that in every act of knowing there enters a passionate contribution of the person knowing what is being known, and that this coefficient is no mere imperfection but a vital component of his knowledge" (Polanyi, 1964, XIV). Freud's methodological fusion of 'Knowledge by Acquaintance' and 'Knowledge by Description' (Russell, 1910/53)—*knowing of* and knowing *about*—had *already* called on the totality of the human response to serve the interpreting intellect.

Freud was acutely aware of the power of words; to Thomas Mann (June 1935) on the occasion of his sixtieth birthday he wrote, an "authors words are deeds." It was no simple quirk of fate that the Goethe prize for literature, rather than the coveted scientific Nobel, was bestowed on him. But psychoanalytic methodology thrust upon the nineteenth century *Weltanschauung* an interpretive science for which it was conceptually quite unprepared. Curiously foreshadowing a post-modernist awareness of the tenuousness of all human understanding and the impossibility of seeking absolute truths, Freud lived his life striving to transcend these human limitations, devoted to a method that enables us to better know ourselves, the roots of which go back to the Socratic 'maieutic' dialogue. A physician/ author reviled as much for his 'daring 'as his 'reductionism,' it is, nevertheless, only a humanistic scientist who could develop a method of healing in which "nothing takes place…but an exchange of words" (Freud,

1917, p. 17). We ought not underestimate the extraordinary effort involved in the formulation of such new abstractions, or minimize the strain in enduring the 'birth-pains' of new insight. (Rapaport 1942.) Freud frequently found actual physical torment in the tensions accompanying his self-analysis and theorizing. Through his letters, we get a palpable taste of the intensely dialectical dynamisms he was caught up in, as well as the vitality of his creative thinking. On November 14, 1897, from Vienna, Freud wrote to Fleiss:

> It was on November 1, a day dominated by a left-sided migraine,. . . that after the frightful labor pains of the last few weeks, I gave birth to a new piece of knowledge. Not entirely new, to tell the truth; it had repeatedly shown itself and withdrawn again; but this time it stayed and looked upon the light of day. (Masson, 1985, pp. 278-279)
>
> . . . and at the end of the same letter:
>
> My self-analysis remains interrupted. I have realized why I can analyze myself only with the help of knowledge obtained objectively (like an outsider). True self-analysis is impossible. . . . Since I am still contending with some kind of puzzle in my patients, this is bound to hold me up in my self-analysis as well. (Masson, 1985, p. 281)

We have not really allowed the intensely *dialogical* phenomenology of the psychoanalytic situation, or the expansion of consciousness that it yields, to suffuse our thinking enough to learn from it what the relevant phenomena for the metatheory truly are. Therefore, we are in danger of further perpetuating a bifurcation of the artistic and scientific faces of psychoanalysis by allowing the schism to take us conceptually and theoretically in different directions. Nowhere in the Freudian opus is the disjunction between metatheory and practice more striking than in his clinical recommendations. Freud's entire explanatory edifice is, in this sense, an attempt to systematize and reconcile metatheoretically, the phenomena and transformational processes he had operationalized in practice. It is striking that whereas Freud has been consistently berated for his reductionism and alleged impersonality, it was, nevertheless, by means of his interpretive sensibilities and intensely discursive powers of translation, that he was able to decipher the peculiar grammar of the primary process and sensitize us to the dynamic forces of the unconscious.

Psychoanalytic situations are semantic fields of a very special kind; in them language is used to translate elusive, non-discursive meanings and unconscious patterns. The analysts observing eye and listening ear attune to meanings that go beyond denotive signification, in ways that are reminiscent of the participatory/sharing that takes place in the appreciation of art. The methodological stance of the psychoanalytic method engages different modes of apprehension, or ways of knowing, simultaneously: observing, listening, feeling, inference, and intuition *all* participate in the emotional/cognitions of this interpretive semantic.

Virtually *everything* that transpires in our semantic fields is taken as a psychical index or sign, of some sort, and hence, as meaningful. In addition to examining communicative phenomena from all metapsychological dimensions (the dynamic, genetic, topographical, structural and adaptive), then, our study will also have to encompass a now vastly expanded range of experiential referents that are considered informative in our discourse situations, many of which are broad projections of affect-states or enactments of both sides of internalized interactions recapitulated at highly undifferentiated levels in the current interchange. I mention this to underscore the importance in our methodology of continuous self-monitoring in order to ascertain that all channels of communication remain open and accessible to awareness. The impact of emotional-transmission, the presentational immediacy of sign, the multidetermined condensations of symbols, and their mediation through psychoanalytic referentiality, are the natural soil of psychoanalytic metatheory, just as the speech and referential forms that shape and reshape our dialogues are the "right categorization" (Goodman, 1984) of phenomena for a systematic study of the *means* of the method.

In order to speak sensibly about our methodology, however, it is essential to specify the particular interpretive purpose to which the method is currently being applied; research, therapy or supervision, since after a certain point, "the technique required for the one opposes that required for the other"(Freud,1912, p.114). Different interpretive goals alter the relationship of interpreter to what is being observed, as well as the nature of the phenomena that will tend to emerge. The morphology of communicative forms came into sharp relief for me while I was observing the supervisory process from the *outside*, at a distance from which the transmissive patterns and unconscious dynamisms emanating from the report and the interchange were more clearly revealed. These forms are much more difficult to identify while directly engaged in the supervisory exchange.

The practice of the method takes place in contexts created by speech; and it is to the inter-active features, forms, processes and phases of our dialogues that we ought to be looking for the phenomena that constitute the scientific basis of the method. For the *scientific* 'datum' must be found and refound, whereas the interpretation of unconscious meanings is contextual, circumstantial, co-constructed, a unique moment of human interchange. It bears repeating; the *scientific* essence of psychoanalysis is *independent* of the material to which is applied (Freud, 1917). Practical application and explanatory principles involve different levels of abstraction. Yet the confusion in psychoanalysis created by the conflation of functional principles and fictional structures — between the mind's *work* and personality dynamisms—endures to this day.

Viewed as research venues, the clinical and supervisory situations become vehicles for examining different types of unconscious communications from within the experiential hub of their interchanges, in the eye of sometimes wordless dynamisms that are engendered in their dyadic and triadic fields. Different forms of communication, that are particularly visible in the supervisory process, exemplify different modes of internalization, different ways of knowing, different degrees of conscious awareness. Studying the reciprocal impact of the forms of interaction themselves from a semiotic lens, traces discrete communicative modes ranging from undifferentiated projective-transmissions to verbalized unconscious meanings.

The great innovation of the methodology, and the potential this work explicitly builds on, is that in its practical implementation of an *interpenetrative epistemology* it opens the door to the possibility of developing a general model of human responsiveness and understanding, a theory of knowledge, built on a holistic theory of mind. By devising a dialogue that could 'enlarge the sphere of the ego', expanding personal awareness, and a methodology that implements a transformation of consciousness, we are now invited to turn the method back upon its own methodology and observe the means by which the mind develops itself. For how we become 'aware,' or, how we come to 'know,' is how the method works.

The yields of such a study must succeed in pulling together, under one system of ideas, phenomena that originate in deep, organic experience, pass through 'psychical' phase, and proceed to conscious awareness through semiotic formulation. The task, quite literally, is the "—construction of a biological concept of mind adequate to the phenomenon itself—" (Langer, 1967, p.74). I believe this is made possible, in part, by a revision of the theoretical gravitational center of our *general* theory of mind, and a return to Freud's "topographical" conception, now adequately reconceptualized in the logical terms of symbolic forms.

Freud turned the eyes of the world inward, stretching the Hellenic dictum "know thyself" to new, dark and unforeseeable depths. At the same time he opened the door to a new semantic that, due to its expanded range of unconscious and experiential referents, will have to adopt a more holistic, metatheoretical framework to account for the full spectrum of bio-psychical meanings accessible to its interpretive purview. Whether this takes us inward, to the individual psyche, or outward, to general forms, it is an approach committed to viewing the human whole, a somato-psychic unity, inevitably intertwined with other vital systems and all organic life. From this perspective interdisciplinary cross-fertilization is virtually a necessity.

The methodological stance introduced by the psychoanalytic method requires of the analyst to 'enter into' a dialogical situation while simultaneously monitoring the self, the other, and the process. In this, and in his pluralistic metapsychology, Freud anticipated the philosophical *zeitgeist* and humanistic science to which we have access today, by one hundred years. This splitting of the observers' referential stance was a radical departure from the traditional 'objectivity' aspired to by empiricism, originating in the fateful Cartesian division of human feelings and reason. The resulting comprehensive use of the self as a reflective-interpreting 'instrument,' was designed to maximize accessibility to the kinds of unconscious phenomena that are to be identified by the method. This analysis of our methodology points to interactive-dialogical phenomena as being of prime relevance to our science of mind. A study of the features, speech-forms and functional-transformations occurring in psychoanalytic communicative fields, becomes an optimal point of entry into a scientific-explanatory framework for 'how the method works'.

From this investigative approach, we will now look at those points of connection and divergence between ourselves and other species, in order to situate human nature, and the nature of the human mind, in the natural world.

MENS NATURANS

> If inherited mental formations exist in the human being — something analogous to instinct in animals — these constitute the nucleus of the Ucs.
>
> S. Freud, 1915, p. 195

> The phenomena with which we are dealing do not belong to psychology alone; they have an organic and biological side as well, and accordingly in the course of our efforts at building up psycho-analysis we have also made some important biological discoveries and have not been able to avoid framing new biological hypotheses.
>
> S. Freud, 1940, p. 195

> There may be a slow accruing of core scientific fact which is relevant to understanding mind,. . . which will ultimately anchor psychology quite firmly in biology without ever making its advanced problems laboratory affairs
>
> S. Langer, 1967, p. 53

Freud's subsuming of his topographical model of mind into a more clinically serviceable model of psychic structures created a theoretical discrepancy at the heart of psychoanalysis that precluded integration of the communicative function of affects. at the start of life. His turning away from the fluid "system Ucs," in favor of reified 'structures' and the dynamic unconscious, led to an entrenchment of psychoanalytic thought in its clinical function, seriously undermining Freud's aspiration to develop a general theory of mind. His sharply divided primary and secondary processes and dark portrayal of the Ucs—a "seething cauldron," likened to an "aboriginal population in the mind" (Freud, 1915, p. 195)—coupled with an "irrational"

Id contrasted to a reality-facing, linguistic Ego, only reinforced the split between soma and psyche that psychoanalysis was intended to mend.

Further ambiguities in Freud's texts stemming from the body/mind dilemma, regarding the precise definition of "psychical phenomena," left the purview of psychoanalytic interpretability open to continual debate. The main distinction Freud drew was between psychical phenomena that issue directly from organic sources and those that are secondarily derived "somewhere behind which the series of organic influences begins" (1916, pp.60-61), a distinction reiterated in the etiological differential he drew between an *"actual"* and a psychogenic neurosis. On the one hand a "psychical" or "mental" phenomenon was required to have a 'sense' or 'meaning'; on the other hand Freud frequently alluded to the "somatic concomitant phenomena" as being what is "truly psychical" (1940, p. 158).[1] This core definitional discrepancy returns to haunt a profession that has gradually moved the clinical method forward—to the treatment of earlier, deeper, more pervasive developmental pathologies—without advancing its metatheory to account for its progressing technique. The investigative method pushes forward, of its own momentum, while the scattered profession proliferates ideological fragmentation.

Whereas we may forgive Freud these early inconsistencies, we have to remain wary of their consequences: with no existing developmental studies, (Piaget was to arrive on the heels of Freud's departure), scant research in the neurosciences and certainly no knowledge of semiotics, Freud's observations of the unconscious brought infancy, childhood passion, conflict, defense, repetition and archetypal constellations of human experience, within the scope of linguistic representation and into the realm of scientific study. But many of these discoveries overlap with fields that have moved on by leaps and bounds since Freuds' time and their advances need to be fully integrated into our metatheory. In word and theory Freud implied that biology is *of necessity* part of psychology; his interpretive semantic brings the biological into its interpretive and theoretical domain. The body, however "energically" interwoven with mind, was central to his metapsychological formulations.

The psychoanalytic listening stance and interpretive technique engages all the senses, taking sensory input as a preconscious signal, always potentially informative of some important aspect of the unconscious, in our situations. "Listening," in this psychoanalytic sense, is not merely an auditory exercise, but an attentional disposition harnessing the entire spectrum of sensibilities and emotional-cognitions that participate in forming preconscious rationality. Such reflections, wrote Langer, as early as 1942, invite us

> ...to tackle anew, and with entirely different expectations, the whole problem of the limits of reason, the much disputed life of feeling, and the great controversial topics of fact and truth, knowledge and wisdom, science and art. It brings within the compass of reason much that has been traditionally relegated to "emotion," or that crepuscular depth of the mind where "intuitions" are supposed to be born, without any midwifery of symbols, without due process of thought, to fill the gaps in the edifice of discursive, or "rational," judgment. (p. 98)

An interpretive semantic that for the last hundred years has been delving into these unspoken regions of human interaction and is now moving toward referencing ever finer, more deeply inter-penetrative patterns of transmission; that is familiar with various forms of tele-mental phenomena as daily occurrences within its dialogues, requires deeper investigation of the functional principles that underlie these profoundly stirring transmissive-processes it has unearthed.

The point is that psyche, communication, and cognition, do not begin where feelings leave off. 'Mind' begins in bodily experience, in sensorimotor modes of apprehension, where feeling and perceiving are one. Meaning-attribution—which is the essence of 'psychical life'—however embryonic, also, begins in "our mere physiological constitution" (Langer, 1942, p. 89). Initially charged with the expressive strength of affect, from the start, human communication involves the *whole* organism. And the role of the body, though gradually subdued as predominant channel for sending, receiving, and qualifying messages, continues throughout life.

It has been more congenial to the profession's 'scientific' identity to shroud many significant phenomena in secrecy, to promote a view of psychoanalytic listening as a "ratiocinative activity" (Makari and Shapiro, 1993) performed before a cognitive backdrop of theory. While this is also true, neither how we listen, nor the multiple functions our dialogues serve, or the kinds of inter-psychical phenomena it engenders, are adequately accounted for by an outdated, excessively narrow view of what human 'cognition' encompasses.

The mediation of experience by signs that *indicate* and symbols that *represent,* is a seamless, synthetic process involving sensory and peripheral activities of the central nervous system as well as cortical, cerebral functions. Everything that is registered and apperceived participates in this ratiocinative, cognizing process; "The power of reason is simply the power of the whole mind at its fullest stretch and compass" wrote Creighton in 1921(p.469, in Langer, 1942 p. 99) and today, the contemporary neuroscientist Damasio (1994) reminds, body and brain are one, emotions bear on cognitions just as cognitions can be brought to bear on emotions. Many processes influencing 'thought' originate in what must be viewed holistically as an organic system. A semantic that necessitates anything but ordinary listening is, therefore, obliged to seek the roots of its "*paralinguistic, kinesic and linguistic*" (Makari and Shapiro, 1993, p. 1001) signifiers nested in their biological soil, just as we would unearth the etymological roots of words through their layers of meanings.

Piaget's(and Inhelder, 1969,1970)'genetic epistemology' and Langer's (1942, 1967, 1972) sweeping philosophical studies of symbolic expression, both definitively anchor the beginnings of thought in the feeling body, Piaget in a primary sensorimotor stage of intelligence, Langer in the direct presentational projection of *ideas* in artistic and ritualistic expression. It is commonly recognized that both cognition and creation originate in sensory, pre-sentient forms of knowledge that are preconscious before they become manifest. Given our sharply divided Ego- and logo-centric model of consciousness and 'rationality,' how are we to postulate an 'idea' that is pre-ideational? A memory that is pre-representational? Meanings that are *pre-*semiotic? The unconscious transmission of patterns of affect, interaction, information? A *bio*psychical field that is porous, interpenetrative, 'telemental'? Even Freud (1915),who advised that psychoanalysis steer clear of dabbling in telepathy, could not avoid a furtive glance at the 'uncanny' and at non-verbal transmissions as legitimate *phenomena* of the Ucs: "It is a very remarkable thing that the Ucs. of one human being can react upon that of another, without passing through the Cs. This deserves closer investigation, especially with a view to finding out whether preconscious activity can be excluded as playing a part in it; but descriptively speaking, the fact is incontestable" (p194)

Once we embark on this closer investigation, however, we find that the field has shied away from a systematic inquiry of this sort of phenomena tending, rather, to hide their appearance in embarrassment. We lack any viable principles within the framework of communication that might legitimize their occurrence and render them less 'mysterious'. At the moment, only Jungians feel at ease writing and talking about these sorts of phenomena thanks to Jung's ideas on synchronicity and his very different views on the possible interconnections between unconscious and conscious. Yet even this school acknowledges the current absence of adequate explanatory principles for the kind of 'numinous' material with which most analysts are familiar. Our theoretical grounding still lacks the conceptual amplitude to integrate these quasi-biological transmissive frequencies within a single system of ideas that would account for a class of communicative phenomena which hover between bio- and psycho-logical functioning.

In Freud's model, the nineteenth century "instinctual drives" took the place of affects as prime movers in human psychology; and today the term 'biological' has been abducted by psychiatry to refer almost exclusively to physio-chemical processes. Both these perspectives bypass the organic centrality of affects as transmissive forces and the vicissitudes of their amplification, diminution, ejection, projection, subjugation, transformation and expression as; a) primary channels of communication and; b) *prime movers* in organismic adaptation and personality structuring.

Later to modulate into more differentiated and nuanced *emotions,* human affects are, at the start, powerfully informative, global physiological states triggering deep and pervasive neuro-hormonal repercussions throughout the organism. How and in what ways affects are mediated — which is closely tied to how and in what ways they were responded to early on — is *central* to the understanding of human psychology. An updated metapsychology of personality development inclusive of this central dynamic would place affect-arousing interactions and their derivatives, no matter how diffuse, at the *center* of transference analysis. Because affects are such powerful interpersonal forces, whether they have been strangled or subverted, their original expression and aim twisted, transformed or forced to turn inward and go under, their derivative dynamisms continue to weave through and permeate communication. These interactive patterns *retain their dynamic impact* and pervasive organic effects whether we are immediately aware of this or not.

Psychoanalytic practice has uncovered the enormous inductive pull to enter into and participate unconsciously in the repetitive reactivation of these inter-psychical patterns by observing our own responses to them. Recorded in interactional units, their reactivation and analysis is used as a means of understanding, reconstructing and modifying the inner world. We have learned through verbal mediation and interpretive negotiation to identify and analyze, rather than to react automatically, when under the influence of the unconscious force-fields they engender. But we now have evidence of still deeper, more diffuse, interpenetrative forms of pattern-transmission, impacting directly on sensory-frequencies at quasi-biological levels of responsiveness, the operative principles of which begin to resemble, if not correspond with, sensibilities triggering automatic action-patterns in other species of the natural world.

It is noteworthy that of only two times in his entire opus that Freud referred directly to animals, he did so in his metapsychological paper "The Unconscious"(1915), when hypothesizing the existence of "inherited mental formations"(p.195) in humans at the nucleus of the Ucs. He must have intimated the possibility of there existing some obscure principles of convergence between ourselves and the higher primates (which he mentions), perhaps at the core of attachment behaviors, a convergence that also highlights the greater cortical divide between Homo Sapiens — the *animal symbolicum* — and all other animal species.

This points to the lacuna in our metatheory this section attempts to fill; namely, the integration of primal and primary sensory-affective modes of transmission into a comprehensive developmental/continuum tracing the mediation of human interactive means from natural (biological) to linguistic (semiotic) forms. The kinds of unconscious modes of communication and inter-penetrative transmissive phenomena that psychoanalytic dialogues uncover necessitate biological principles as part of our explanatory framework. To this end, it is helpful to spend a moment tracing the evolution of our own communicative development and comparing and contrasting it with that of other species.

Compared to other neonates, phylogeny equips the human infant with precious little other than a loud signaling system and a prodigious brain. While most young are mobile only minutes after birth, and moving nimbly shortly thereafter, the prolonged immobility and complete dependence of the human infant renders a cluster of attachment and communicative behaviors of paramount importance to survival. Endowed with heightened sensibilities favoring the senses of greatest survival value, other animals also inherit sets of fixed-action-patterns that are timed and released at various maturational stages in close pairing with environmental triggers. We, in contrast, arrive with very few such predetermined links and start out with crossmodal sense-reception —or synesthesia — a predisposition for pattern-recognition through all sensory channels, which makes for infinite variability of response.

Gifted with formidable imitative and recall abilities, the human baby more than compensates for its physical dependency by using faculties that rapidly develop and reinforce the distinctive mediational skills around which mastery and socialization, or *adaptation*, center (Morris, 1969). Rapidly, through the profoundly assimilative and integrative tendencies of the human nervous system, subtle coagulants of 'signification' take shape: there appear intentional sounds and deliberate gestures of indicative reference, request, interest, response, as well as disinterest, impatience, aversion, distress, disgust. Long before we have learned to use language, the dialogue has already begun (see Werner and Kaplan, 1963; Bruner, 1983).

The biological roots of this dialogue begin, as with other species, in phylogenetically inherited natural signaling expressions that are programmed subcortically in limbic nuclei of the brain. Our species is endowed at birth with a readiness to read and express a handful of differentiated facial expressions with widespread organic and behavioral manifestations signaling internal states and affect dispositions to which we react viscerally. The autonomic nervous system of members of a given species is genetically programmed to respond in like fashion to affect-signals from its members.

(Basch, 1983) It is this "autonomic mimicry," or contagion, a reflex-reaction (not *yet* identification), that underlies the origins of affect-resonance, a later more evolved and decentered capacity to 'empathize' with another's emotional experience. Affects and affective behaviors are best defined as "*somatic* responses to the intensity of stimulation of the nervous system, and not to the content, quality, or symbolic significance of the stimulus" (Basch, 1983, p. 107). While this primary interactive mode will become infinitely overlaid and convoluted by the interpolation of acquired signs and symbols, our primal responsiveness to sensory-affective input — immediate, involuntary, organismic — does not go away, no matter how subverted or subdued its expressions become. The emotional-signal will continue to impact viscerally, at undifferentiated levels of experience, or when attention is oriented toward these porous levels of interpersonal resonance.

Clearly, if these basic expressive-patterns have been selected during evolution for their survival value, their vital communicative purpose and interpersonal function, at the outset of the human encounter, must be of enormous consequence to adaptation. It is probably at these deep subcortically-wired functional levels, where the activation of communicative and attachment behaviors originate, that we will also find nuclei of the interpersonal glue that cements group formation and bonding processes; that elicits group thematic-convergence phenomena; that generates cultural expression through the dramatic and creative arts in theatre and ritual, and that predisposes humans toward social, national and ultimately ideological affiliations.

The biological substrate of the 'psychical' is part and parcel of its subject matter (Langer, 1967); affects and not 'instincts' are the biological soil of human psychology, key motivators, core organizers and disorganizers of experience. Life begins in bodily experience; in sensory-motor modes of attunement. However disguised, the biological substrate continues to participate in most human interchange and psychoanalytic dialogues reengage, investigate and work-through, this somatic base. This work points toward an integrated theory of affects and emotional expression that correlates with the method of therapeutic change.

Feelings and felt-expressions are the currency of the first exchange as well as prime instruments of early conditioning; and unconscious dispositions pass easily into a psyche that is at first porous, open, exquisitely receptive to transmissive projections. Habituation abbreviates processing time and hastens response; quickly we learn, and we learn to remember. Animals are programmed for stereotypical reactions; humans mediate experience and modulate response. Animals continue to act in patterns, humans begin to feel and think in patterns. Evocative recall turns into recollection; verbal recounting linearizes and sequentializes thought. Narratives are born: the uniquely human time-factored and time-factoring, storying mode of cognition has begun. (Marschack, 1975)

For all species with complex nervous systems the brain is a master coordinating instrument, integrating sensory stimuli from within and from without and directing interactions with others. Ultimately it is the functional anatomical structure of this organ, serving the nervous system, which determines the kinds of response-patterns and interactions that are possible between an organism and its environment. The human brain is essentially a "signal-processing organ coordinating the activity of all systems of the organism as well as its own" writes Basch (1976b p. 394). Only humans have developed cortices that enable the mediation of experience and modulation of response by thought; and only the human brain features specialized regions forging circuitry that generates interconnections *through its own activity* creating a synergistic functional structure that works much like an orchestra, by coordinating the ever changing contributions of many different parts of a whole. Imagine a symphony — or better still a symphonic score — and you have a picture of the complexity, the multilayered compositional quality of human meanings and communication. Language, in this formation, does not always carry the main melodic line and subcortical channels of transmissive frequencies, the *basso continuo* of our polyphony, remain vital organic pathways to affect-responsiveness and gut reactions.

Of the basic senses — touch, smell, taste, hearing, and sight — vision will become the most highly developed in humans. Sensorimotor schemata retain the intensely diffuse, multisensory input characteristic of primary undifferentiated modes of apprehension; they also provide patterning for the perceptual set, or visual 'Gestalten,' predisposing us toward what we 'see' and how we interpret it. Sensorimotor schemata are gradually, and only partially, superseded by selective distinctions mediated by the linguistic eye and, since all cognition tends toward re-cognition, the indelible neuropsychological imprint of primary sensorimotor patterns leaves deep and lasting traces reverberating throughout personality structure. As a primary *mode of apperception*, however, the sensorimotor gateway continues, throughout life, to be the "common pathway for physiology, communication theory and psychology" (Basch, 1976b, p. 4).

We start out with only slight variations on the signaling theme; animals with fixed action-patterns, humans with malleable affect-patterns. But almost immediately the fundamental differences that set us apart promote divergent development: the mere fact that we are supremely attuned to registering our caretakers' *unconscious* attitudes; to identifying the expressive features of the human face, each of which become meaningful to us in association with the particular *feelings* they have induced, and that we will retain this interactive experience in terms of its *pattern,* must be quite significant for how our minds develop. The fact that we are phylogenetically programmed to react viscerally to a set of expressive signals that are *already differentially signified* through facial configurations must also be consequential in the evolution of a brain that develops its functioning around retaining and abstracting increasingly complex and condensed forms of signification. In effect, we are genetically predisposed by the very characteristics of our primary signaling system toward the reception and retransmission of signifying forms: "A mind that works primarily with meanings must have organs that supply it primarily with forms," reasoned Langer (1942, p. 90). The primary 'patterns' we observe are facial expressions, meaningful to us because they are registered by inducing *feelings*. A template pairing feelings with meanings is set, and *"...feelings have definite forms, which become progressively articulated"* (Langer, 1942 p. 100). Logically, we could not "conceive significant form *ex nihilo*" but only "*find* it, and create something in its image," reasoned Langer (p. 251). The phenomenological world of the unconscious and what are broadly referred to as 'fantasy' and 'imagination' are created by these 'formulations.'

This tendency toward "abstractive construing," or pattern-making, is functionally operative in the primary interaction of *perception* and *emotion* in memory, as processed by hippocampal and amygdaloid structures in the limbic system: "If we consider an event as made up of a confluence of sensory inputs...the highest order of perceptual abstraction of these sensory inputs together with an emotional association are presented to the hippocampus for processing...." writes Winson (1986 p. 29), and of the same process Basch (1976b) writes "Abstraction implies the encoding of the essentials of the form of an event" (p. 405). This spontaneous unconscious process of formulative abstraction is part and parcel of cognition, so it appears that "thc conditions for rationality lie deep in our pure animal experience—in our power of perceiving, in the elementary functions of our eyes and ears and fingers" (Langer,1942, p. 89).

One might view this advance toward conceptual abstraction through any representational medium as a basic principle of mental evolution, applicable to all symbol systems. This implies that the growth of human intelligence and deepening of thought can occur by using any symbolic "grammar," and that the significant mark of its higher forms will be the increasingly condensed, conceptually complex, quality of its manifest formulations. Speech, in this conception, is the practical, interpersonal expression of a more general human tendency compelling humans everywhere to depict, notate, enumerate, narrate, compose, ritualize and otherwise give *meaningful shape* to life events and experiences which are then remembered and "seen" in terms of these organized constructs. Human cognition tends toward economizing thought- and meaning-patterns through condensation and abstraction, a tendency that has produced the panoply of sign-systems with which we are all familiar.

The power of "regarding everything about a sense-datum as irrelevant except a certain *form* that embodies it" results in the ability to recognize a "concept in any configuration given to experience, and forming a conception accordingly" (Langer, 1942 p.72).[2]

"Form" or 'expressive-shape' as *signifying*, is *a priori* in humans, inherent in our bare constitutional endowment, and we react physiologically, emotionally to its impact. "Physiognomic perception," a term fallen into disuse, referred to this pronounced sensitivity to gross expressive features, a sensibility which predisposes toward "seeing-and-feeling" as our first intuitive mode of *understanding.* Wordless, sensory, morphological, 'expressive projections' may be fashioned, amplified and transfigured through many diverse symbolic media, their registration requiring engrosed participation for their full impact and meaning to be grasped. The *primal sharing* of this emotionally-sentient mode of human expression subsumes cognitions of a special kind. But the *signifying principles* that underlie such morphological forms of meaning operate via very different, more direct, sense-pathways than do other forms of reference. They depend on a particular, de-differentiated mode of participatory-attunement, an attentional-disposition that predisposes toward organismic-resonance, the effect of like on like.

When understood as our primary interactive means, 'Emotional expression' becomes the first communicative-mode along a bio-semiotic continuum reflecting the functional evolution of communication as a mirror of 'mind'. This bio-semiotic progression—from felt/unconscious through working-through to verbalization and consciousness—is recapitulated in micro- and macro-genetic sequences in clinical process as the unconscious becomes conscious. If we view this primary mode of "expressive interaction" as a *psychical* phase in a continuum that transitions from biological to semiotically mediated modes of interaction, we are justified in inferring that there may be preceding stages, still deeper, characterized by finer sense-registrations that operate along the lines of biological signals. Reik (1948) pointed out that we receive impressions, now imperceptible to humans, that can be traced to our evolutionary past: "The sense of direction in bees, the capacity of birds of passage to find their way, the sense of light in insects' skin, the instinctive realization of approaching danger in various animals," he wrote, "all bear witness to sense functions with which we have almost no human conceptions to compare." (p. 137) We know that bees dance their instructions in the air, bird's pattern the skies in travel formations, frogs swell to menacing proportions and peacocks flare flashy feathers in sexual enticement; intraspecies communication, throughout the natural world, is transmitted and registered directly through sensory-channels involving the whole organism. The value of acknowledging the continued presence of these vestigial, *pre*-psychical modes of interaction is that it alerts us to the possibility that their deep, sensory-pattern registrations are still impacting on us all the time.

We can tease 'psyche' apart from her bodily, biological substrate only conceptually through the schematic aid of a hypothetical continuum. But because our methodological mandate is to interpret *all* human meanings, many of our referents will originate, or certainly cross-reference, with bodily, even organic, expressions. Most of these emerge directly through physical manifestations and various types of projective enactments. Psychoanalysis identifies and signifies these, salvaging from a sea of peripheral stimuli and organic noises, a whole range of such 'meanings' by redefining their sensory codes as unconscious signifiers (Makari & Shapiro, 1993).We *give* meaning in our situations to bodily communications. Psyche is thereby *created* out of soma, or reintegrated, via a semantic field in which unmediated and masked transmissions are registered, investigated and responded to interpretively. The body is taken as a primary channel of *unconscious* meanings and enacted communications and their negotiated understanding is carried into the linguistic fray of the dialogue. In this way, our method transforms not only the *means* of expression but also the *nature of that meaning.* Infact, our semantic field is so penetrating that it puts us in touch with unmediated interactive frequencies emanating from organic and pre-linguistic elements that suffuse the verbal line with multiple levels of thickly-layered, highly condensed messages.

Any excessively dichotomizing conception that splits this bio-psychical continuum, without providing explanatory principles of mediation, necessarily undermines our theoretical integration of all forms of meaning. A developmental study beginning with emotional expressions provides viable foundations for a comprehensive bio-psycho-social model of communication built on interactive phenomena that span from organic and natural expressive-transmissions, to symbolically mediated abstract verbalizations, providing semiotic principles of reference and dialogicality underlying their transformations.

It is language, of course or, more precisely, **symbolization,** that marks the great divide between us and every other species. Not only does its advent provide an immensely efficient and more exact means of communication but it ushers in discursive thought from which propositional logic, causal reasoning and the examination of fact may follow. It is important, however, to keep in mind that language is the verbal expression of a deeper more spontaneous, unconscious process of *dynamic* *schematization* that has been going on all the time. This unique trait of human intelligence, which functions much like a drive, typically operates by organizing global, diffuse sensory experience into signifying *patterns*, progressing toward the increasingly differentiated and condensed symbolic abstraction of *ideas*. But despite our indebtedness to language for the dexterity of our cognition and for that uniquely human of traits, the stream of consciousness, which is our constant companion, we pay a hefty price, emotionally, for our awareness.

The bifurcation of human experience into inner and outer, wordable and subliminal impressions, and the consequence of this for psychic integrity and awareness, is a subject already well trammeled. Because language is closely paired with socialization it precipitates a split in human experience between what is true to the self and what is indoctrinated by the environment; what is, and can be, spoken about and what must not be uttered; between what is seen and said, and what is truly felt. By its very objectifying and denotive tendencies, language limits the scope of our thoughts and communications to what can be fitted into its prepackaged signifiers and proscribed sequencing. It is most unsuited to the simultaneous representation of multiple processes or the transient quality and morphology of feelings.

It is especially not helpful, then, when examining communication developmentally, to separate what are initially intricately interwoven facets of total organismic-functioning that, in great part, continue to be dynamically interwoven throughout life. Perception, emotion, cognition, locomotion; interactions between impulse and action, feelings and speech; image, meaning, and memory; the relative balance between effectance and affiliative needs, attachment and individuation, reality testing and identification, all, are negotiated simultaneously and in idiosyncratic ways that are shaped by the unique meeting of temperament and environment, in the singular circumstances and dynamisms of first encounters. All the while the steady growth of the semiotic function, the gradual mediation of experience through the use of sign and symbolic vehicles, unfolds its predictable developmental sequence: out of a pre-verbal dialogue of expressive and indicative looks, gestures and sounds, first single words, then language will appear to configure our perceptions and habits in particular ways.

In early development, the emotional ebullience and shared immediacy of our primary communicative mode is modulated by words: the fluid spontaneous responsiveness of the whole sensorium becomes increasingly subdued and differentiated, outward expressions retaining only faint traces of earlier modes, the rest funneled neatly into culturally tamed, conventional codes. We grow accustomed to the speech forms and referential habits of those around us: language fixes for us in awareness primarily what we have been shown, while everything else, the multipaletted sensory-rich cognitions of our felt life and its unique, subjectively tinged values, fall by the wayside of awareness, or go under. The dynamisms of personality style and psychic-structuring evolve out of an amalgam of private experience woven through the fabric of social veneer. Of all species, only humans develop an inner and an outer face; a linguistic profile with an emotional shadow. These discrete modes of life-experience and the disjunctive effects they have on the human psyche have already been amply discussed. Both Freud and Langer, from different perspectives, examined their diverse forms of knowledge, Freud referring to them as the **primary** and **secondary processes**, Langer as **presentational** and **discursive form**. The attributes that characterize the primary mode were identified and carefully listed by Freud (1900) in terms of "mechanisms" that become 'bound' by the linguistic processing of the secondary mode; they were described by Langer (1942) in terms of the self-limiting properties of **discursive** vs. the expressive power of **presentational** "forms." Freud and Langer had obverse views of the Ucs; Freud saw a "seething cauldron," Langer the wellsprings of creativity. Language, for Freud, constituted *the* rational vehicle of thought and reason, Langer pointed to the specific weaknesses in the properties of discursive form which yields only a particular, narrow *kind* of thinking. Conceptually, 'mechanisms' and 'forms' belong to different paradigms; yet the phenomena under discussion are the same.

Despite Freud's (1900) recognizing that the nucleus of the dream 'thoughts' employs cognizing faculties of the *whole* mind, and despite Langer's (1942) statement that "The recognition of presentational symbolism as a normal and prevalent vehicle of meaning widens our conceptions of rationality far beyond the traditional boundaries..." (p. 97), neither integrated the far-reaching implications of these assertions into a general theory of knowledge that takes the communicative *and* significative function of affects as its starting point, a move that leads logically to the *close pairing of feelings and thought*. Although each identified the presence of ideas in this *emotionally sentient* form of knowledge — Freud in the interpretation of dreams, Langer in her analysis of art and ritualistic symbolism — and both sought biological roots for psychological shoots, neither anchored *emotional-cognition* in the biologically differentiated affect-signal that is our primary mode of responsiveness,[3] as a primordial template of 'meaning'.

Consequently, we have inherited a somewhat dichotomous picture of 'psyche' (with connotations of 'lower' and 'higher') its *organic* fibers insufficiently knitted into a unified theory of mind. Clearly it is theoretically imperative for a *science* of the 'unconscious' to integrate these disparate physicalist and philosophical conceptions into a single system of ideas. Neither pathogenesis nor art nor cognition *alone* suffice as starting points for a comprehensive understanding of human nature, and our study will have to yield a synthesis. The construct of a continuum from natural to mediated forms serves us better in this integrative endeavor and accommodates the indisputable fact that "ideas" and "understanding" are both *unconscious* before they are formulated through verbal mediation. We alone, among all species, are able to exploit verbal form for communicating and thinking; the trajectory from natural expression to florid speech and abstract thought, however, is not without its obligatory phase-transitions and referential passages. Cognizance of symbolic and referential process is quite central to our understanding of the quality of psychoanalytic listening and interpreting.

A developmental study of human interactions thus becomes a window through which to observe the transformative microgenetic-process of verbal signification and the effects of this type of mediation on mind. Given our methodological focus, we can also examine the mediation of unconscious to consciousness by observing our own shifting modes of responsiveness as we adjust our attunement to different organizations of meaning along this continuum. Once a functional hierarchy has crystallized, it is important not to confuse function with form but to understand that human meanings are always an amalgam of interrelationships and compromise-formations between multiple unconscious threads issuing from different developmental levels. In fact, each functional-organization that can be isolated along this continuum may yield highly sophisticated and abstract ideation, if we are receptive to its form of expression—a lesson we learned from dreams that, in themselves, are neither more nor less "primitive" than their dreamer. But if we remain unattuned, or unresponsive, to the frequencies transmitting a particular kind of information, we will neither register its forms nor understand its messages. A sophisticated understanding of human meanings has to take into account the functional organization in which a particular form is being used.

To understand the unconscious interplay of words, feelings and enactments that manifest transferential material—the *sine qua non* of the psychoanalytic method—it is necessary to 'enter into' the field of interaction, using oneself as a 'receptive transmitter.' The different forms of unconscious communication and transmission elicited by this attentional stance and its interpretive aims, reach undifferentiated regions of human inter-action for which we have no adequate terms or concepts. Insofar as these interpenetrative, transmissive phenomena are fairly common in our situations, and appear with some regularity in dreams, it is reasonable to infer that as a species, we are phylogenetically programmed with particular sensibilities that are finely tuned toward affective-cues. These biological, pre-semiotic phenomena require biological principles of functioning to understand them. 'Drives' took the place of 'emotions' as primary dynamic forces in Freud's metapsychology, creating a conceptual schism between the human psyche and human communication and an enormous split between theory and practice in his metatheoretical framework. But his interpretive semantic, and its primary methodological goal, effectively unifies the two. Reintroducing 'emotional expression' as our primary mode of interacting, within a *communicative system* governed by principles of semiotic mediation, brings together the practical and theoretical faces of depth psychology. The purpose of this section is to integrate biological principles of communication into our predominantly linguistic framework

The morphological perspective provides the missing metatheoretical dimension from which to develop a comprehensive model of human communicative means tied to modes of attunement that encompass the pre-psychical, biological substrate. Morphological principles also stitch seamlessly into formulative principles of semiotic and referential mediation.

The intuitive recognition of meaning in emotional expressions of the human face, I believe, functions as a template predisposing us to physiological responsiveness to the signifying impact of 'form.' Out of this primary foundation can be derived principles of meaning and communication the most basic of which have to do with perceptual and intrapsychic *differentiation* and *separation,* and the develop-'mental' leap resulting from the use of *mediated vs. natural* modes of communication. Conceived in this way there are no sharp breaks between physical, psychical and 'mental' realities, only "thresholds where mentality begins, and especially where human mentality transcends the animal level, and mind, emerges" (Langer1942 p xix). Instead of dichotomies, this conceptualization, proposes *phases and phase-transitions.*

Perhaps this is the crux of why, even toward the end of his life, Freud felt that he had failed to fully grasp the "nature of the psychical." 'The psychical' is not a 'thing' to be grasped by reifying grammars; it's nature is fluid, a multidimensional transitional *passage* in an ongoing stream of sense-registrations ever building on one another, wedged, as it were, between biological, unconscious and mediated, conscious experience. One essential quality of this phase is that it manifests through *presentational projections* the expressive records of which are recognized as having meaning only to those who are receptive to their modes of appearance. Words affix significance to these condensed psychical meanings, but only to certain aspects of them and only in partial and very limited ways, as one would momentarily freeze an image from a single frame of a moving picture or halt a musical passage to review a single bar with only parts of an orchestra. The richly hued, multidimensional, combinatorial palette of unconscious form is far too varied, subtly nuanced, swiftly shifting and complex to be captured, in its entirety, by discursive form.

And here again we meet with one of the profoundest of human dilemmas: the splitting in two of our social nature by a linguistic mode of communication and conventions of discourse that leave out, or eclipse, a vast array of *felt*-registrations, while our primary mode remains highly sensitive and responsive to these interpersonal cues. In order to 'tune in' to these transmissive-frequencies and be able to identify them linguistically we have to remain both receptive to, and aware of, their subtle interpenetrative modes of informing.

The most important thing to note about this, aside from the multilayered quality of all human interchange, is that different forms of information are registered in different ways; for the primary mode the *quality* of "being felt" is already an index of meaning, whereas for the secondary mode the act of "naming" is a first step. The primary *transmits* connotational patterns of feeling *directly*; the secondary *communicates* information *sequentially*.

The fundamental difference, then, between these two semantic domains, in terms of *responsiveness,* lies in their discrepant modes of informing: expressive meanings of the primary mode touch us directly by evocation and induction whereas communications of the second inform by indicative and denotive *reference*. Each captures and delivers discrete aspects of human experience and sentience but differs radically in the mode of transmission. The primary mode is uniquely capable of conveying intangibles such as degrees and qualities of mood, the tempi of emotions, the nuanced morphology of feelings, in fact, the whole panoply of sense responses that constitute the emotional undertone of interactions. The linguistic mode, on the other hand, demarcates, denotes and points to material and conceptual "things"; reification and sequencing are its trademarks. The primary mode is capable of capturing simultaneity in time and fluidity of process, the secondary operates by placing one thought after another and stringing them like pearls, constructing causal chains, logical reasoning, narratives of value and belief.

Psychoanalysis is the first interpretive semantic to integrate the two by using the latter to interpret the former. And a good part of the difficulty is inherent in problems of translation — there has to be fluency in the transposition from one form to another. Words can only describe sequentially what the primary mode conveys instantaneously. Basch (1976b) likened this to the problems in translating poetry; "That which can be denoted gets translated, but connotation, the capacity to effect total transformation, is lost" (p. 415). Citing Hall (1966), he emphasized how rules of conduct, culture and relationship are learned through unspoken messages: we signal attitudes, intents and feelings through nonverbal activities of the body, for which speech-content is often just a "background noise behind which the relationship unfolds…" (p. 416). Basch (1976b) went so far as to say that psychoanalysis is not really a discursive cure because, in its method, speech is used only "to promote a transformation through interpretation" (p. 419), a point that is worth considering.

In order to stay within a conceptual paradigm that accommodates principles of form and transformation, I suggest the terms **morphic sentience** to conceptualize this primary nonverbal, perhaps unspeakable, way of knowing, and **morphological apprehension** (morphe: form. apprehend: to seize, arrest, perceive, understand.) (Concise Oxford Dictionary 1958, 4th ed.) to define its de-differentiated mode of emotional-*understanding.* In addition to sprouting a number of useful derivatives such as morphic-mirroring, morphic-echo and morphic-matching, to define a number of clinical interventions that might so far lack identifying terms, the aptness of this terminology, for these types of meaning, within the general framework of communication, will shortly become clear. In seeking to understand the nature of 'mind' through a developmental study of modes of human interaction, we would begin in the expressive body of infancy, at the very inception of life, from where we can "trace them to their sources below the psychological levels, and perhaps conjoin two sciences in a single system of acts…" (Langer, 1942 p. 65).

To cast this integrative understanding into a theoretical construct it is necessary to discard the illusion that 'thinking', 'understanding' or communicating are 'cerebral' activities. For the certainty that 'mind' emerges out of broader, organic, sensory-sources is a ponderous obviosity to anyone who has had a childhood. We might, at this point, turn Descartes' famous schismatic dictum "I think therefore I am" around to "I feel therefore I *understand*," but we have yet to articulate a sufficiently comprehensive theory of human sentience to back this up. Theory, observation and practice, however, come together under one system of ideas in a psychoanalytic study of communication that also fills the metatheoretical void left by insufficient consideration of the communicative function of affects as *signals* at the start of life.

The convergence between ourselves and other species in nature is to be found in the automatically-activated *physiological* character of the signal response-pattern. In animals this operates exclusively by contagion (and remains fixed) whereas in humans it becomes overlaid by mediated responses while continuing to operate unconsciously through induction.

These vestigial, deeply porous modes of pattern-transmission and registration, emanating from the biological substratum, continue to induce unconscious 'replications' and 'repetitions' until their impact is mitigated by conscious awareness. To seek out viable *principles* of communication that encompass organic, undifferentiated modes from deep strata of functioning, it is helpful to borrow some interesting new ideas from our neighboring field of biology. They come from the renowned English biologist Rupert Sheldrake (1981, 1988, 1991) who, in three incisive volumes, has proposed a trenchant evolutionary hypothesis of "formative causation," suggesting that self-regulating systems at all levels of complexity, including organisms and societies of organisms, are organized by the habituating processes and goal-oriented properties of "morphic fields."

Sheldrake's work is the culmination of a major shift in developmental biology evolving out of the holistic spirit of the 1920's when the nature of biological inquiry turned away from the study of molecular "mechanisms" toward the discovery of their principles of organization. Around this time developmental biologists had begun thinking about biological morphogenesis in terms of embryonic, or **morphogenetic fields** (Sheldrake, 1991), an idea that has now been widely adopted. Like the known electromagnetic fields of physics, which are conceptualized as regions of influence with inherent holistic properties, morphogenetic fields within and around vital organisms are believed to attract members of a given species to their developmental or inherent growth potentials (p.109). Living and developing organisms would thereby inherit not only genes but also morphic fields (p.112).

Morphic fields would account for a kind of collective memory from which "each member of a species draws and to which it in turn contributes" (Sheldrake, 1991, p. 110) and which, outside of genetic principles, is modeled on the actual forms and patterns of behavior of previous members that inherently draws toward maturational goals: "As in the science of magnetism and electricity souls were replaced by electromagnetic fields, by a comparable step in biology, entelechies were replaced by biological fields"(Sheldrake, 1991, p.109). The likelihood of a behavioral form or pattern being taken up and followed to habituation depends on the frequency with which it is practiced, and the fields are viewed as the means by which such habits are built up, maintained and inherited (p. 109).

In this framework, **morphogenetic fields**—only *one* kind of morphic field specifically concerned with the physical maintenance and development of organisms—are capable of generating habits that are followed and established through repetition. The forms of learning and memory that influence morphic fields depend on **morphic resonance** a process based on similarity, the effect of like on like through space and time. Morphic resonance is not affected or diminished by distance; it does not involve a transfer of energy but of *information* (p. 111) and is best defined as an intraspecies mode of information-transmission transcending time, place and geographical boundaries. Sheldrake's (1991) hypothesis enables Jung's idea of a 'collective unconscious,' or Freud's phylogenetically inherited Id, to be viewed not only as human phenomena but as part of a more general natural process. In effect, it proposes that the regularities of nature be understood as governed by a mixture of inherited and acquired *habits* maintained by morphic resonance, a factor that includes humans and the human mind, as part of its evolutionary design. Testing his hypotheses, Sheldrake predicted that "patterns of thought should tend to occur more readily the more they have happened before" (p.128) with results yielding considerable evidence that this does indeed occur. Again, Jung's concept of *a priori* ideas, the primordial image, the archetype, would fit into this mold.

The notion and properties of fields, incidentally, fits equally well with the new science of networks and the dynamic architecture of their growth, proliferation and impact.

The idea of biological fields, morphological in character, capable of generating and transmitting information within their regions of influence, is very appealing to those of us in psychoanalysis who are interested in studying the constitution of unconscious processes of communication. If this hypothesis joining form and energy in transmissive-frequencies can be generalized as a *principle* of intraspecies communication, it ought to be applicable not only to animals of instinct but also to those of symbols. It is in this sense that I propose applying the idea of **morphic resonance** to human **semantic fields**, conceptualizing these as spheres of awareness and new ideas that are spread through discourse by specific referential and dialogical activities that gradually expand the domains of human consciousness, behavior and knowledge. These fields would be set in motion and operate through verbal exchange, generating semantic spheres .But their maintenance and advance would simultaneously be fueled by deeply unconscious, collective, biological patterns of nonverbal transmission. In this conception, almost all human affairs are understood as operating simultaneously at multiple levels of interaction — like many channels — from which the linguistic, probably due to its denotive properties, is usually selected as the most dominant.

Modern science and contemporary physics have now transcended the old atomistic, mechanistic world view; rigid determinism, and the "hard, inert atoms of Newtonian physics" have dissolved into force-fields and invisible regions of "vibratory activity," writes Sheldrake(1991, p. 5). The breakdown of space/time as separate dimensions and the idea of 'fields' of energy existing in many different forms have virtually supplanted the formulas of force and matter of the science of the Freudian era from which, it is embarrassing to say, our "temporary" metatheoretical "scaffolding" is still molded. Scientific methodology itself has become probabilistic, nonlinear, chaotic, its discourse given to constructing domains of inquiry among many possible perspectives; from many quarters the murmurs of a major paradigm shift are gathering momentum.

Delivering first a sharp critique of the still prevalent mechanistic world view, Sheldrake (1991) astutely points out that contemporary science is now pushing to the threshold of a new synthesis, beckoning toward a potentially more unifying, holistic and naturalistic world view. Writing at the twilight of a century of massive change, when what was thought to be a vacuum is "found to be pulsating with vitality and energy"; when particles and antiparticles spring into "virtual existence" out of space; and at the dawn of a "communication" era when protons and electrons are viewed as "quanta of vibration" (pp. 87-88) writes Sheldrake, "The invisible, organizing powers of animate nature are once again emerging in the form of fields" (p. 5).

Psychoanalysis is such a preeminent *semantic* field; its powerful new referential orientation — "the unconscious" — and innovative interpretive method awakening us, and the culture whole, to the world of "psychical" reality. Basch (1976b) drew attention to the fact that the value of the discoveries pertaining to psychoanalytic discourse are part of a broader philosophical movement toward structuralism and general systems theory which gained ascendance in the middle of the past century, while Schöen (1986) also traced different epistemological visions inside the psychoanalytic movement itself to a more fundamental shift in twentieth century thinking from *objectivism* to *constructvism*. But what has less frequently, and not forcefully enough, been pointed out is that this was *implicitly* Freud's philosophical position. He could not otherwise have devised the scientific methodology, or practiced and advocated the loosely-receptive, nonjudgmental, multiperspectival interpretive stance that is its requisite, were this not the case. Psychoanalysis heralded and is still, philosophically, at the epicenter of a major, gradual epistemological transformation, and its founders' methodological insights foreshadowed the whole sway of *relativism*, the harbinger of a new synthesis ahead. The vector of this trend is best delineated in Goodman's(1978) words, himself an important voice in this mainstream of philosophical thought that began when "Kant exchanged the structure of the world for the structure of the mind, continued when C. L. Lewis exchanged the structure of the mind for the structure of concepts, and now proceeds to exchange the structure of concepts for the structure of the several symbol systems of the sciences, philosophy, the arts, perception and every-day discourse. The movement is from unique truth and the world fixed and found towards a diversity of right and ever conflicting versions of worlds in the making" (p. x).

In effect it was Freud and only Freud among those forming the psychoanalytic movement of his day who could sustain the ambiguity and multiperspectival interpretive and theoretical scope required of the world of the 'unconscious'. Ultimately he stood alone, forging a path in the dark without the benefits of guidelines or glare of doctrinal headlights. Curiously, Freud has been ensnared by the very limits of the conceptual language and science of his day — against his own beliefs and writings — devalued for a metapsychology that by its 'provisional' nature openly declared the very conceptual deficits he decried. Freud's scientific genius is placed at the heart of a controversy in which the dominant epistemology, and malformed metatheory it helped misshape, have obstructed our view of what psychoanalytic methodology discloses. For our part, we have lacked the wisdom to submit our method to a rigorous methodological analysis.

The extraordinary value of psychoanalytic methodology lies in the exquisite fit it provides between method of inquiry and the nature of the phenomena under observation. The interpretive stance requires a sustained, controlled partial breakdown of the subject/subject division in order to gain access to what cannot be identified or made 'sense of' by other means. Because this division is itself, in part, generated by discursive form and reinforced by conventional speech codes, the method adopts a highly specialized, complementary listening stance for its highly specialized interpretive purposes. This mutual fit between the communicant's speech-form, the dialogues purpose and the interpreter's referential perspectives, together, generate psychoanalytic **semantic fields**, wherein unconscious phenomena and *psychical* meanings rise to prominence. Unwittingly, these regions of *interpsychical* connection have also revealed forms of transmission that are 'mysterious' only insofar as they have yet to be understood within the framework of viable principles of human interaction. Psychoanalysis takes these non-linguistic transmissions, repetitions and manifestations *as communications* and, by translating them into words, stretches language beyond the confines of discursive form. It does this by splitting the participant/observer's *experiencing* self from the *referential* self and linguistically joining the two. This methodological stance, paired with a primary 'referential perspective' oriented toward everything 'Unconscious', generates a new *way of knowing* that is ideally suited to the interpretation and research of the human psyche.

Freud's approach was never objectival but *dialectical* to the very core, as we saw in the previous section. Pathways of personal inquiry and insight are more effectively pursued through a human dialectic, since "we can know our own subjective depth as much by scrutinizing the meaningful objectifications 'expressed' by other minds, as by introspection. In complementary fashion, self-scrutiny may give us clues to the penetration of objectifications of life generated from the experiences of others." wrote Turner (1981, p. 14) in a Diltheyian vein. Ours is a multimodal listening stance, mediating input from all sensory channels, integrating information through visual, emotional and linguistic modes of attunement: we simultaneously observe exemplifications, experience evocations and enactments; feel projections and inductions; and listen to ideational, conflictual content. Out of this interplay of form, content and response *within* contextual process, we strive to understand the individual, personal unconscious. But in order to identify these multiple currents of transmitted, enacted, and communicated material, theoretically, we have to be familiar with their diverse forms.

This is why a psychoanalytic, developmental study of communication inevitably becomes a springboard for metatheoretical revisions, even a platform for their implementation.

Freud stumbled on a refined, exquisitely fecund instrument of psychological investigation. His discovery brought forcefully to the fore that we can ourselves become agents of our own transformation by showing, with Darwin, that "organic species and individual minds are fundamentally modified by the processes in which they partake" (Whyte, 1960, p. 49). Unfortunately, the physicalist orientation defining "science" in his day failed him completely when he turned to it for concepts of form, organization, pattern and meaning; the simultaneity of polyvalence and multidetermination; the dialectical mutuality of interaction and recursive embeddedness; and the phasic, spiraling progressions of slow change and labored transformation that are the dialogical, process-phenomena of the psychoanalytic method. Freud found himself caught in the middle of what Whyte (1960) referred to as the "great transformation" (p. 49), a slow shift in philosophical and scientific thought that is gradually moving us away from "*static toward process concepts*" (p. 49), a paradigm revolution that is spreading but is by no means complete.

When we refer to clinical psychoanalysis as a 'process,' we actually mean a *dialogical* process. But the tendency of language to reify, and of the human mind to exploit this concretization, has made a "thing" out of process itself, obfuscating the fact that to study process-phenomena *scientifically* is to identify their features, forms, phases and stages, the nature of their combinatorial elements and properties, in relation to each other and to their unfolding. Like music, dialogue is complex, multi-leveled, temporal, fluid, always moving forward in time, influencing cumulatively, the present building on the past, the past reiterated in the present, tumbling, spiraling, leading forward, ever forward.... As with all living processes generated by people meeting for a purpose, the journey is organic, dynamic, fluctuating, expanding and contracting, its tempi ebbing and flowing, energies synchronizing and desynchronizing, its qualities shifting, changing, always a becoming, transiently rising to awareness and fluidly passing away....

Psychoanalysis is not a medical 'cure' but a *dialogical process*, its psychological impact and therapeutic effects based on re-experiencing, working-through and acquired insight, an emotionally laborious, reflective journey that cannot be delegated or handed down as 'information' but has to be traversed personally. There is here no inherent division between the process and those participating in it; the nature of the cure and nature of the analysts' understanding and wisdom. Ideally, the disposition of the psychoanalyst is that of a thinker not a healer. I am inclined to agree with Reiff (1962) when he says that a "cure cannot be achieved without an exemplary presence"(p. 29), as much due to the banality of imitation as to the fact that *psychoanalytic* insight can only be arrived at by guidance from someone who models and embodies, in practice, its *modes* of understanding. There is here, again, no division between form and content: the process *is* its material, the collaborative effort and its internal creative processes having much in common with the aesthetic experience (Beres, 1975) and the kinds of criteria that matter in the analysis and appreciation of art.

For all of this, psychoanalysis has always met with enormous resistance; as a science it is discredited altogether. This has less to do with its true scientific merit than that its multiperspectival, participatory epistemology and dialogical practice did not fit 'scientific' protocol. Yet the fixity of the fields' problems and the acrimonious rifts that appear endemic to its constitution belie deep-seated resistances that are played out at practical and communal levels but that may have even deeper roots. Notoriously unwilling to look dispassionately at what we would rather not see, psychoanalysis holds up a mirror reflecting aspects of human nature, and the flimsy foundations upon which many human convictions stand, that have transformed our psychological vision and cultural discourse. These represented both cherished illusions and hidden facets of human nature from which the species has recoiled for centuries via externalizations, projections and expedient, if fictive, divisions. The resistances that it unleashes at multisystemic levels are deeply entrenched in a world view that placed the seat of our superiority in 'rational', linguistic faculties, implicitly dichotomizing spiritual and instinctual dimensions, debasing the body along with the rest of the non-sentient animal kingdom. The confines of this ancient edifice are with us still as are many of the prejudicial, moral codes upon which it was erected. We ourselves are the creators of this charter of conceit, proliferating mythic divisions that provide refuge for longstanding attitudes of dominance and control that continue to sanction our abusive entitlement to 'master' and usurp all other species and exploit the natural world.

Such apertures as the psychoanalytic lens afford enlarge the conceptual awareness and scope of human responsibility in ways that are so profound, suspect and, as yet, unclear, that it calls forth enormous defenses. By challenging the remaining bulwarks of our tacit assumptions and conceits, it threatens to dismantle the remnant partitions that are the last stronghold of an old, Cartesian world view. In more ways than one, psychoanalysis awakened us from this slumber: at personal levels we have had to encounter the enduring soil of primitive affects, primal fears, cherished illusions tied to archaic longings; at communal levels we have been called to question the very foundations of linguistic structures that conceal hierarchies of power and codes of control; at epistemic levels psychoanalysis challenges implied divisionary dichotomies between subject and object, emotion and thought, science and art, forging links between animals of nature and those of culture, disclosing a continuum between signal and sign, the enduring resonance of biological sense along with the semantic symbol of significance. With its liberating, free-associative speech, designed to dislodge the self-limiting constrictions of conventional discourse, and its phylogenetic dimension, psychoanalysis threatens to reach those vestigial regions where animals and humans meet, as different species, diversely endowed, yet biological species nevertheless, dwelling within, and as part of, natures fields.

The greening of the human psyche makes plain that dialogue is its garden, grown from the seeds of a primary dialectic, our root human condition. As with all living, organic things, the imprint of its past encounters lie fossilized in the deep tissue of its structuring forms; it tells the history of itself as do the rings inside a tree, or the geological layers of the earth's crust. Like all dynamic forces of nature, the power of diadic dialogue on the human psyche is immense and, depending on how it is used, can yield regenerative, benevolent or catastrophically destructive results. Perhaps this is why those after Freud who intimated the enormous potential of this new process-science often pointed to the threat it posed as well: "Psychoanalysis," wrote Loewald(1970) is "as dangerous and as promising an undertaking as atomic physics, depending on how we use this emerging power of understanding the formation, composition, decomposition, and reorganization of the human psyche" (p. 50).

Curiously eschewing parallel biological concerns with growth, maturation, evolution and the morphological shifts, which would appear to be the natural subsoil for a study of mind, psychoanalysis took the path of physics instead. Yet psychoanalytic dialogues are based on processes of recapitulation, dissolution, restructuring and redevelopment, akin to morphological regeneration and growth. Including the morphological dimension into our metatheoretical propositions provides the missing link in a conceptual framework that joins natural, presemiotic forms with semiotically mediated modes of interaction while opening an empirical window to the observation of communicative forms as indices of bio- and psycho-social processes.The phenomena that are of relevance to the science of psychoanalysis are these dialogical and semiotic processes of the therapeutic and supervisory situations, the latter which, as Levenson (1994) pointed out, operates at a higher level of abstraction. There is much to be gained by approaching the study of dialogue as a living, dynamic, organically-transforming process that can harness natural tendencies toward psychological integration, consciousness and maturation. A study of communicative forms and dialogical process can be the starting point for a radically different conceptual lens through which to reconstitute the foundations of our theoretical propositions, taking psychoanalysis into a paradigm of pattern, transforming interchange, meaning and communication.

Freud opened the door to a new interpretive semantic—primarily a means to better understand ourselves—which, it is now clear, will have to adopt a more naturalistic, organismic/developmental, epistemic framework. What it now needs, in Loewald's words (1978), "might not be a new 'language' but a less inhibited, less pedantic and narrow understanding and interpretation of its current language leading to elaborations and transformations of the meanings of concepts, theoretical formulations, or definitions that may or may not have been envisaged by Freud" (p. 193). By its recognition and exploration of our timeless "psychical reality" it foreshadowed post modernist sensibilities; and by its loose unprejudicial attentional disposition it reveals that efforts to dominate are incompatible with efforts to *understand.* At some profoundly primordial level the *intent* to understand is equivalent to an act of love.

Where there is no antithesis between science and art, and the inquiry "consistent with our view of art, poetry, and other activities of no material gain," wrote Rapaport (1966), our investigative method is an unparalleled, scientific interpretive instrument. From the perspective here espoused, then

> ...the human mind in all its fullness is itself an expression of natures essential being. And it is only when the human mind actively brings forth from within itself the full powers of a disciplined imagination and saturates its empirical observation with archetypal insight that the deeper reality of the world emerges. A developed inner life is therefore indispensable for cognition. In its most profound and authentic expression, the intellectual imagination does not merely projects its ideas into nature from its isolated brain corner. Rather, from within its own depths the imagination directly contacts the creative process within nature, realizes that process within itself, and brings nature's reality to conscious expression. Hence the imaginal intuition is not a subjective distortion but is the human fulfillment of that reality's essential wholeness, which had been rent asunder by the dualistic perception. (Tarnas, 1991, p. 434)

SECOND MOVEMENT
HUMAN INTERACTIONS

THEME & VARIATIONS

Theory and concepts, and the material of experience to which they pertain, are inextricably intertwined. In psychoanalysis it becomes increasingly clear that *interactional* processes — those that are intra-psychic and inter-psychic ones, and these two in their interactions — are the material of investigation, epitomized and highlighted in the psychoanalytic process. It is for that reason that this interactional situation itself is the subject matter par excellence. It provides the best experiential basis and testing ground for our theories.

(H. Loewald, 1980 p. vii)

INTRODUCTION

From the dawn of human life, within the matrix of a primal dialectic, begins a uniquely human form of interaction. An infant's involuntary movements and noises are responded to by someone who begins inferring and interpreting their "meanings" and reacts accordingly. The nexus of this exchange already contains the mutual shaping, the search for sense and intent, and the building of trust and understanding, that form the basis of intimacy in human interchange. The vocabulary of this primal language is bathed in sounds and movement-patterns of handling, holding, soothing, gazing, cleaning and feeding, awash in the sensory qualities of physical and emotional expressiveness. Inherently bi-directional, the exquisite mutuality of this primary biological fit is epitomized in the reciprocity of lactation which simultaneously feeds the baby while benefiting the mother as it forges the most powerful and formative of human bonds. Whether ministrations were warm, tender, playful and vocal, or tense, despondent, silent and detached, will leave lasting traces in the anlage of experience, swaying natural dispositions toward or away from the human encounter as currents of a river propel its waters this way or that.

Development will progress in a direction that moves away from the mirroring matrix of this intimate orbit toward increasing self-regulation, autonomy of movement, locomotion, action and thought. And the human environment provides for this incremental maturational-individuation by furnishing communicative foundations and programming a lengthy, multipronged educative, acculturation process, spanning several developmental stages, that is designed to equip the young adult for autonomous living.

Learning to communicate verbally is at the very heart of this entire process. And our offspring enjoy privileged access to language that is facilitated by a steady stream of linguistic input from those around them, subsequently reinforced by the community and society at large. Very early in the enterprise, notes Bruner (1983), children participate in the management of joint attention, inferring meaning and intent, learning referential acts, negotiating procedures and reciprocity, and in so doing are "learning the ways of the culture as well as of its language" (p.11). Identifying four cognitive endowments — "means-end readiness, transactionality, systematicity, and abstraction"(p.30)—that provide the enabling interactive conditions upon which language acquisition builds, Bruner (1983) emphasized, "Linguistic conventions and standard forms do not leap full grown from the egg," but are "usually slow transformations of initially primitive or 'natural' procedures that become socialized in negotiation"(p.69). These interactional sensibilities and skills evolve out of general, non-linguistic exchanges that are implicitly cultivated in routinized formats and play situations that form the communicative subsoil of the early milieu: "predicting the environment, interacting transactionally, getting to goals with the aid of another, and the like," are all processes that have to reach requisite functional levels *before* language can serve to "specify, amplify and expand distinctions" (Bruner, 1983, p.30) which are there even without words. Language becomes a tool for interpreting and regulating the culture, and "The interpreting and negotiating start the moment the infant enters the human scene" Bruner (1983, p. 24).

But changes in form of communication are also spurred by innate, progressive pathways that follow certain timetables and are subject to critical periods: language, for instance, appears at a particular time, in a particular sequence, and in response to environmental exposure. The advent of speech brings correlate changes in mentation: relationships between speech and thought are such that language is capable of radically transforming the nature and quality of experience. Carried inward, speech traces an ongoing internal, private commentary that will subsequently go under while continuing to influence and regulate many aspects of the personality.

During early development, communications and events are assimilated according to available cognitive structures and phase-appropriate modes of thought, a factor that creates implicit disjunctions between a situation and how a child construes it. Furthermore, experiences are filtered through highly idiosyncratic temperamental dispositions and developmental needs: turbulent passions sway behaviors toward compromise-formations sowing seeds that are precursors for defenses already visibly taking shape. At the least differentiated levels the *whole* domestic ambiance is introjected; its rhythms, routines, odors, menus, dynamic patterns of interaction, vocal tone, style and duration of utterance, facial and postural expressions, habits of holding and touching, approval and rebuke, unconscious attitudes, modes of affect-regulation and impulse control, its movements, gestures and glances… are *all* taken in wholesale.

Children learn how to behave, what to say and what to hide, by imitation and by how they are responded to; and both the response, its emotional-tone *and* how it felt, are introjected as a unit. In this way, codes of conduct, cultural values, and unconscious family dynamics are all transmitted through communicative interactions that become increasingly funneled through linguistic exchanges. And while, the restraining power of superego-precursors have, undoubtedly, been influencing behaviors long before the advent and internalization of speech, it is nevertheless the auditory admonition, the specifically *vocal* character of the superego, that enables it to plant a tenacious grip on personality controls, unlike the ego ideal which, self-created, has more visual or imagistic qualities. "In this way," wrote Freud (1940), "the super-ego continues to play the part of an external world for the ego, although it has become a portion of the internal world" (p. 206). Although Freud's pioneering observations did not encompass semiotic or semantic processes, his dynamic, structural model indicates a sophisticated appreciation of the impact of internalization through his construct of the superego:

> Throughout later life it represents the influence of a persons childhood, of the care and education given him by his parents and of his dependence on them — ….And in all this it is not only the personal qualities of these parents that is making itself felt, but also everything that had a determining effect on them themselves, the tastes and standards of the social class in which they lived and the innate dispositions and traditions of the race from which they sprang — …."

> (p. 206) It could be viewed that "...the external world, in which the individual finds himself...represents the power of the present; that his id, with its inherited trends, represents the organic past; and that the super-ego,...represents more than anything the cultural past..." (p. 206) And so, he concludes, the superego "...unites in itself the influence of the present and the past" (p. 207).

Most of early development takes place in communicative contexts and through communicative interactions; as Rapaport (1951) pointed out, communication is the "quintessence of socialization." Recalling Shilder's (1924) words, he added, "Socialization is not an acquisition of man, he does not learn it in the course of his lifetime. It is a fundamental implication of his nature: it unfolds as he matures, but it is there from the beginning" (p. 449). For this reason it is well nigh impossible to separate 'communication' from 'psyche,' so closely have the two grown up together.

Major theorists from Janet to Freud, Piaget to Vygotsky, have tackled the important question of how the inner world takes shape, each stressing and focusing on different facets of this process. The internalization of patterns of interaction and communication is a fundamental principle of development, the essence of which is that during development children begin adopting internal attitudes toward themselves that were initially used by others in relation to them. The genesis and formation of psyche take place gradually through an interactive matrix that for the child is initially undifferentiated. Laced with sensory, kinetic, vocal and visual cues, tied to *somatic* modes of introjection, all these sensory signals are assimilated unconsciously. The *individual* psyche grows out of incremental *differentiations* between self-and-other. Its character and constitution will derive from the meeting of natural disposition with the attitudes and behavioral codes underlying key relationships during formative years. Similar ideas where expressed by Loewald (1962, 1970, 1978b):

> The concept of internalization, as the essential process in intrapsychic structure formation or,...in individuation, presupposes neither the subject-object split nor the assumption of a separate

> psychic apparatus or organization, however primitive, from the beginning; it posits an original field or matrix, the mother-infant unit, within which individuation processes start. If one thinks in terms of an original undifferentiated phase of psychic life, this then would refer not only to id-ego as intrapsychic potentials, but equally to the psychic undifferentiatedness of psyche-environment, of internal and external. (1970, p. 290)

Loewald, was pointing toward a developmental orientation that understands psychic structuring in relation to planes of increasingly *differentiated* functional organization, an idea also developed by Gedo and Goldberg (1973).

But the missing piece to this developmental puzzle and one that has, thus far, been neglected, is the symbolic function itself, both an instrument and a result of *differentiation.* Without knowledge of the principles and implications underlying the developmental line of symbolization (Aragno 1997), with its concomitant advances in separation-individuation and changes in the quality of social and internal life, theoretical integration is incomplete. Symbolization (Aragno 1997) follows a slow developmental course closely tied to affect-regulation and verbalization, interwoven with representational capacities, objectification, and innate cognitive preparedness. The advent of the semiotic function indicates a developmental readiness to use differentiated signifiers to name, denote, and indicate things, but the assignment of meaning, and its psychological effect, is contingent, and will impact, on overall functional organization. Complete referential distance between signifier and signified, which is requisite for a truly *symbolic* relationship, must await considerable development and functional differentiation—the two go hand in hand—so that language and words are not used by three year olds in the same way as they are by thirteen or thirty year olds. Piaget (1969, 1970) made this amply clear: by taking a biological perspective in studying infant and child development he realized that "no symbol by itself supplies operative meaning, but that, on the contrary, the meaning and meaningful use of symbols is subordinated to available operative structures," (Furth 1970). Different levels of operative functioning in the use of language imply different organizations of meaning even *within this symbolic system*, a factor that is extremely important to psychoanalysis and its instrumentation of speech. This progression of 'meanings' and inherent ideational advance, cannot take place without the dialectical soil of discourse to help promote its higher symbolic organization.

For the better part of development, and in most learning situations, this gap generates what Vygotsky (1978) called the "zone of proximal development," loosely defined as the distance between actual level of independent problem solving and potential level as determined by problem solving with guidance(Vygotsky,1978 p.86). Viewed by Vygotsky as a fundamental principle of cultural development, the idea of an inherent learning or developmental **region** allows one to consider not only what learning has already taken place, but also what learning is just beginning to occur and is still in transitional or formative stages. The zone of proximal development, which subsumes socio-cultural, semiotic and referential aspects, encapsulates those processes whereby what has been experienced socially, on the inter-psychological plane, becomes internalized and structured intra-psychically. I am not alone (see Wilson and Weiner, 1992) in viewing this as an eminently useful concept for psychoanalysis — in the analytic process, but also in supervision and throughout psychoanalytic discourse — because it invites a detailed situational analysis tracing the particular interactional forms and semiotic processes involved in this transition inward.

Vygotsky's (1978) concept serves effectively as a tool for studying the *specific* impact of different situations and relationships, a task to which Piaget (1962) had also turned, suggesting; "It is therefore not 'social life' as a whole that psychology must invoke, but a series of relationships established in all possible combinations between individuals of distinct levels of mental development, and as a consequence of various types of interactions (coercion, co-operation, imitation, discussions, etc.)" adding, "Though obviously social life plays an essential role in the elaboration of concepts and of the representational schemas related to verbal expression, it does not in itself explain the beginnings of the image or the symbol as they are to be seen in deferred imitation or in the first imaginative games of the one year old child"(p. 4). The confluence of many endogenous and exogenous streams, originating from different aspects of experience and organismic functioning, converge during early development, condensing sensorimotor and perceptual schemas as well as innate imagistic and *signifying* tendencies of the human psyche.

Vygotsky's decidedly social and semiotically based model of internalization, pivots around the close interrelationship between learning and development. From a Vygotskian (1978) perspective, higher mental or specifically *human* psychological functions, originate in processes of socio-cultural exchange. Therefore cognitive *and* psychical structuring comes by way of the social use of semiotic tools; conventional signs, numbers, various notational and verbal symbol systems. The internalization of social interactions in terms of the character of their semiotic forms is quite central to Vygotsky's approach. The key to understanding the development of higher processes of mental functioning is in the modifying effect on human action of the sign carried inward: "A sign is a means for influencing behavior," wrote Vygotsky (1960) "either ones own or another's:...it is a means of internal activity directed toward the mastery of humans themselves. A sign is inwardly directed" (p.125 in Wertsch, 1985, p.78).

Vygotsky's (1978) main ideas on internalization, as spelled out in *Mind and Society*, can be subsumed in the following three key points: a) an operation that initially took place in external interactions is reconstructed and begins to occur internally; b) higher functions originate in actual relations between human individuals; an interpersonal process is transformed into an intrapersonal one (or an interpsychical situation becomes intrapsychically structured); and c) the transformation of an interpersonal process into an intrapsychical one is the result of a long series of developmental events....the transfer inward is linked to changes in the laws governing their activities; they are incorporated into a new system with its own laws (pp. 56-57).

As a psychological instrument, language has the capacity to radically transform mental functioning;[4]

when introduced into a mnemonic process, for instance, it brings about a fundamental change in that function and consequently also in the nature of experience and behavior; "by being included in the process of behavior, the psychological tool alters the entire flow and nature of mental functions. It does this by altering the structure of a new instrumental act..."(Vygotsky, 1981a, p. 137, in Wertsch, 1985, p. 79). Vygotsky's genetic law of cultural development invite a detailed analysis of the specific situational features and communicative processes that engender a sphere of potential development and become the basis for the transition from an interpersonal exchange to its intrapsychic structuring — an approach that is especially congenial to the study of the semiotic and speech processes of psychoanalytic contexts.

I am drawing attention to the fact that in the genesis and formation of psyche, those very semantic and semiotic forms, speech habits and patterns of interaction that were learned and internalized early on, partake of the nature and dynamic constitution of what we refer to as 'psychic structure'. Vygotsky (1978), a social psychologist, wrote, "The history of the process of the internalization of social speech is also the history of the socialization of children's practical intellect," (p.27), while Loewald (1970), a psychoanalyst, stressed the internalization of *interactions*; "What become internalized, are not objects but interactions and relationships" (p. 291). Again, these two aspects of psyche – cognition and object-relations – are inseparable from the nature of the interactions that took place early on, and the history of these experiences is encrusted in a psyche that will subsequently reveal both in communicative form and style. This trajectory of theoretical thinking, initiated by Loewald (1970), emphasizes the interactional origins of psychic structuring and reality:

> a theory of mind, of the psyche as it shows itself to psychoanalytic research, should start with the hypothesis of a psychic matrix within and from which individuation proceeds. In this regard I have tried to describe parallels between the psychoanalytic situation as a novel force field and earlier fields of psychic forces within which differentiated and autonomous psychic entities and structures arise and develop (p 229).

Communication will parallel and reflect this increasingly differentiated, symbolic functional organization. And through an array of subliminal expressive and indicative nuances that complement, embellish, sometimes contradict and always qualify the verbal line, it will continue to reveal information from unconscious, sensorimotor sources of which the speaker is totally unaware.

Given this enduring multistratal and multimodal quality of human experience it is important to keep in mind that different modes, or levels, of assimilation play a considerable role in all new 'learning'. Greenspan's (1982) organismic-developmental model takes this into consideration: it proposes three forms of learning and awareness tied to *pre-representational* and *representational* cognitive capacities. Three, hierarchically organized, principal levels of learning are posited characterizing — **somatic, consequence** and **representational-structural** learning (p. 661) — each of which accounts for different aspects of human experience and all of which continue to operate throughout life. These are viewed not merely as maturational milestones but as organized levels of learning, suggesting that there may be different forms of awareness, from barely distinct sensations to fully organized feelings and ideas, all of which remain open to change through experience: "Awareness is not an exclusive function of the highest level of central nervous system functioning but involves the entire body" (p. 667). Greenspan concluded there may be a hierarchy of levels of awareness paralleling the three basic levels of learning, all of which are in constant interplay with each other. [Others studying the nature of psychoanalytic learning, particularly, Rapaport, 1960; Piers and Piers, 1965; Ornstein, 1964, 1967; have also noted different modes of learning].

This conceptualization converges with many of the ideas that are proposed in this work. Greenspan, however, chose not to address the "complex issue of conscious and unconscious awareness'" (p. 672) thereby omitting the dimension that is most central to a psychoanalytically informed model. The piece that is left out is the same that most have neglected, namely, the impact on experience and knowledge of *specific* semiotic mediations and referential processes. This crucial dimension, with all its various ramifications, will be taken up again at various points in the situational analysis of psychoanalytic contexts (chp,3). Suffice it to say at this juncture that the *potential* for becoming consciously aware is co-developed through the dialogical progressions which also seal in, as it were, the additional *awareness of being aware* that is characteristic of, and unique to, psychoanalytic dialogues.

But processes involved in becoming aware cannot be divorced from what one is to become aware of, both of which involve verbal acts of referencing and symbolization. As Vygotsky (1978) noted, the mind is not so much a complex network of *general* capabilities; learning processes do not affect *overall* capacities, but rather exercise a variety of particular abilities to focus attention on specific things in particular ways: "This leads to the conclusion that because each activity depends on the material with which it operates, the development of consciousness is the development of a set of particular, independent capabilities." (Vygotsky, 1978, p.83).

The whole impressionable climate of early development is so completely imbibed in communicative interactions that it is impossible to tease apart what has been structurally welded together, from the beginning. Once we appreciate what this means, we can better understand the value of a method that by its specialized speech forms, interpretive semantic and contextual objectives — that is by dialogical means alone — succeeds in having the experiential past unfold *in vivo*, re-externalized, before our very eyes. By virtue of its historical/genetic perspective, its quasi-experimental qualities (we observe shifts in awareness taking place in minute to minute exchanges), and transformational goals, it provides the slow process conditions that are ideal for broad-spectrum psychological inquiry and change. Certainly, it is *the* method for studying the genesis, ontogenesis and "fossilized" forms of psychical structure that express character traits, behaviors, and the inner world.

The technique, method and theories of psychoanalysis, though premised on the analytic inquiry of the personal unconscious or the individual mind, were operationalized by Freud, in relational or *interactional* terms, through interpretive activities that simultaneously encompass the self, the other, and the two in relation to each other, as the dialogue unfolds. The unit of investigation in psychoanalysis is therefore the *single* mind but the method works by establishing an "inter-psychical" semantic field wherein an interpretive dialectic, implicitly generated between two people, leads to the contextual phenomena that form the foundations of psychoanalytic processes. As preeminent vehicles of the clinical method, transference and resistance are phenomena that arise in interaction: as Loewald (1970) emphatically stated, they are basic "interactional phenomena of psychic life, and...no psychoanalytic investigation is possible without their making their appearance and being taken into account" (p. 287). Whether we consider the psychoanalytic situation as a "novel interpsychic field" (Loewald, 1970,

p. 285) or simply as a "conversation," as did Freud (1926), the conditions that set in motion psychoanalytic processes have proven to be the "arena *par excellence*," (Loewald 1970) for observing the "underlying principle activities that enter into the organization, maintenance, and growth of the individual mind" (p. 293).

It follows that a psychoanalytic study of communication, comprising an analysis of its own communicative forms, will be an extension of the study of mind. If we see in psychoanalysis what Freud (1914) saw, "a science erected on empirical interpretation" (p.77) then we will approach our study of communication from all metapsychological perspectives and from the vantage point of integrating communication into our metatheories.

The central theme of this entire movement is the idea that a psychoanalytic investigation of communicative processes must take the inception of human interactions as its starting point and, from this genesis, will trace its ontogenetic course and forms from all metapsychological perspectives. Communication interweaves with all aspects of 'mental' and psychological development continuing, throughout life, to be an instrument of processes by which higher forms of symbolic, functional organization and knowledge can be reached. A specifically *psychoanalytic* study of communication therefore will not favor a purely "linguistic" or even a "speech" orientation, but will enter into, and become part of, the "bi-personal" (Langs,1976) field it generates, in which biological and psychological processes continuously interdigitate.

Communication is polysemic, polyvalent, polyvocal: through it can be identified different types of meaning, different semiotic and referential forms, the impact of identifications and internalizations, including the behavioral codes, beliefs and traditions of that culture, that family and that society in which the historical formation of that individual psyche developed.

Suffice it to say that although we may tease apart what is tightly knit in nature, the complex interdigitation of a number of different developmental lines in early development can only be understood in terms of a dynamic synergy of them all. Neither an exclusively socio-*or* psycho-linguistic approach suffices when examining an interpretive process that reaches beyond manifest linguistic meanings to unrepresented experiences tied to the subverbal soil. Only the integration of many dynamically interconnected semiotic and a pre-semiotic organizations of meaning, paralleling a hierarchy of communicative modes, provides a sufficiently comprehensive and complete picture.

The idea that psychoanalysis is inherently an ideal method for researching the dynamic processes of communication echoes the ideas of Rapaport (1951), Searles (1955), Rycroft (1958), Basch (1976b), Peterfreund (1980), Freedman (1971), Freedman and Steingart (1975), T. Jacobs (1993), and Shapiro (1991), to name only a few authors whose works point toward the need for further investigation of communication in the psychoanalytic and supervisory situations. A similar interest was pursued by the early analysts Ferenczi (1919), Reich (1933), Reik (1940), Deutsch (1947, 1952) and Gostynski (1951), to point to those who also approached the subject from an organismic perspective.

The three essays that follow, like variations on a theme, are designed to provide the conceptual underpinnings for using communication as a mirror of psyche. Like thematic introductions, foreshadowing the full development of melodic lines to follow, each section examines and integrates communication into each of the five metapsychological dimensions, and the last recasts the current pluralistic 'versions' of psychoanalysis into the language of discourse. In this way I begin to implement the broad, conceptual revisions from which the theoretical foundations of this work emerge. This exploration will uncover what can be drawn from using communication — in all its sublinguistic, transmissive, enactive and symbolic forms — as a metatheoretical point of entry for understanding how the genesis, formation, and subsequent regeneration of the human psyche through a dialogue, takes place. Far from a mere veneer on the analytic surface, approached in this way, communication becomes the living soil of deep interactive phenomena exhibiting a multifarious web of unconscious roots, as well as the stems, leaves, buds and flowers of bio-psychical processes, of intrapsychic makeup, and of the enormous transformative power of dialogue to impact on mind.

FROM SIGNALS TO SYMBOLS: THE MEDIATION OF NATURAL EXPRESSION BY SEMIOTIC MEANS

> Our consciousness of the perceived world yields us an objective system, which is a fusion of mere data and modes of thought about those data. Whitehead, 1927, p. 37

> The whole progressive genesis of conceivability, the evolution of human thinking in all its complexity, lies in the divergence of these forms. Langer, 1967, p. 81

In this section I present a highly simplified and abbreviated version of what has been exhaustively examined and more fully developed in "Symbolization" (Aragno, 1997). The following provides a simple outline of the developmental principles and corresponding forms of reference and response, underlying the functional differences between basic semiotic forms.

Our species lives in a world of signifiers: signs and symbols orient our perceptions, bridge our communications, sculpt our ideas. With their help we envision our creations, plot our course and record our discoveries; they embolden our strategies, impact on our relationships and determine the quality of our inner life. Those realms of meaning and reason and imagination that we define, quite rightly, as uniquely "human," are just that, thanks to the organizing function of the *sign*, the use of which generates fundamentally new and qualitatively different forms of behavior, communication and thought. However much the formal customs of conduct and gesture, value and belief, differ from culture to culture, the ability to behave adaptively, to balance inner and outer realities and, ultimately, the difference between mental order and disorder, rests on the fluid status and functional stability of the symbolic function.

The whole fabric of human experience, the potential and realization of human modes of thought, of higher forms of understanding, abstraction and selective response, are predicated on the developmental steps and subsequent interweaving of these different forms. No general theory of mind or of communication is complete without a thorough understanding and integration of the logical principles underlying their diverse organizations.

Stages in semiotic mediation may be thought of as qualitative shifts along a continuum: each transitional phase is influenced by and evolves out of those preceding it, epigenetically, and each produces radically different modes of experience and organizations of thought. The stages crystallize into more or less organized levels forming the hierarchical organization that characterizes multileveled functioning. One is struck by Freud's perspicaciousness in this regard, when, in "The Unconscious" (1915), he noted:

> …analysis shows that the different mental processes inferred by us enjoy a high degree of mutual independence, as though they had no communication with one another, and knew nothing of one another. We must be prepared, if so, to assume the existence in us not only of a second consciousness, but of a third, fourth, perhaps of an unlimited number of states of consciousness, all unknown to us and to one another. (p. 170)

This observation is quite accurate: although these are not so much "states" of consciousness as organizations or *forms* of consciousness, each derived from different referential forms yielding significantly different types and degrees of awareness. However, like many of Freud's ideas belonging to the topographical model, this one, also, was obfuscated and abandoned for lack of a viable conceptual framework within which to develop it.

In my 1997 interdisciplinary study of the ontogenetic stages of symbolization, I attempted to provide a detailed developmental template for a model of mind accounting for the mediation of unconscious to conscious through transpositions in semiotic form. The same linguistic, mediational sequence and obligatory referential progressions are recapitulated whenever something is brought to conscious awareness. In addition to generating a genuine paradigm shift—from metaphors of energy to principles of form—the theoretical underpinnings of this model provided the pivotal concepts for **process, phase-transition** and **transformation** that were missing in psychoanalytic meta-theories. It thereby provided an explanatory basis for the therapeutic action of the clinical dialogue and a conceptual prism through which to examine the particular referential and speech activities by which *overall,* higher symbolic functional organization is achieved.

It was this epistemological and developmental perspective that yielded observations of the shifting morphology of communicative forms in supervision, in essence, a live viewing of diversely evoked, enacted or verbally mediated modes of reporting and exploring clinical material. This same perspective, also in supervision, provided a direct lens for indices of progress in psychoanalytic thinking through the supervisee's increasing ability to objectify the process. Improvements were characterized by a reversal in the ratio of reproductive 'showings' to 'tellings' paralleling greater referential distance, clinical acuity and verbal articulation. One of Freud's pivotal clinical precepts regarding the inverse relationship between action and thought — 'what is not remembered will be repeated' — is well borne out by the logical principles of this framework.

The transpositions in reference and semiotic-form underlying many key psychoanalytic dialogical processes reflect mediational shifts along a semiotic continuum that can be understood as recapitulating in micro-sequences what in ontogenesis occurs serially, producing transformations in awareness that are "linked like stages of a single process" (Vygotsky, 1978, p. 46). Accordingly, each advancing progression revisits the phenomenological experience to which its form is tied, along an increasingly denotive continuum moving from somatic (Ucs) expression, through indicative reference and naming (Pcs.) to fully symbolic, verbally articulated thought (Cs). Formal organizations, or phases-transitions, along this continuum are observable, and other psychoanalytic researchers have also traced its course through various movement indicators (see Freedman, 1971; Freedman and Hoffman, 1967; Freedman and Steingart, 1975; Freedman and Grand, 1985, 1997).

In speech and everyday exchanges signals, signs, and symbols intermingle and mix, each weaving its strand of meaning into the overall sense. Most importantly, the differences between these semiotic forms are universal; their phylogenetic course in human evolution can be traced behind an ontogenetic developmental sequence that yields different modes of thought and awareness. The ways in which their levels and organizations impact on meaning, understanding and consciousness, and their logical progressions, are general phenomena of mind generating universal principles of communication. These are applicable to all dialogical, linguistic activities, but most particularly to those specifically harnessed by psychoanalytic processes, for which they provide explanatory foundations.

Curiously, the field has failed to recognize the importance of this bio-psychological model, despite the fact that it provides theoretical grounding for the central operative and transformative activities of psychoanalytic dialogues and a venue for testing many of its central therapeutic hypotheses; as Vygotsky (1978) noted, "The history of the development of the higher functions is impossible without a study of their prehistory, their biological roots, and their organic disposition" (p. 46).

We look to ontogenesis to analyze the macro-sequential stages in the mediation of natural expression by verbal semiotic means. Human learning usually results from a combination of organic preparedness coupled with environmental input in interpersonal exchange, so that the social climate of early development provides the conditions by which "*children will grow into the intellectual life of those around them*" (Vygotsky,1978, p.88). Similar processes ensure the trans-generational transmission of culturally-determined habits, beliefs and universal taboos; "Behind this childhood of the individual," wrote Freud (1900) "we are promised a picture of a phylogenetic childhood—a picture of the development of the human race, of which the individuals development is in fact an abbreviated recapitulation influenced by the chance circumstances of life" (pp. 587-588).

For a reconstruction of this phylogenetic heritage I turn to the renowned and controversial anthropologist A. Marschak (1972). Through his detailed studies of the notational markings and artwork of early Homo Sapiens, Marschak surmises a vast amount of communication, although not of an entirely vocal or semantic nature, that would have been expressed, recognized and understood, requiring near human brain functioning for its use:

> Once voice and brain had evolved to the point where the hominid could utter symbolic words, these words would not in the early stages, have been used as *defined* symbols, abstracted in meaning, as we define words today....On the contrary, it would seem that the words would...have been used *as part* of a communication of meaning that could be understood only within a process, or relation, or if they referred to a process or relation....To understand the evolution of language one must therefore understand the scope of the visual-kinesthetic, non-verbal, cognitive aspects in hominid communication. (pp. 117-118)

Prehistoric forms of early-human communication would have been of a special kind, involving concepts and processes in time and space consisting of symbolic, storied-communications of their time-factored meanings. These meanings, in turn, would have expressed particular and specialized knowledge of such things as local geography, the skills, customs and culture of the particular hunting group and habits of the animals they hunted: "To the extent that 'story' was involved," writes Marschack (1972), "communication and knowledge were *beginning* to be abstracted and therefore to be generalized as 'cultural coin,' capable of being inherited..." (p. 117). When they appeared, words would have been *supplementary* in these communications, perhaps accentuating and specifying nonverbal content that would always have carried meanings more pressing and more inclusive than could any word. Experience and knowledge would have been context-bound, not yet generalized information regarding animals or seasonal changes at large; words would not have been truly symbolic, yet, but would have referred directly and concretely to the tasks, processes or relations pertaining to a specific place and time.

Another important factor in early human communication going beyond matters of 'meaning' or 'understanding' to proto-conceptual and mnemonic cognitions...

> ...concerns the nature of what is meant and understood. It includes memory and the capacity for comparison, for learning, for mimetic and kinesthetic understanding, for synthesizing and abstracting relational concepts and concepts in a time-factored geometry. This evolved, hominid communication would include the capacity for expression and recognition of feelings and "states." Because of this complexity speech would have been only one aspect, perhaps simultaneous, of that broad evolving, non-verbal process involved in communication and symbol-making
> (Marschack1975 p117).

Marschack's (1972) important message is that words and language emerge out of broader, more basic, species-specific symbolizing tendencies that are already active at early pre-verbal, sensorimotor levels of intelligence. During development the first referential acts are shared and gestural; sensorimotor learning (Piaget and Inhelder, 1966) takes place predominantly through the "unspoken preceptorship of significant models" (Basch, 1977, p. 234). Indicative, denotive, expressive and evocative gestures and intonations result from mimicry and imitation, in a dialogue in which one member of the dyad, the adult, operates at symbolic levels while communicating and, sometimes, communing also in signaling or sensorimotor terms. Once the child is capable of pairing name with person, word with thing, and can pronounce this utterance audibly this has resulted from a dynamic, dialectical matrix that has been cultivating these prelinguistic foundations in functions that are first fulfilled "primitively if abstractly" (Bruner, 1983, p. 31) through preverbal means: "...there is a wide, changing, developing, and diverse interplay of meaning, understanding and recognition between mother and infant *before words* are used intelligibly...and this pre-verbal interplay includes the communication of relatively complex 'storied' meanings" (p. 119)

The initial one-word sentence of infancy contains an entire scenario of such storied-meanings. Like the "name" that calls a presence to the inner eye, the single word of childhood floats in a connotative sea, adrift in a tide of evocative sense-associations. Likewise, in all probability, for the word-using adult *Homo Erectus* for whom, Marschack (1972) infers, "naming" would have subsumed a whole complex aggregate of contextualized and storied-meanings:

> The spring flower that we today call by some Latin classifying name, early man might have named, "he, yellow after the snows." The complex of meanings in this simple statement would have included for that hunter in that culture a recognition of the round of years, the dearth of winter, and the spring thaw and flood. Within the local knowledge it might also have had reference to the spring coming of the great herds or flocks of water birds in the time of "he yellow." The name, then, implied reference to a "story," to a *relation or process* which was understood, teachable, and communicable. It was a recognition with meaning in time and space. (Marschack, 1975, p. 119)

This, then, is what is in a name! In addition to the extraordinary condensation and multiplicity of implied meanings that gather within the single word, naming is an immensely efficient act promoting increased order and focus to sensorimotor experience (Basch, 1976b), affecting perception, memory, communication and cognition: "...the notion of giving something a *name* ...the vastest generative idea that ever was conceived"(Langer1942 p.142), its impact, quite possibly, having modified our species' mode of living, feeling and thinking within a few generations. Semiotic activity of any kind performs specific organizing functions that result in fundamentally different, mediated, more controlled forms of behavior. The word's denotive specificity and organizing power is a leap beyond any gesture — indicative or expressive—its use ushering in an entirely new, distinctly human form of thinking and communicating, and an increasingly *psychical*, or 'signified,' inner life.

Words are like prisms, capable of refracting different meanings; their underbellies face deep, sensorial root-associations, their sense open to the whims of context and use. In this light "meaning" is merely a potential, materializing in organic acts of linguistic exchange, so that "In living speech this meaning is only a stone in the edifice of sense" (Vygotsky, 1934, p. 305, in Wertsch, 1985, p. 124). We marvel at the metaphoric foundations, the plasticity and malleability of language, that it can shrink or expand to meet the user's intellect and needs while providing the means for stringing along a running commentary of life experience, the stream of consciousness, silently, steadily wording everything.

To trace the ontogenetic progression of verbal symbolization is to stumble again on certain basic processes of differentiation and internalization: the words first function is social, and how it was initially used socially will be reflected in how it begins to operate internally. Language carried inward also becomes an instrument of self-regulation and thought: concepts are born of words. Speech is the public face of a medium with private and subterranean functions deeply interwoven with perception, emotion, cognition, identification and action, so that *"... as soon as speech and the use of signs are incorporated into any action, the action becomes transformed and organized along entirely new lines"* (Vygotsky, 1978, p. 24). One cannot understand the impact of semiotic mediation, spoken or thought, until the functional dynamisms of the *whole* organism are observed and degrees of differentiation and self-awareness are figured in. In order to fully integrate the therapeutic role of language into an explanation of the psychoanalytic process and cure, our metatheory has to encompass the functional impact of sign-use and symbolization. The theory has to account for the *specific* semiotic and referential activities that our dialogues set in motion and the transformative nature of the ways these are actualized in our interpretive processes.

The logical principles of semiotic forms are broad, overarching metatheoretical principles that underlie different functional organizations of meaning, modes of thought and the phenomenology of human experience and awareness. These formal principles are woven through the process at many levels: their metatheoretical, explanatory value is articulated at very high levels of abstraction. For this reason it is important for psychoanalysts to be aware of their development and distinctions.

The development of the symbolic function flowers in an interactive field that is vitalized or devitalized according to the nature and quality of early care and interchange. Its *operative* functioning, however, is always contingent on sufficient anxiety-free experience (or adequate anxiety-regulating mechanisms), since intense anxiety wipes out the space wherein the symbol is born. A deeper understanding of the functional interrelationships between various developmental lines early on is therefore central to psychoanalysis, particularly with respect to the vicissitudes, use and channeling of symbolization. Spheres of sophisticated symbolic functioning may not be immediately apparent if we look only at verbal activity. This is a *crucial* point in the analysis of artists with early talents whose predominant symbolic articulation may have matured outside of the verbal, communicative field, and another important reason for understanding development as uneven, discontinuous, the dynamic expression of unique, individual endowments meeting adaptive needs in highly idiosyncratic ways;

> ...child development is a complex dialectical process characterized by periodicity, unevenness in the development of different functions, metamorphosis or qualitative transformation of one form into another, intertwining of external and internal factors, and adaptive processes which overcome impediments that the child encounters.
>
> (Vygotsky, 1978 p.73)

Simply put and in developmental sequence; humans move from natural signals to increasingly mediated expressive and indicative gestural and then verbal signs, to the ability to use fully differentiated denotive verbal symbols. Only the latter are capable of abstracting conscious knowledge. The marked formal and functional differences between these three imply different types of reference and meaning, different modes of experience in communication, which elicit different kinds of response. These are their differences. **Signals** alert; their transmissive function to induce reactive response; the distance between signal and signalizer is nil, the two are one, hence the expressive form and intensity of signaling behaviors *are* what they "mean." Due to this non-referential character, signals incite physical reaction not ideation: the signal can only mean itself; action is its currency. **Signs**, on the other hand, are more differentiated and discrete, by their indicative or denotive reference they point to, single out, identify, and draw attention to. But unlike the symbol, which is fully differentiated from that which it stands for, the sign-function still partakes in some way of that to which it points or shows: its referential distance is therefore greater than that of the signal but not sufficient to incite *conception*; signs announce their objects, whereas symbols lead us to *conceive* of them (Langer, 1942). Only the **symbol** proper and *symbolic* referencing is truly ideational, of the mind: the symbol filters and frees experience from the senses, becoming a vehicle and instrument of thought by representing not the "thing" itself but the "idea" and meaning of that to which it refers. It is this complete differentiation between symbol and experience that lifts mental functioning to a higher plane.

Signification and symbolization then belong to two functionally distinct semiotic organizations, although sign and symbol are in constant interplay during everyday exchange. It is important here to dispel a common misconception among psychoanalysts based on the assumption that if something is verbalized it is automatically 'symbolized'. First of all language is a sign system before it functions symbolically, and secondly, there are many forms of language that operate at non- and proto-symbolic levels, particularly at the height of transference or parallel process enactments. Functional shifts toward the kind of thinking that indicates advances from the sign to the symbolic use of language and higher organizations of mental functioning occur during development, primarily by means of the youngster's own mental activity and through participating in dialogues that provide a 'zone of proximal development. Speech, language and especially learning are not conflict free functions, but heavily implicated dynamic expressions of the whole personality. Infact, they are readily contaminated by defensive and identificatory processes that calcify through habit into interactive patterns that potentially interfere with symbolic thought, learning, reality-testing and intelligence itself. The implications of this appear to me to be enormous considering that a parent that relates and communicates to a child primarily through symbolic organizations of thought will implant radically different modes of speaking and thinking than one that is predominantly posturing through linguistic signals.

The functional shift from the **sign** to the **symbolic** use of language is major in development and at any time again thereafter, when this same semiotic sequence—identifying, naming, processing, and abstracting—is reiterated. This context- and subject-specific progression of symbolization generates far-reaching transformations in the nature of thought and awareness and, in psychoanalysis, also of *overall* functional organization. Becoming aware of 'something' consciously always implies semiotic progressions and linguistic referential activities that in the psychoanalytic semantic include verbalization and working-through of repressed and deeply unconscious experiences that are still functionally tied to organic, or signal and proto-sign, levels of organization. Our semantic is unique in giving verbal reference to essentially non-indexical meaning-forms as well interpreting the repressed.

The semiotic and referential processes of identifying, naming and working-through of the deep unconscious bring denotive clarity to otherwise amorphous experience and enacted patterns. In terms of referential forms, as Goodman (1985) has noted, denotation runs in the opposite direction from evocation which involves "production of a feeling, memory, idea...and so is to that extent not a referential relation at all" (p. 65). The referential stages of the interpretive process in psychoanalytic dialogues generate "actual reorganization of relevant aspects of brain function" to use Gedo's (1995) words, whereby "cortex and midbrain collaborate to provide better control" (p. 353). In a continuum from action to verbal abstraction, it is easily demonstrable that verbal symbolization promotes order, self-regulation and higher levels of autonomous functioning and thought.

The intricate fabric of meaning in human interchange is an amalgam of all three, signals, signs and symbols; but only the symbol, complex, condensed *and* conceptual is capable of subsuming and abstracting meanings carried by all three. The analyst in the analytic setting is not so much an arbiter of reality as the bearer of a symbolic order, striving against inordinate regressive forces pushing for reenactment, to restrain, reflect, re-member and work-through, instead.

For both analyst and analysand the semiotic progressions leading from unconscious experience to conscious insight are reached by the similar routes although each has a different role and purpose in the analytic space. Therapeutic activity includes the analysts facilitating and the analysands acquiring the ability to curb impulse, tolerate tension, observe, reflect and work-through. This progression, repeated over time and along many thematic threads, gradually moves the whole functional organization toward higher levels of symbolic articulation where language is transmutative of action and words acquire "a peculiar degree of autonomy" (Loewald, 1978/1980, p. 190). For analysts it is the degree to which they have quickened the ability to simultaneously identify and objectify unconscious dynamisms operating in the current process combined with the technical arts of timing and wording interventions; for analysands, it is the ability to enter into the process and use analytic interventions to identify, differentiate, work-through and reflect on unconscious meanings and experience. The semiotic sequences produce both self/object differentiations *and* verbal symbolization: therapeutic gains are felt along interpersonal and cognitive/intellectual lines, for it is assumed that a more differentiated psyche is less likely to act-out repetitive or defensive patterns in displacement.

Acquiring "conscient mentation" as (Loewald, 1978, p. 199) referred to it, or raising the whole cathectic level as Freud conceptualized it, is a *referential* process, integrative and maturational only insofar as it advances capacities for self-observation and reflection, joining affect, memory and word, in working-through *while communicating this to another*. The therapeutic task of the analyst and the interpretive challenge of the transferential encounter is to "differentiate or re-differentiate thing-presentation from word-presentations" (Loewald 1978/1980 p. 190), to disentangle current experience from its signal/affective template, a linguistically generated individuation that simultaneously yields personal integration and autonomous thought. As I emphasize throughout, it is not verbalization *per se* that is mutative, but the fully differentiated *symbolic* use of language to objectify and abstract specific unconscious derivatives. Only a certain *kind* of talking comes from the kind of thinking reflective of the fully differentiated objectification *and* integration of various levels and aspects of personal experience.

It was Freud's (1914) genius to take action as remembrance; to understand displacement and enactment as unconscious forms of narration and to provide the conditions and referential perspectives for interpreting the contamination of present experience by unbidden incursions from the past. Tensions emanating from the momentum set in motion by this therapeutic method, and the regressive pull against which it meets, generate the often explosive forces and dynamic distress that characterize the special features of psychoanalytic processes. To devise a method that replaces action with words "ties together the past and the present, the id and the ego, the biological and the psychological" (Loewald, 1973/1980, p. 88) as well as generating a semantic field wherein the transformative stages of symbolization are exhibited *in vivo* through shifts in communicative form. It must be noted, however, that the semiotic processes that have to be catalyzed whenever the unknown is made knowable tend, as Freud cautioned, to meet with massive resistance.

The idea of an epigenetic continuum from natural to semiotically mediated communicative means in which hierarchic organization does not preclude functional continuity of earlier modes yields a biopsychological approach to the study of human communication that concurs with Freud. In this infrequently cited Appendix B of his seminal 1915 paper "The Unconscious," he specified:

> It is probable that the chain of physiological events in the nervous system does not stand in causal connection with psychical events. The physiological events do not cease as soon as the psychical ones begin; on the contrary, the physiological chain continues. What happens is simply that, after a certain point of time, each (or some) of its links has a psychical phenomenon corresponding to it. Accordingly, the psychical is a process parallel to the physiological—'a dependent concomitant.' (p. 207)

'Therapeutic action' consists in linking unconscious meanings with words. This passage from physiological expression and proto-signific behaviors to semiotic phases of increasingly clarified verbalization is actually traceable and its sequences can be logically exhibited according to developmental principles of symbolization. The fundamental insight regarding the interpretation of meaning in human interactions to be derived from these formal principles is one of communicative matching (morphic matching) or attunement.[5]

An awareness of the *kind* of response that is called up tells us of the current mode of experience (and functional organization) of the speaker. Therefore, in psychoanalytic semantic fields, the *nature or quality* of the response that is stirred in the analyst is informative in and of itself, the interactive equation being, signals *incite*; signs *indicate*; and symbols *invite* conceptualization.

The mysteries of human awareness are not so mystifying when studied in the language of dialogue, reference and symbolization. Principles of reference and meaning tied to different semiotic forms dictate their own formal laws and sequences of translation insofar as signals must be *signified* before their meanings can be articulate, signs must be identified before their current *sense* is understood, and symbols must be unpacked for their condensed meanings to be interpreted. While the semiotic function itself is indicative of the beginnings of symbolizing (or 'mental') activity, it only provides the *potential* for conscious articulation to occur, it is not yet *functionally* (or psychically) fully symbolic. The symbolic act requires further abstraction to create the *concept* or *idea* of that to which it refers. What qualifies a symbol *qua symbol* is its complete referential distance from what it stands for. Only when the function of words is to call up "ideas" and not the "things" themselves, can we speak of *symbolization* proper. Language is the only semiotic system pliable and precise enough to provide distinct vehicles for referencing a broad range of human experiences; and only language, therefore, contains the breadth of sense-potential *and* conventional fixity of word-meanings for its use to result in a true 'marriage of minds.'

In this section I have presented an organismic-developmental approach to higher mentation. Transpositions in forms of knowledge and communicative means are due to increasingly symbolic formulation, a process that is recapitulative in both a functional and formal sense, in terms of the microgenetic steps in semiotic mediation leading to verbal denotation and conscious thought. Attaining consciousness is neither unitary nor continuous but an uneven, discontinuous and dynamic affair, spiraling rather than linear in design, and both content- and context-specific. The discussion interweaving onto- and phylo-genetic processes of the early part of this essay suggests that the expansion of human awareness and knowledge grows by generating new referential fields that themselves produce new linguistic terms and discourse leading to new domains and dimensions of awareness. By its investigative focus on the human unconscious, psychoanalysis generated an entirely new semantic field that in its interpretive situations reveals also how new knowledge is acquired. This supports Freud's (1900) early conviction that "...psycho-analysis may claim a high place among the sciences which are concerned with the reconstruction of the earliest and most obscure periods of the beginnings of the human race" (p. 588).

The analytic situation brings into play a number of potentially therapeutic interactive modes of interchange all operating simultaneously, at different levels and in different ways, some of which are echoed in the supervisory setting. It is precisely from this multistratal, multidimensional quality of human communicative experience that I derive my musical analogy. Laws of musical harmony are based on stable tone-relations and combinations governed by different keys and tempi and structured according to formal compositional rules that yield the myriad infinitely varied sound effects that we call music. Similarly, underlying human communication are stable principles of semiotic forms that govern different modes of experience, communication and knowledge, that when composed in combinatorial relationships yield that thick tapestry of conscious and unconscious meanings the threads of which we are here attempting to disentangle.

CHANNELS OF COMMUNICATION

> While it has always been clear that defenses can limit and cut down communications by destroying channels of communication, closing them or causing them to be clogged up, we must now add just as clearly that communication, keeping channels of communication open (and it seems to be one of their rules that disuse tends to make them close up or cease to exist), limits the spread of defenses and their effects on channels of communication and consciousness. Here again we must remind ourselves that though we tend to think mostly in terms of verbal, conscious communications, we are talking about the nonverbal and unconscious communications also.
>
> (Rapaport, 1951, p.448)

Psychoanalysts listen, but also look and feel; we are attentive to the errant glance or word, the dissonant tone, fleeting grimace, aware of discordant themes, repetitive metathemes, the discrete but persistent signal. We operate in contexts with a deepened understanding of what is significant and are required to register and refer to an expanded range of transmissive stimuli. More than words qualify as signifiers in our semantic and becoming adept at exploring the unconscious means learning how to record and respond to meanings that are ordinarily beyond the reach of consciousness.

An effective training analysis has opened and reopened intrapsychical and interpersonal channels of communication and in our practice we continue to sharpen sense-acuities and strengthen these passageways. We learn, in short, that the body speaks; posture, gesture, gait and gaze, breathing and speaking rhythms, movement patterns and general muscle tonus are all direct, expressive transmissions of inner states and interpersonal dispositions. Unconscious meanings emerge at the interface of word and expressive action, the one qualifying the other. To us, they signify the psychical:

> The minutest movements accompany every process of thought; muscular twitchings in face or hands and movements of the eyes speak to us as well as words. No small power of communication is contained in a glance a persons bearing, a bodily movement, a special way of breathing. Signals of subterranean motions and impulses are being sent silently to the region of everyday speech, gesture and movement. (Reik, 1948, p. 135)

Written by the author of "The Third Ear," among the early analysts, Reik (1948), in particular, was sensitive to this kinetic underlay of subliminal expressiveness, the "language of eyes and gesture" (p. 136). He was not alone: F. Deutsch (1947, 1952), also an ardent observer of soma in relation to psyche, stressed that "Whatever happens in one part of the body is reflected in the whole body and is integrated into the functioning of the whole organism. This is true of the simplest as well as for the more complex processes" (1952, p. 196).

The nonverbal, to which this essay will also continue to refer, is certainly an important channel of communication. But this essay takes up a theoretical challenge that originates in Rapaport's 1951 brief paper by the same name.[6]

I am indebted to it for seedling ideas that seemed to be well worth revisiting and for which a developmental framework for the study of communication seem most apposite. Rapaport (1951) was looking for a concept that could subsume psychodynamic and interactional phenomena as well as those areas neglected by id and ego psychology such as ego-development, processes of socialization and the impact of culture. He wondered if the concept of 'channels of communication', might not "serve as a concrete avenue to the study of the psychodynamics of interpersonal relations, for the study of which the only major concepts we have so far are those of transference and identification" (Rapaport, 1951, p. 449). And he suggested relating it directly to defensive blockages that interfere with the expression of topic-sensitive or emotionally charged verbal exchange,

He defined the concept thus: 1) whenever a person can communicate a particular kind of feeling or thought, we can speak of the *existence of a channel of communication* pertaining to that type of content; 2) whenever existent channels of communication for certain types of thoughts or feelings can be used with a particular person, we will speak of an *open channel of communication*, whereas when such content cannot be communicated, we will speak of a *closed channel of communication*; 3) when censored or intolerable information is sent through a channel of communication, we will speak of a *closed channel of communication* (paraphrased from Rapaport, 1951, p. 443). By this loose but clever recasting of defenses and resistances in interactive terms Rapaport (1951) proposed to explore: (a) whether this would allow us to look at defenses from the angle of communication rather than intrapsychic dynamics; (b) whether this idea could provide a conceptual avenue toward a systematic examination and treatment of defenses; (c) whether the "slogan science of interpersonal relationships," could be reduced to its actual substance, namely, psychodynamic interactions, by means of some conceptual equivalence such as that of defenses and "channels of communications," as here defined (paraphrased from Rapaport, 1951, p. 443).

Certainly what actually takes place in a well conducted therapy is that defenses manifesting as resistances, both to the situation itself and to becoming consciously aware, are gradually dissolved through analytic work thereby opening up a variety of new intra- and interpersonal channels of communication. In a therapy that is going well channels of communication are constantly being pried open, others unclogged, reshut, reopened, tended to and kept open through use. The primary purpose of verbal interventions that clarify, interpret, and integrate transference/resistance material in analysis, reasoned Rapaport (1951), is to present to the "patient's external perception" (p. 447) a "new significance" (p. 443), or to draw attention to something that could not otherwise have been observed or brought to consciousness via introspection alone.

In this brief yet incisive paper, Rapaport's (1951) exploratory foray into communication subsumed both the interpretive activities of clinical psychoanalysis as well as the semiotic processes that are operative in its mutative action. Examining emergent contextual experiences in terms of these being repetitions stimulates the resurgence of memory traces linking past with present, affect with word. Time and temporality are dimensions marked by linguistic form, unknown to the unconscious; the wording and working-through of repressed affects and thoughts militates against further defensive blockages, transforming these psychic strata into molten substance, a verbal account, that can be uttered to and heard by another. Rapaport (1951) was pointing to the need for a major revisionary exercise; that of transplanting our concept of intrapsychic dynamics to the interactional/dialogical stage where they manifest. He recognized that human communication is the "most varied, rich, and condensed source of external perceptions, and therefore its role in safeguarding the reality principle, the secondary process, and reality testing cannot be overestimated" (pp. 447-448).

With respect to the above mentioned attributes it is virtually coterminous with functions of the 'ego'. Internalization, defenses, language, secondary process thought and reality testing, are all aspects of ego functioning, developed through interactions that were shaped, mediated and molded by the impact of the early milieu. Methodologically, the most direct experiential referent of the psychical that we have is communication, in its multidetermined totality.

According to the developmental model here espoused, condensations from multiple dvelopmental lines crystalize into hierarchic stratifications that operate in dynamic synergy to yield a current "psychic organization." This incorporates the traditional idea of a hierarchy of defenses, each layer created to modulate more primitive affect/drive impulsions, so that "a continuum of affects extends in all shadings from massive affect attacks to mere signals or even signals of signals" (Rapaport, 1953/1996, p. 507). Linked together by innate disposition, drives, affects, and motivation, form a tightly knit dynamic triad operating from the very core of the personality. The pathways taken by defenses during development, whether to trammel, suppress, transform, or divert original aims, are always convoluted and complex, and tracing them an arduous, if essential, aspect of analytic labor.

In general, the less textured and effective the hierarchic modulations the greater the intensity of affect outbursts: on the other hand the more rigid or excessively tight the controls the more impoverished, both in intensity and variability, will affects become. A richly hued and well mediated emotional life appears to be the mark of a "strong ego" (Rapaport, 1953/1996, p. 507).

Traditionally psychoanalysis viewed affects as an "archaic discharge syndrome," capable of supplanting "voluntary action under certain conditions" (Fenichel, 1945, p. 43), the expression of innate disposition and ego weakness. Strengthening the ego facilitates "control over them" whereby they can be "released" in "tamed forms of anticipatory signals" (Rapaport, 1953/1996, p. 507). The unmistakable stigma of emotions as primitive 'disharge valves' rather than as communications, created a theoretical blind spot: consequently defenses against drives and defences against affects are viewed as following similar routes:

> Drive discharge is delayed and becomes action using thought as preparation, and the tension dammed up by delay is discharged through the safety valve of affect discharge. But affects do not remain inborn discharge channels used by dammed-up drives as safety valves: they too partake in the development sketched: they become progressively tamed. (Rapaport, 1953/1996, p. 506)

Nowhere in this early conception was there room to articulate the now well established fact that affects are *not* archaic discharge valves but the expression of our primary mode of communication and therefore intimately tied to a core self-experience. Whether their modulation took place through suppressive strangulation or via verbally mediating empathic interactions will have great, even fundamental, consequences for the entire sway of personality development. Degrees of attuned responsiveness, as well as personal attitudes toward emotions of early caretakers will be instrumental in how the vocabulary of this primary language will be learned. Two divergent avenues, that of defensive suppression versus semiotic mediation, will result in dramatically different outcomes in relationships and in life adaptation.

The manifestations of "tamed" affects are extremely diverse, textured according to highly idiosyncratic compromise-solutions and because their "taming" occurred through early interactions, the residues of their patterns are woven through communication itself. The analytic loosening and working-through of introjections and often layers of defenses constitute the woof and warp of our dialogical cloth. We observe defenses parrying communication itself, blocking interactions, counterfeiting their content, concretizing words, splicing feelings from thoughts, language from meaning, or otherwise inhibiting and stymieing the verbal articulation of topic-sensitive or deeply covered affectively charged material.

A typology of defenses along a developmental continuum from least differentiated to more intrapsychically structured, would be helpful, a rough sketch of which follows: toxic interactions at the most archaic, undifferentiated end of this continuum would result in massive withdrawal and avoidance patterns; the earlier the defense the more widespread its effects, the more pervasively will it permeate the entire encounter and the more impenetrable will it appear. We recognize immediately a powerful cluster of core "narcissistic" defenses blocking access to a fragile self, their formation indicative of impairments in the establishment of the very first filaments of interpersonal links. Among defenses indicative of very early interpersonal lesions I would list wholesale projective/introjective mechanisms and tendencies toward massive avoidance, withdrawal or dissociation; slightly later would evolve primitive splitting of affects, object representations and ego states, wholesale identifications and identification with the aggressor, dissociative flights and reversals, and modulated forms of avoidance, denial, undoing, rationalization and partial identifications, all defenses that impact severely on cognition and reality testing. Higher level defenses, often organized around conflicts, would include repression, displacement, isolation of affect, ambivalence, undoing, rationalization, and more adaptive defenses against impulse and affect modulation. With respect to this developmental program, in my opinion, Freud's original list of catastrophic anxieties — fear of dissolution, loss of object, loss of the object's love, and superego anxiety — still holds.

Grouping defenses according to broad developmental criteria (such as degrees of differentiation) and considering resistances in terms of their impact *in interaction*, provides an experience-near template for different qualities of interchange and proposes different intervention strategies for different stages in the treatment. The earlier and less differentiated the organization of a defensive constellation the more diffuse its inductive potential, the less easily is it accessible to the observing ego and the less do words appear to serve effectively as communicative bridges. Even when a viable alliance has been painstakingly created, genuine self-reflection and the symbolic articulation of insight are but distant ideals, in such cases, and the establishment and maintenance of a bond already a major achievement.

Dedifferentiation dissolves or decomposes higher levels of functional organization where brittle defenses are operative, hence, clinical regressions tapping archaic levels of the personality may risk arousing primitive, potentially overwhelming affect-states linked to intolerable feelings of helpless rage and vulnerability, preconsciously associated with envy and shame. Unless the working-through of these massive affects (encoded as undifferentiated states) can take place, such individuals will remain encapsulated, sealed in impenetrable bubbles that are designed to protect a fragile, seedling self with crumbling self-esteem. It seems clear that conflictual ideation, and the interpretation of conflict may not, initially, be of primary importance to this kind of psychical structure or, more generally, at preoedipal or preverbal phases of regression, but that other kinds of verbal interventions, over time, can help regenerate primal interpersonal ties.

Rough as it is, a developmental typology of defenses and associated resistances renders an experience-near dialogical concept such as that of communicative channels all the more interesting. The tier-like quality of defensive strata, each successive layer of which must be carefully probed, explored and worked-through, suggests how crucial it is for analysts to remain attuned to multiple levels of the personality, all communicating simultaneously often in contradictory ways. What cannot be communicated explicitly will be expressed implicitly and what does not emerge through direct verbal communication will slip in covertly through nonverbal channels. In this sense the concept of 'channels' also refers to diverse modes and dimensions of human communication — i.e., the somatic/affective, the gestural/expressive, the enactive/behavioral and linguistic, etc. — each of which, to different degrees and in different ways, contributes to the full unconscious composition of any interchange. We can conceptualize a continuum of such modes each tied to a particular expression of meaning, all of which, including the somatic and emotional, can be brought under the sway of conscious control: "The kinesic, the tactile, and the olfactory channels are just as subject to regulation as is the audio-aural," reminds Birdwhistell (1970, p. 57) the renowned scholar of structural kinesics. The analyst's sensitivity and attunement is technically paramount in this. In order to register, refer to and *use* unconscious resonance, analysts have to maintain *all* channels of interaction attuned and accessible to verbalization since continuously re-presenting ideas helps to undermine repression. (Rapaport, 1951)

In this respect, the importance of the training analysis cannot be overemphasized. Sensibilities can be cultivated or blunted, their use disciplined and refined or stunted and suppressed. To do effective analytic work today, analysts have to have thoroughly visited and familiarized themselves with the deepest recesses of their own unconscious and become thoroughly conversant with the nonverbal dimensions of a semantic that has vastly expanded our referential awareness. Once conversant with this unspoken vocabulary, analytic listening *is* multileveled, polysemic, polyreferential, deep, hovering evenly between a spectrum of registrations that corresponds with a spectrum of communicative forms. This implies an ability to cross-reference information that is registered from different sensory sources and semiotic levels and an awareness of the different kinds of meanings that issue from each of these transmissive organizations. Because sensorimotor input continues to participate in the processing of interpersonal experiences, using the induction of transient somatic and emotional states is an important source of unmediated information.

In view of the above, an updated definition of the term "channels of communication" would refer to; 1) intermodal cross-referencing that links different facets and kinds of personal experience and thought; 2) appropriately mediated communications flowing from each of these modes between oneself and others; 3) the modulation and mediation of affects by verbal means; 4) easy interplay between primary and secondary process thought; and, 5) the ability to interpret bodily expressions and to translate sensory input and intuitive inference into linguistic communication.

That all these modes and channels continue to interweave with one another makes for the polyphony of informative cues that emanate from conscious and unconscious aspects of communication. All human interactions grow increasingly condensed and polyvalent as their symbolic complexity increases; what may not be expressed through one channel will emerge via another.

To grasp the phenomenology of these multiple channels entails tracing their ontogenetic roots and developmental transmutations. At the dawn of life, affect and communication form a single expressive unit: modulations of this basic biological signal system depend on degrees of parental attunement or misattunement. What results are hybrid patterns of interaction to which both parties contribute "...on the unconscious level, the parents response is not directly to the child's affect state as such, but to the affective state generated within the parent by his or her autonomic response to the infant's appearance and behavior" (Basch, 1983, p. 108). It is the parent's job to read and respond empathically to their infant's messages and to become increasingly adept at translating their child's communications into words; and it is again, the parents, who will determine which facets of experience will become represented and referred to, what kinds of communications will carry their negotiations into verbal exchanges and which are to be left out. Affects are the nexus around which primary adaptive compromise takes shape and the organizing matrix around which character structure is built. Those to which the parental environment can respond with adequate containment and verbal referencing will potentially become organized, modulated and integrated; those to which it cannot respond acceptingly will find alternate routes or go under.

The parents' own personality disposition, character style and psychological defenses are, of course, woven into early care-giving exchanges and later communicative patterns. These very interchanges, along with their subliminal cues, unconsciously patterned rhythms, typical topics and conversational style, are the transmissive soil for the direct introjection of similar defensive and stylistic patterns. Parental character traits and unconscious needs are picked up and responded to unconsciously by their exquisitely attentive and impressionable offspring with truly dramatic impact on their own psychic structuring.

As the shadow of early objects descends over the ego so does the stamp of family, education and culture contribute to the shaping of character. Contexts define and people determine the nature of the subjects that are spoken about: behavior follows word, conduct as stiff or as free as situations allow. Parents limit what can and delimit what cannot be said: children, equipped with words, move into their heads. For the child, only what is identified and verbalized or otherwise *verified* is real: those feelings, thoughts or 'things' that are not spoken about remain unspeakable.

All of this emphasizes the impact of communication on psychic structuring. "Intrapsychic structure" is intrinsically constituted by the nature of our early interactions. Expressing similar ideas, Loewald (1970/1980) wrote:

> I would venture to suggest that differences in parental attitudes and child rearing have something to do with differences in neurotic development,...I am reasonably convinced that such factors,...play...a far greater role than was recognized in the analytic work of earlier days. In a large number of families, many problems of psychosexual development and growing up tend to be pushed under the rug,...often because of the parents' own personality restrictions and uncertainties, their tendencies to evade direct confrontations, prohibitions, and injunctions, but no less to evade the more open, unabashed expression of their .own love-hate involvement with their children and of their own emotional-instinctual needs and urges. Such trends tending to diffuse, repress and suppress clear-cut feelings toward their children as well as in their children, may have some bearing on the diffusion and spread of neurosis over the total personality development, resulting in what we call character neurosis. Defenses would become more insidious in proportion to the insidiousness and blunting of instinctual life and affect expression. In such measure as there is less unhampered and unselfconscious communication, negative and positive, with ones children, there is perhaps less "trauma"....The occasions for symptom formation would be lessened." (pp. 306-307)

Psychoanalysts are required not only to identify and interpret a broad range of meanings for which only the slightest behavioral indicators are consciously accessible, they must also try to establish fluid interconnections between different strata and kinds of personal experience and between different forms of information. The many channels of this referential hierarchy have to be open and receptive during analytic work and, like the multi-hued palette of the artist, the analyst's apperceptive repertoire, richly and skillfully exercised. The dialectic thereby engendered, as Loewald (1970/1980) pointed out, is such that "Internal communication, on which self-understanding is based, and communication with another…are inextricably interwoven" (p. 280).

Psychoanalytic dialogues generate bi-directional, interpsychical fields wherein less differentiated, more permeable modes of interaction exert a quite extraordinary reciprocal impact. At these profound levels of mutuality where interactions touch preoedipal and nonverbal forms of experience, communication revisits those deeply empathic channels experienced in the better-than- average early communion between optimal mother/infant pairs. The analyst's job, however, is to function at higher levels of symbolic organization; to consistently stand for this higher potential to which every interpretive intervention points and to which the analysand's responses will eventually reach. Like a good parent, the analyst practices reflective understanding and integration while facilitating its achievement by communicative modeling. Insights achieved through sustained verbal interactions function as integrative bridges for analysands who thereby acquire referential habits that promote continued self-reflection. Used in this way, language may well operate at secondary process levels but because its referential range has now embraced the vast territory of primary process meanings, their sharing, in and of itself, provides verbal mirroring which is an integrative experience for the whole personality. It ought not be overlooked that while the communicative medium may be linguistic, key metaphors used by analysands can be picked up and used by analysts in ways that allude to, resonate with and refer to, subverbal meanings: "While verbalization is the prominent means of communication (and this itself…involves far more than the uttering and hearing of words and sentences), the range of communicative interaction is vast." wrote Loewald (1970/1980) ranging from "the most intimate mutual understanding and empathic merging to high abstract dialogue and argumentation" (p. 286).

Analytic attunement translates into technique through the availability of this whole spectrum of interactive channels and the ability to move fluidly between them. In a controlled context where meanings are drawn out and funneled through words, speech acquires quite formidable powers and communication can serve to reach, mend, mirror, repair, reconstruct, and even create new channels of connection, just as ancillary venules can sprout from arteries that are clogged in order to speed vital blood-flow to the heart. From the matrix of this intense dialectic, communication not only investigates and clarifies emergent material for the analyst, it does so for the analysand, generating and consolidating connections that alter the nexus of psychic processes.

The dialogical interchanges that interpret and promote working-through of what has never before been articulated create new referential channels actually forging new brain circuitry, what Gedo (1995) refers to as "novel…arrangements in the nervous system" (p. 334) i.e., learning new cognitive and communicative skills. Effective interventions encompass far more than the analyst's words. The psychological restructuring that results from sustained participation in a dialogue that works toward translating different kinds of unconscious of experience into words alters the emotional core of ones identity. This, I believe, is what Basch (1976b) means when he says that the patient actually acquires a different sense of self, or becomes a "different person," and that speech, in psychoanalysis, is used primarily to promote this deep symbolic transformation.

Shapiro (1991), on the other hand, would approach words and feelings from the opposite direction, proposing a linguistic analysis. His answer to the requirement in psychoanalytic therapy that feelings be nominalized is to apply a linguistic analysis to illuminate the "range of effects that language has on…complex affective states" (p.321). Shapiro(1991) understands the unique phenomenology of the psychoanalytic dialogue as a "subcultural experience"requiring special linguistic consideration in order to account for data derived from; 1) its contrived communicative patterns; 2) the theoretical underpinnings of a method including dynamic unconscious mental functioning, and; 3) free association and transference as special cases of discourse (summarized from p. 346). According to Shapiro we have to account for the unique role of affects in these three areas, each of which is embedded with linguistic significance that can be informative in understanding how language facilitates emotional expression and comprehension within the special context of an analysis. A purely linguistic approach, he maintains, gains depth and meaning by adding to it how unconscious dimensions impact on the symbolic organization of verbal form, forcing linguistics "to include affective valence in its definitional parameters" (Shapiro, 1991, p.346). As he has elsewhere (Shapiro, 1970, 1979, 1980), Shapiro provides fertile integration.

Central to Shapiro's (1991) thesis is that words are far more than mere labels appended to feelings and thoughts but rather that their selection and form, their tonal deliverance and placement along the verbal line are important indicators of the quality, nature and meaning of those feelings to which they refer: "*words in use,*" he emphasizes, "are our most parsimonious means of rendering inner personal, subjective experience."(p. 324). For Shapiro, even grammatical structure bespeaks underlying wishes or intents so that affective import and meaning are spun into the linguistic fabric of verbalization: "Syntactically, we notice the subject-object vectors of feeling. Semantically, we note the representational valence of affects as part of word definition" (p. 321).

Emphasizing the fallacy of drawing a sharp line between feelings and thought ["The latter distinction between cognition and emotion is quite artificial and fraught with confusion" (p.324)] Shapiro (1991) draws attention to their convergence in the analytic situation through the common pathway of transference speech-behaviors which, once identified and explored, place affects within a "syntactic field" (p. 328). Regarding the pitfall of dividing emotional and verbal expression into two separate domains, Shapiro points to the value of a tripartite analysis of symbolic forms that considers the logical and functional differences between signals and signs as affective triggers and emotions which, on the other hand, are symbolically organized and defined by words."Linguists use a feature analysis as a way of defining symbols" (p.332), he writes, including affect as part of a word meaning. Moreover words themselves have dynamisms and are not interchangeable in their ability to mobilize emotional reactions; "Feces is different from shit. Masturbation...different from 'jerking off'" (p. 332) I would add the former *denote* what they stand for; the latter *evoke* it, a difference in referential form illustrative of the ways language and body interweave.

Citing the example of bilingual patients whose use of a particular word in their second language evokes no emotional response, while expression in the first language brings with it strong emotions, Shapiro (1991) notes that this example "provides simple evidence that emotions are linguistically as well as cognitively bound to sentences and complex thoughts" (p.333). Psychoanalysis cannot consider affects simply from their overt expression or merely from a physiological perspective. He advocates the need for a modern, interdisciplinary approach in order to gain in-depth understanding of how affects are linked to conflictual constellations of ideas and the words expressing them. From this perspective, it is less about a translation from one channel into another, than a fusion and integration of the two.

With respect to bilingual examples, in a paper on "The Accessibility of Early Experience through the Language of Origin," Aragno and Schlachet (1996) found, similarly, that verbalization *per se* was not enough for those whose analyses were conducted in a second language—they had to be the original words of childhood. In the context of discussing the nature of early internalizations and clinical problems encountered with bilingual analysands who recalled and recounted but without any affective involvement, we wrote:

> ...the memories of such experiences themselves are accessible and can be put into the words of another language, but these are words devoid of associative triggers leading to the emotive soil in which the affective roots of these memories lie. In other words, although it may be denotive in communicative value, the second language does not conjure the vibrant hues and emotional urgency embedded in the sounds of the first intensely charged vocables, nor does it reflect the rich connotive web of sensory meanings and primary attachments of which our unconscious underlay is constituted. (p. 25)

Like Shapiro, we sought theoretical grounding within a framework of symbolization and the logical differences between signals, signs and symbols. Ours, however, was a strictly developmental approach, correlating language-use with age of experience in terms of proto- or fully symbolic organization; certainly many words, names in particular, function as signals before they pass into symbols, and language itself is primarily signific — a system of signs — before it functions in truly symbolic form. Childhood experiences are embedded in the undifferentiated physio-affective phenomenology of presemiotic organization, their registrations encoded unevenly in sensorimotor modes tied to the very sounds, smells and interactions of which the original language was an integral part. The associative underpinnings of these early experiences are linked to the linguistic contexts of the developmental stage in which they were internalized and become meaningfully rearoused and emotionally worked-through via that original language.

The premise is that words are first learned as indicative signs that *equate with* rather than *represent* the object to which they refer. Operating with the immediacy of signals and signs, rather than the more differentiated and abstract quality of the fully symbolic vehicle, therefore, initially they directly evoke or *present* rather than *re-present* what they stand for (Aragno 1997). In these forms of organization mnemonic fragments cluster around sensory-emotive associations that function like *signaling* triggers implicating the entire organism. The vocable, in this case, holds valence for its very sound, as part of a global reaction carrying the emotional charge of the whole interpersonal and contextual milieu of its encoding. Second languages, acquired when greater differentiation and higher symbolic organization has been achieved are, by their very nature, pallid by comparison. Without deep roots reaching into the emotional turf of childhood they do not command the same emotional rekindling that is requisite for complete working-through.

The psychoanalytic process is, in great part, designed to reconnect many disparate aspects and channels of connection within oneself and between oneself and others. Vestiges of each dominant mode of experience during development is interwoven and condensed in complex ways, and new avenues of communication are created through material that appears through projections, enactments and conflictual or conceptual ideation. Often it matters less *what* is said than *how* it is recounted. The associative flow of the clinical monologue is thematically organized but representationally uneven, textured through and through with contributions from different stages of development and different facets of the personality alternately evoking, inducing, illustrating, enacting, narrating and commenting on meanings that appear layered above the earliest, deepest, and most persistent dominant themes.

The more I delved into these complex, interrelated components of communication and development, the more difficult it was to tie their strands together into a comprehensive whole. The difficulty is compounded by the fact that much research is highly specialized, focusing on only one facet rather than on interfunctional relationships between parts to the whole organism. In sifting through the literature I found myself flooded with details and jargon of which I could make little use that provided an overload of irrelevant material. In gathering information on developmental processes that are recapitulated in analysis, I found it more and more difficult to provide integration and synthesis against a swelling tide of irrelevant data. The psychoanalytic approach is implicitly holistic, biological *and* psychological, by its very nature grounded in *select principles* of development that correspond with functional processes and events of the clinical method. The developmental vectors of affects, recall, language, symbolization and communication cannot be studied separately from total personality reorganization, from a psychoanalytic perspective.

Information that *is* relevant, as background reading to psychoanalysts, can be culled from the important works of Tomkins (1962, 1963, 1979); Izard and Tomkins (1966); Izard (1971, 1977); Plutchick (1980, 1984); Plutchick, R. and Kellerman, P., eds. (1980); Eckman (1973, 1977); Eckman and Oster (1979); and Eckman, P. and Friesen, W. (1969, 1974); in the realm of affects. These works offer in-depth studies of the biological origins, forms, categories, physiology, cultural, and cross-cultural expressive features of affective behaviors. Founded on Darwin's (1872) spearheading study "The Expression of the Emotions in Man and Animals" subsequent investigators have deepened and broadened our understanding of the adaptive purposes and functioning of the communicative repertoire with which we begin life but have not approached them from a psychological perspective in terms of the impact of their mediation on the entire personality, their potential transformations and continued importance throughout the lifecycle.

To look for answers in growing cognitive, semiotic and socio-cultural competencies, the important contributions of Piaget (1937, 1952, 1970); Piaget and Inhelder (1969); Werner and Kaplan (1963); Bruner (1964, 1969, 1973, 1983); Vygotsky (1978, 1981); and Gardner (1982); have been of particular interest to me. Much can also be gleaned from the anthropological literature on communication in the works of Hall (1959, 1969); Morris (1967, 1978); and especially from Birdwhistell (1952, 1970) and Bull's (1983) studies on kinesics and communication, both important, perhaps even essential, additions to the traditional body of psychoanalytic literature. But it is in the research of N. Freedman (*et al*) whose focus for over twenty-five years has been the study of the most central issues in listening, communication and symbolic processes in the therapeutic encounter, that the most valuable data can be found. His psychoanalytically oriented research fulfills the promise of those initial, halting steps in movement observation begun by early analysts such as Ferenzi (1914); Reich (1933); Reik (1948); Gostynski (1951); and, particularly, Deutsch (1942, 1947, 1952) who similarly were interested in better understanding the external, kinetic indicators of internal psychological phenomena.

These early analysts approached their subject from the perspective of expressive motor or 'non-verbal' behavior and, through the lens of topographical, structural and genetic dimensions, Gostynski (1951) drew attention to the necessity for a developmental approach to the study of "gesticulatory behavior" (p. 318). In coining the term "analytic posturology," Deutsch (1947, 1952) was attempting to open avenues for observing organismic involvement in the expression of unconscious, dynamic motives and the ego's integrative activities when regulating voluntary and involuntary movements. He too detected a developmental course paralleling the achievement of insight in analysis, but went even further, delineating several broad dimensions of kinetic activity reflecting dynamic patterns, tension- and anxiety-regulating processes, and movements associated with internalized object relations and thought processes.

Deutsch (1947) analysis of bodily movements in conjunction with verbal expression was an initial attempt at integrating component-messages issuing from the whole organism; "There is no more favorable experimental setting than analysis for resolving a symptom complex into its constituents and among these the postural pattern appears as signal and symbol during the analytic process, preceding, substituting or accompanying verbal expressions. It is not possible to understand the pattern before the meaning of the elements in the configurative pattern is known" (Deutsch, 1947, p. 197). Deutsch (1942, 1947, 1952) considered the observation of 'postural patterns' to be an integral facet of analytic attention supplying information regarding psychodynamic as well as cognitive advances in the course of analysis. He noted that the progress could be assessed by the appearance of small movements which can be analyzed along with verbal content These "involuntary movements...are not a substitute for insight but often accompany acquiring it...," he wrote, "Postures emerging in analysis seem to be the product of a developmental process similar to psychological development" (Deutsch, 1947, p. 212) an observation to be verified by Freedman's research on symbolization. Although couched in the terms and theoretical orientation of his time, Deutsch's seven year study of postural behaviors during analysis anticipates the systematic study of the sources and meanings of movements as indicators of psychological process that flowers in Freedman's work.

I am neither a fan nor proponent of quantified research in psychology, however, Freedman's studies focus on interactive phenomena taking place in live clinical encounters, considering various patterns of kinetic behavior exhibited by both interlocutors as indicators of listening, registering, symbolizing and language-construction activities. His research accomplishes the difficult task of identifying, coding, scoring, and systematically tracing observable kinetic markers of interactive assimilations and internal semiotic processing, providing evidence for correlations between the two. Video-taped sessions are studied examining non-verbal behaviors during communicative sequences revealing phenomena that provide additional evidence for intimate connections between movement and cognition, imagistic and internalizing activities, pointing to kinesic behaviors as objective 'measures' for processes underlying clinical listening (Barroso and

Freedman, 1992). For well over two decades, Freedman and his colleagues have fed a steady stream of papers presenting the yields of their findings into the psychoanalytic community from an approach that has culminated in the most recent (to-date), an advanced study of the therapist's assimilation of a patient's transference and differentially symbolized or desymbolized countertransference (Freedman and Lavender, 1997).

Sustained, systematic research in the field of kinesics and kinetic behaviors began with the publication of Birdwhistell's "Introduction to Kinesics" in 1952. In this original study of gestures were the first indications that kinesic structure paralleled linguistic structure and that contextual studies of movement revealed a formal kinesic system that is astonishingly like words in language (Birdwhistell, 1970). Advocating the need for the location of natural contexts of occurrence for the study of human behavior, Birdwhistell's studies of movement and communication culminated in his "Kinesics and Context" (1970) a series of essays on body-motion communication based on the conviction that movements are a learned form of communication, patterned within a particular culture, which can be broken down into an ordered system of isolable elements. Through his detailed research he devised a system of transcription for coding hundreds of body movements and established the idea of structural kinesics as a parallel to structural linguistics, drawing attention to the social significance of bodily cues in relation to encoding and decoding, even defining communications.

Unlike Freedman's approach, which draws a clear distinction between non-verbal *communication*, in which body movements are part of a code that is decodable by a listener, and non-verbal *behavior*, in which motor acts are indicators of processes at work within the organism, the structural and sociological schools take *all* non-verbal cues as being the product of learning, in which "…the study of situational context, interpersonal relationships and culture become the prime focus of investigation" (Bull, 1983, p. 24). Structuralists and sociologists argue that learned forms of communication must be interpreted and understood contextually.

Freedman's work, on the other hand, is psychoanalytically sophisticated growing more and more focused on the clinical interchange over the years; the kinetic act is observed as a gauge of assimilation and differentiating processes, as well as a manifest component of listening and thinking,

"...kinetic behavior is not only communicative but also representational"; it is "not only concerned with the transmission of information but also points to the body's participation in the symbolizing process. The appearance of movement, then, may become regulated not only by context but by the individual's personal repertoire of available symbols" (Freedman, O'Hanlon, Oltman and Witkin, 1972, p. 239).

In papers analyzing movement behavior from psychodynamic, cognitive, affective, linguistic and attentional perspectives, Freedman and Hoffman (1967); Freedman (1971); Freedman, O'Hanlon, Oltman and Witkin (1972); Freedman, Blass, Rifkin and Quitkin (1973); Freedman and Steingart (1975); Barroso, Freedman, Grand and van Meel, Jr. (1978); Freedman, Barroso, Bucci and Grand (1978); Freedman and Grand (1985); and Barroso and Freedman (1992); provide observational data documenting the contributions of gesture and body movements to cognitive steps in symbol formation, imagistic ideation, speech production, and different "levels" of listening. Their research confirms the idea that body movements are not only reflective of interactive processes but are also channels for observing those activities we refer to as "mental." Even listening exhibits different forms of receptivity in which "actions of the body provide a source of information for the objective behavioral study of the listening process" (Freedman, Barroso, Bucci and Grand, 1978, p. 159).

In "The Bodily Manifestations of Listening," Freedman, Barroso, Bucci and Grand (1978) present their theoretical orientation and method for the "kinesic-linguistic analysis of listening-speaking sequences" (p. 160). They introduce the concept of "kinesic strategies," constellations of body movements accompanying different modes of listening that either "promote" or "retard" listening (p.159). To demonstrate that "body movements are indicators of the quality of listening..." (p. 159), Freedman *et al*, (1978) provide cumulative evidence that during talking, body movements reflect organismic participation in processes of information filtering, decoding, and of symbolic representation, making kinetic activity a possible "...signpost or indicator of the kind of listening that is taking place" (pp. 159-160). Freedman's observations address the outward manifestations of attention-gauging processes including internalization, differentiation and associative activities in communicative sequences; they also observe diverse forms or classes of enactive and tension-regulating movements reflecting information-processing and language construction themselves. In this sense their body of research documents an observation noted earlier, namely, that body movements 'live' in two environments: one is the interpersonal sphere, where they may be viewed as an aspect of the transmission of information. The second might be termed the kinesic-symbolizing context; where movements are embedded in a series of inner experiences, states of consciousness, imagery, organization of thought, and the construction of speech (Freedman and Steingart, 1975, p. 355-356). These two broad movement spheres subsume those multiple dimensions of movement patterns prefigured in Deutsch's (1947, 1952) studies reflecting both interactive *and* intellective processes.

From video-taped interviews of children and adults, Freedman's team delineated another construct they called "*Kinesic Internalization*" (1975) operationally defined by particular hand movements which, they observed, occur frequently and almost universally during discourse. In their further analytic breakdown of *kinesic internalizations* they identified two discrete classes of hand movements, one in which image representations or actions are motorically enacted, another in which the hands are used to regulate body tensions in forms of self-stimulation. They correlate these body motions with the internalization and assimilation of sensorimotor schemata and the formulative steps in concept and language articulation. Dividing these hand movements into two broad categories — *object*- and *body*-focused — and relating these to assimilative and cognitive processes, Freedman's studies distinguish between enactive and tension-regulating behaviors as these alternate in any communicative situation. "In enactive behavior the body is used to represent, depict or simulate the figural or relational aspects of the physical object world — the shape of things, their kinesthetic, tactile or even abstract properties, which are given motoric expression albeit in often highly condensed or only subtly noticeable form" (Freedman & Steingart, 1975, p. 357).

These object-focused, enactive hand gestures, matching with rhythms of speech, tend to move away from the body and are complementary to verbal communication. Generally Freedman and Steingart (1975) identified three kinds of enactive integrations in object-focused activity: subordination, supplementation and substitution (p. 358). In body-focused movements, they identified various forms and levels of tension-regulating, soothing and self-ministrating hand behaviors touching the body surface. Body-focused movements are continuous and appear to be unrelated to speech. They seem, rather, to be instrumental in creating an optimal "tensional and perhaps attentional state that either facilitates or interferes with retrieval, assembly, and organization of thought" (Freedman and Steingart, p. 352). These authors again identified three broad levels of tension-regulating movements defined by their forms of self-stimulation, which range from diffuse and unpatterned to discrete and circumscribed, and are intrinsically related to the individual's information-processing capacities.

Throughout Freedman's work there threads a consistent interest in symbolization. His investigation of communicative interactions emphasizes the body's participation in the symbolizing process; by implication, this incorporates the trajectory of language- and thought-formulation. The observation of movements accompanying speech affords an opportunity to "gauge in *statu nascendi*, as it were, the molding of experiences into symbolic form" (Freedman, O'Hanlon, Oltman, and Witkin, 1972, p. 239). Occurring at the beginning of phonemic classes, movements partake in syntactic planning, in grammatical structuring of spoken sentences, or may depict the expression of feelings and imagery which are only partially articulated verbally (p. 239). Kinetic involvement appears to be part of the organism's effort to establish a referential relationship between what is being experienced and some symbolic form, gestural or linguistic, in which to denote it.

This kinesic-accompaniment has its roots in early phases of development and represents the vestiges of archaic, sensorimotor modes of information-processing and interpersonal distance- gauging, which continue to be active in the present. In the child, hand activity is an important mediator between the objective, outer world and subjective, inner experience. Piaget's accounts of the sensorimotor stage are replete with descriptions of hand and limb participation in successive levels of sensorimotor schema formation. In Freedman and Steingart's (1975) view "What is internalized, and carried throughout life, are the somatic, sensory, and motor operations of early childhood which confirm the existence of an object, and regulate tension and perhaps attention." (p. 361). It was assumed that these early somatic forms of cognition were superseded by more complex, linguistic or symbolic elaborations of thought (p.361), however, in these studies, Freedman and Steingart (1975) suggest that the persistence of physical movement in adult communication not only serves a complementary function to language but might also have a dynamic significance of its own. In the case of enactive and tension-regulating activity, early sensorimotor schemata, they suggest, become increasingly short-circuited and integrated; "...enactment and tension-regulating behavior constitutes somatic information-processing activities necessary for the establishment of meaning" (p. 359) since the coordination and integration of sensorimotor organization prefigures cognitive competencies involved in the structuring of classes and relations.

In a 1985 discussion of "shielding," Freedman and Grand introduced the concept of *associative organizers*, hypothesizing that "a matrix of bodily sensations and motor experiences, rooted in the coenesthetic and vestibular experience of earliest childhood" (p. 355) persists in the associative act of all analysands. Even in the most mature adult dialogue, they write, the regulatory and organizing impact of this sensorimotor nucleus continues to exert a structuring effect on communicative processes (p.355). One facet of this process is tied to the most rudimentary, pre-imagistic, unconscious psychic-organization, the other to the act of verbalization.

Freedman and Grand (1985) identified two associative organizers representing behavioral anchoring points in a developmental sequence during clinical interviews: "*shielding,*" the first, functions to define boundaries between inner and outer worlds and presumably originates long before the acquisition of symbolic capacities. The second, a "*transforming activity,*" is concerned with reflectiveness and meaning-generating processes which function as preparation for the construction of language (p. 356). Observations in clinical settings led to inferences and abstracted ideas which could be verified in other contextual domains since shielding and transforming serve the important functions mentioned above in any associative narration. Optimally, they oscillate rhythmically throughout the associative process. The concept of associative organizers evolved from the cumulative data of fifteen years of recorded studies in which Freedman and Grand (1985) developed coding for the analysis of verbal channels of communication, as well as codifications for kinesics and non-verbal channels.

Further hypotheses regarding kinetic expression as indicative of degrees of psychological differentiation, and the idea that movements are part of symbolizing thought processes, are tested and discussed by Freedman, O'Hanlon, Oltman, and Witkin in a 1972 paper entitled "The Imprint of Psychological Differentiation on Kinetic Behavior in Varying Communicative Contexts." Taking the variable of field independence, these authors questioned whether an individual's capacity for symbol-formation was in some way related to the dimension of psychological differentiation, asking specifically whether motor behavior in the communication of adults reflects greater or lesser differentiation. They hypothesized that more object-focused or speech-related movements were to be expected of more differentiated individuals and more body-focused movements of less differentiated individuals (p. 240). They found no simple correlation between object-focused (speech-related) and body-focused movements in relation to degrees of differentiation but rather as indicative of a particular cognitive style. Their conclusions point to the stylistic and cognitive roots of gestural behavior, challenging those schools that attribute kinetic expression exclusively to culturally determined, learned behavior.

These researchers, further, found sources of motor expression to be generated by the *"effort to represent"* (p. 254) and formulate thought, and also in *"the effort to reach"* (p. 256) — an attempt to establish contact with the object of communication. Of particular interest was their observation of persistent and continued body touching in an interview that ought not to have warranted such a response. They viewed this unwarranted transposition of body touching gestures as indicative of negative object experiences and the internalization of such representations. With ontogenetic roots in the matrix of the mother-child relationship, body-touching or self-stimulation, seems to be an indicator of negative interpersonal experiences.

Among human infants and baby primates self-stimulation is a behavioral phenomenon seen in response to object loss, separation and mourning. In adult communication it is frequently paired with gaze avoidance, reduced vocalization and hesitancy, all indicators of inversion and withdrawal from the object. "Persistent body touching in the absence of an injuring object is a prevalent phenomenon in clinical practice. It is the stuff of psychotherapy research" write Freedman, O'Hanlon, Oltman, and Witkin (1972, p. 257) conjecturing that it has long been assumed that depressed individuals behave as though faced with indifferent or cold objects regardless of how empathic or warm the environment might be.

In the most recent (to-date) of these empirical studies of communicative and kinetic processes, Freedman and Lavender (1997) point the video camera toward the therapist and focus on tracing nonverbal indications of fluctuations in attention and receptivity during clinical listening. Observing the same therapist at work in a 'not-so-difficult' versus a 'difficult' session, they identified three relatively distinct modes through which the analyst experiences the patient: 1) *empathic attunement*, is associated with rhythmicity, by which they mean concordant movements indicative of optimal attention and receptivity; 2) the *symbolizing countertransference*, is marked by transitory arhythmicity, which refers to momentary lapses in attention, sleepiness or compensatory over-engagement; and 3) the *desymbolizing countertransference*, manifests in continuous arhythmicity, indicative of a disruption of optimal receptivity or breakdown in the clinical stance, with increased shielding from the interaction in attempts to restore an imperative, inner "working space" (p. 81). Their delineation of these three distinct listening responses, they write, captures their view of countertransference as a "variegated phenomenon that may be experienced by the analyst as a potentially constructive inner dialogue of subjectivities" (p. 97). They stress that as indices of listening, bodily actions are "amenable to empirical documentation" representing a bridge that serves to both "express and regulate" (p. 83). To address the tricky question of when and how the therapist became aware of his/her physical reactions and could use them as informative signals of the process, they took a view from "within and from without" concluding that although these parallel perspectives were often complementary, it is the point at which the two converge that is revealing:

> Sometimes bodily actions are mute, discernible only to the outside viewer, yet sometimes they become loud and take center stage. When the mode of empathic attunement is operative, interactional synchrony occurs between listener

> and speaker; absorbed in the story, the listener does not know he or she is moving. But, in states of symbolizing countertransference (and most certainly in the desymbolizing variety), the analyst senses his pulse, posture shifts, breathing, and even fidgeting....Awareness of the body becomes an important signal in the process of disembedding from the downward pull of the countertransference. (p. 100)

Psychoanalytically informed research integrating body movements with the study of listening and symbolic processing is valuable to psychoanalysis because it reinforces an organismic approach to the study of mind. Moreover Freedman's focus of interest — kinetic expressions of listening, information-processing and differentiation, symbolization, language-construction and speech — are of particular interest to those who share a theoretical orientation based on principles of symbolization. At times, epistemological problems appeared to seep into the interpretation of this data, permeating the language used to identify and describe conceptual distinctions such as those between 'inside' and 'outside'.

Freedman's research is grounded in the empirical protocol of experimental psychology which tends to fractionate phenomena, start out with a hypothesis and then test its validity via measures of quantified data. Much of his systematic research, and the conclusions he draws there from, provides ample corroboration for my own informal observations and more generalized and abstractly conceptualized theoretical constructions. The yields of both, I believe, definitively demonstrate that the foundations of attention, assimilation, referencing, symbolization, thought and linguistic formulation, emanate from, and correlate with, observable bodily manifestations.

Many of the early analysts were interested in pursuing the study of non-verbal behaviors in relation to mind/body expressions. It is all the more surprising therefore that the field has not sought to integrate more information from kinesics and body-movement studies. The implications of neglecting the nonverbal in the overall training experience and particularly in the training analysis, has been raised by T. Jacobs (1994). His criticism, that data issuing from the non-verbal realm is under utilized, is apt, given that experiences from the personal analysis and supervisory situations lay lasting foundations in all areas of professional functioning. As Jacobs (1994) states, minimizing the importance of the nonverbal and the scant attention given to it in training has broad repercussions in technical deficiencies that are then handed down from one generation to another. Focusing on verbal material to the virtual exclusion of concomitant bodily expressions, the young analyst "develops a scotoma" (p.742) for those transmissions emanating from somatic channels: "Having experienced little understanding and effective interpretation of his own non-verbal communications in analysis, and having been exposed to little teaching about the subject in supervision or in courses on technique, he can be expected neither to appreciate the importance of the non-verbal dimension in analysis nor to develop competence in working with it" (Jacobs, 1994, p. 742).

As an analytic candidate, Jacobs (1994) comments, fresh from a residency in which he had been exposed to the import of nonverbal communications in psychotherapy through the work of Scheflin (1963, 1968), he had tried to include such observations in the material he presented to his supervisors. The responses he received were mild interest from some, very little from others, while most were clearly eager to move rapidly to verbal process, this material representing what was "truly analytic" and comprehensible (p. 760). Similarly, I have participated in supervisory group discussions where the prevalent focus was on "verbatim transcripts," in which nonverbal communications of all kinds — even the expressive embellishments that give emphasis and meaning to speech — were systematically ignored or undervalued. My drawing attention to the intimate connection between the form of the supervisee's commentary in relation to the dynamics of the material being recounted, and copious questioning of the emergent expressive features, were frequently not understood as being relevant to the content of the "clinical process." I grew to understand this logocentric focus on the spoken or written word to be a major resistance to receiving the supervisee's or the patient's *unconscious* projective and enactive transmissions in their entirety.

Jacobs (1994) comments on the different modalities, various levels, and complexity of communications within the analytic situation, noting that we are only just beginning to investigate this relatively uncharted area calling for a new approach to our listening and how we think about what we are observing (p.761): he writes, "From this perspective, the exploration of the non-verbal dimension in analysis constitutes one of the few remaining frontiers. It is an area that promises to yield information of great value — information that will not only enrich our understanding of our patients' verbal communications, but of the entire analytic process" (Jacobs, 1994, p. 761).

Yet the relative neglect of our para-linguistic and nonverbal vocabularies as important sources of psychological information is, in my opinion, reflective of broader issues. The problems we are still facing are perceptual and conceptual reliquiae of deeply embedded epistemological traditions that perpetuate divisions between what ought to be understood as *organismic* phenomena. At the sensorimotor core of the central nervous system, body *and* brain, participate in the transformation of sense-impressions into meaningful stimuli. It seems evident, at least to me, that since Piaget we are obliged to recognize the centrality of the body in the evolution of thought, intelligence, understanding, and the use of language. Freedman's studies seem to confirm that these processes begin, are reflected in, and continue to be generated and expressed, through various bodily channels.

In conclusion, it strikes me that this exploration of the concept of "channels of communication" has taken on the rich complexity and referential breadth that, I believe, Rapaport (1951) intended. His speculation that it might be possible to look at intrapsychic dynamics and defenses from the angle of channels of communication in interactions as "conceptual equivalents" (p. 443) of the "psychical," is well borne out by the above. In fact, such a shift does more; it brings our methodological center-force "the analysis of transferences as resistance" into the phenomenological field of human interactions and discourse as it renders obsolete the epistemologically flawed conceptual division between inner and outer, physical and psychical, body and mind. In a semantic of unconscious transmissions and meanings, manifest form is not only the expression of unconscious process and experience, it is coterminous with it. The notion of mind as "inner" and body as "outer" is a hindering remnant of dualisms that are an impediment to understanding the interrelationships between form, content and meaning, in human communication. The body not only participates in the psychical, it *exhibits* it. Gesture, movement, tone, posture, rhythm, intensity, expressiveness—how word-meanings deliver their sense—are the direct, observable indices of the unconscious, of personality dynamics, internalizations, and of what we refer to as "mental" process.

The human nervous system continuously filters stimuli, assimilating different kinds of information registered through multiple sense channels simultaneously. And the whole organism participates in their selection and organization. Residues of earlier more diffuse modes of assimilation persist, underlying higher more explicit strata of verbal exchange, their muted signals subtly interwoven with sign and symbol through the form and content of human discourse. Emotion and cognition overlap and merge to converge in forming highly condensed, multidetermined polyvalent expressions. Internalized interactions and defensive maneuvers encrusted into habitual communicative patterns and style echo and re-echo the past in present process. To those listening to the unconscious, the body speaks; to the trained eye, the mind's body mirrors psyche.

THE PSYCHOANALYTIC SEMANTIC

Its Five Metapsychological Dimensions and Nine Referential Perspectives

> We have no way of conveying knowledge of a complicated set of simultaneous events except by describing them successively; and thus it happens, that all our accounts are at fault to begin with owing to one-sided simplifications and must wait till they can be supplemented, built onto, and so set right.
>
> Freud, 1940, p. 205

> I believe there is, or can or should be, one psychoanalytic theory that should be differentiated from nonpsychoanalytic theories of human mentation. This theory, which is psychoanalysis, will contain all elements considered necessary and sufficient in the combined theories.
>
> Rangell, 2000, p. 452

The pluralistic confusion in our field today rings like the cacophony of a mutinying orchestra with players from each of the principal instrument groups all simultaneously playing a different tune. Where rigorous epistemological rethinking was called for there has, rather, been undisciplined fragmentation. Along with the continued exclusion of metapsychology from contemporary discourse and a "decline of intellect and insight" (Rangell, 2000, p. 457) the digressive dynamics of 'dissent, discredit and divide' — already evident from the beginning — have now overridden the integrative impetus of a young science still attempting to define its relevant data and translate this into a cohesive body of theory.

We are a conglomerate of clinical models, incomplete, derivative *versions,* of a master-method the full scientific implications of which are obscured by fragmentation. Partial truths substitute for whole truths (Rangell, 2000, p. 455), tangential findings replace radical revisioning, while this fractionistic tendency has increased rather than reduced the gap between method and metatheory. The field's dispersion drains focus from the more difficult task of bringing together principles of theory, method and a now vastly expanded investigative process, into one viable conceptual framework. As Frank (2000) commented, although diversity and discussion may yield progressive thinking, the "cacophony" of voices currently issuing from at least a dozen (or more) different points of view (pp. 174-175) has stymied rather than furthered our theoretical progress.

In my opinion, these segregate "schools" of analytic thought are nothing more than offshoot clinical "genres" derived from component elements of an interpretive master-method that contains them all. None of these versions, however, is a complete "theory" since a genuine theory is required, at the very least, to subsume and possibly even explain the operative principles underlying a vast range of relevant phenomena.

In response to Franks' (2000) "clarion call for synthesis" (p.177) the following proposes a recasting of our definition of "schools" into the vocabulary of discourse using the concept of *referential perspectives* to re-define our multi-perspectival interpretive methodology.

One of the paradoxes of the post-modern era is that the more we know the more we have come to realize on what flimsy ground this knowledge rests. Genetic epistemology and constructivism have ineluctably shown that versions of reality are structured according to cognitive stages/abilities and fashioned by cultural signs, symbol-systems and language-categories: we know what has been singled out for us by words. Underlying the sweep of this zeitgeist there has been a subtle rapprochement between the interests of philosophers and psychoanalysts both of who are concerned with the effects on mind of putting things into words: how language shapes reality. Whereas both acknowledge the centrality of language in the formative conditioning of human experience, philosophers look on this as an epistemological devise whereas psychoanalysts use it as an instrument of integration. Both, however, agree that the semiotic structures and referential categories that language provides creates our realities and our consciousness of them. The human mind is incapable of knowing a world that is not crafted from its own instruments: all understanding is ordered by the limits of our intellectual capacities and semantic categories. There is no subjective experience or 'object' independent of our definition of it; "All human understanding is interpretation," states Tarnas, (1991,p. 397): we make worlds with words, writes Goodman (1984), in the same way that "we see a constellation, by putting its parts together and marking off its boundaries" (p. 42). Cognition is intimately tied to perception, and both are constructed from an amalgam of what we re-cognize and how language has defined it for us.

Major advances in human knowledge leading to new consciousness essentially spring from new symbolic abstractions; these, in turn, open up semantic windows that spread new awareness through dialogue and discourse. Methodologically, psychoanalysis embodies these activities of semiotic mediation as its end and instrumentation and, given its interpretive processes and goals, it also provides an investigative avenue for observing the constitutive stages in the development of consciousness. As early as 1942, Rapaport alluded to the possibility that a psychoanalytic theory of thinking might lead to a marriage between philosophy and psychology by discovering the "psychogenesis of the modes of apperception" (p. 106) in connection with Kant's autonomous categories of pure reason. In one of many later attempts to integrate metapsychological formulations with contemporary knowledge of cognitive process Rapaport (1959b) asserted that the task was predicated on breaking down the "perception-cognition dichotomy" (p. 780) as well as being able "to express both process and structure variables in terms of a single dimension" (p. 779). The field did not pursue investigations guided by Rapaport's perspicacious theoretical directions leaving the systematic study of unconscious thought processes to other disciplines. If it had, it would have found that the microgenetic stages of verbal symbolization provide such a structuralizing process and that many other answers converge on the unique features of semiotic and referential activities particularly 'working through' which, in joining affects with verbal expression, leads to the kind of personal transformation associated with radical, structural change.

It is not surprising then that philosophers turned to the exploration of species of reference, interpretive strategies, and the analysis of discourse semantics to understand the nature of our constructs. In my opinion, psychoanalysis generated a new semantic through its commitment to investigating unconscious phenomena, processes and meanings, a semantic which has become increasingly polyperspectival to accommodate the multiple dimensions of the 'unconscious' that have come to light through its method. Finding the right categorical concepts for a semantic that encompasses the polyperspectival "nature of the psychical" then becomes our primary concern; "For if we make worlds, the meaning of truth lies not in these worlds but in ourselves — or better, in our versions and what we do with them" (Goodman, 1984, p. 38).

The word **semantic**, from the French *sémantique* (1887) originates in the Greek ***semantikos***, significant; ***semanio***, meaning; and ***semeion***, sign; and relates to meanings in language. At one level semantics is concerned with the nature, structure, historical development and changes of meanings in speech forms: at another it is the scientific study of the relation between signs or symbols and what they refer to or denote, and of the psychological and sociological aspects of human behavior as it is influenced by the use of these linguistic signs and symbols (Webster New World Dictionary, 1966 ed., p. 1324).

The hallmark of the psychoanalytic semantic is its experiential nature and those navigating its waters must be willing to *enter into* its bio-semiotic fields as part of the 'objectification' of the data. This is the new revolutionary dimension of Freud's methodological stance: an 'attuned' or 'participatory-objectivity' with respect to referential perspectives and interpretive purpose: in psychoanalytic discourse the semantic function of the word "unconscious" is *part of the perceptual medium*, a filter permeating and pervading the entire interpretive purview. This semantic leap that launched our inquiry into the human unconscious continues to challenge the very limits of discursive form and in this sense psychoanalysis is a semantic anomaly in that it requires that we process sensory/emotional/mnemonic and highly charged *qualities* of personal and inter-active experience through the limited vocabulary of a linguistic medium. 'Quality' of experience is central to this task and becomes an important, objectifiable, source of information, because *quality* of experience begets ideation which is a *significant datum* in this realm — a signal, sign or symbol, expressing the meaning of what is going on in the organism.

The new range of phenomena to which psychoanalysis gained access provided the referential means to put the dynamisms and pulse of the inner life into words. But due to the simultaneous presentation of its referents – that it is *compositional* rather than sequential – words, and even verbal form, are often simply inadequate for its ineffable attributes. With its spurts and fluctuations of thought, state, emotion and mood; its interplay of imagery, fantasy and meaning; it's universally narratized archetypal themes; the unconscious is also the creative wellspring of 'representation' and art. Langer (1942, 1967, 1972) went to glorious lengths to emphasize that language is by no means our only articulate medium, that "not every sort of semantic can be brought under this rubric" (1942, p. 94). "The eye and the ear," she reasoned "make their own abstractions, and consequently dictate their own peculiar forms of conception" (1942, p. 91). Like Freud before her, she noted that the "laws that govern this sort of articulation are altogether different from the laws of syntax that govern language" (1942, p.43), their most impressive difference being their mode of transmission. Linguistic meanings accrue successively and are understood cumulatively: meanings that present their elements simultaneously impact in much the same way as does art which requires a willingness to participate, or *enter into,* its aesthetic domain.

The psychoanalytic semantic is currently governed by five supeordinate metapsychological dimensions (the topographical, genetic, economic, structural and adaptive) and by what are here defined as nine dominant referential perspectives. Each of these dimensions of the unconscious (which may be likened to an instrument group in an orchestra) considers itself an independent "school" and produces its own 'theoretical' fulcrum and clinical/ interpretive orientation. None of these, in my opinion, provides a comprehensive enough set of underlying theoretical principles and all ignore the requisite articulation of psychoanalytic phenomena along all metapsychological dimensions. The "unconscious," is here understood as an umbrella term for many different processes and phenomena all operating simultaneously, outside of awareness. The principles of multiple-function and multidetermination embody this composite, multidimensionality of the psychical, while the concept of *referential perspectives* provides a term to denote the multiple interpretive facets of the unconscious now encompassing the current status of knowledge in our field. I am suggesting that a poly-perspectival, or multi-referential, theoretical conceptualization is, and always has been, essential. The psychoanalytic method operates at many different levels concomitantly bringing various modes of learning, internalization, and communication, into play. In addition to the bio-semiotic field thereby engendered the following lists the dominant referential perspectives to which, in my opinion, contemporary analysts caught in the complex medley of the field's current thinking, refer, either directly or indirectly:

(1) **The unmediated distant-past** and (2) **The unmediated recent-past**; are formally related in that both are expressions of experiences that have been assimilated in presemiotic, sensorimotor modes and are organically/ emotionally registered without semiotic (verbal) mediation or cognitive processing, the first structures a pre-representational, basic core that sets a primary anlage for patterns of interactive experience; the second refers to subliminal registrations of the recent past, as in the parallel process. The former is heavily infiltrated by drives related to early attachment, the latter to current motives and goals.

(3) **The dynamic unconscious**; or the secondarily repressed, which generates unconscious "content" and is formed by the motivated forgetting of thoughts, feelings, and complex meanings, generally due to conflict.

(4) **The creative or System Ucs**; such as we have evidence of in the construction of dreams, creative products and expression in all art forms and the adaptive compromises of everyday life.

(5) **The Archetypal and Collective unconscious**; refer to those deepest reaches of the psychical that are associated with Jungian psychology. The postulation of inherited instinctual patterns of behavior forming part of the

common heritage of humankind stems from a recognition of certain recurrent, primordial mythical motifs and archetypal constellations that cannot be fully explained in terms of repression or through the narrow confines of individual experience and development. Due to their universality and the extraordinary power they wield over patterns of fate, they call for deeper, biological, or even phylogenetic, explanatory principles akin to Sheldrake's (1988, 1991) ideas on morphogenetic fields. For Jung the archetypes are simply the forms instinctual constellations assume, so that "The collective unconscious contains the whole spiritual heritage of mankind's evolution, born anew in the brain structure of every individual" (Jung, 1971, p. 45). It would be a mistake to think that these ideas were antithetical to Freud's. Freud's cognizance of how much light psychoanalytic investigation can shed on phylogenesis has been insufficiently recognized: already in 1900, he wrote; "...psycho-analysis may claim a high place among the sciences which are concerned with the reconstruction of the earliest and most obscure periods of the beginning of the human race" (p. 588).

(6) **Introjects, Identifications and Internalized Patterns of Interaction** from the distant past constitute that part of the personality, including the voice and attitude of the superego, that form habitual ways of being, communicating and relating. The shadow of primary objects falls early and long over the ego, coloring many behavioral attitudes, beliefs, communicative patterns, and personality traits, so that "...the character of the ego....contains the history of these object-choices" (Freud, 1923, p. 29). This unconscious aspect of the personality is formed through relational experiences during development, however, interactive patterns laced with unconscious dynamisms may also be assimilated from the recent past and transmitted in

another context, as we observe in parallel process reenactments.

(7) Created during development out of the meeting of natural disposition with the quality of early care, the precursors of later more stable and rigidified **Psychological Defenses** form early, determining both the type of compromises and subsequent character style. Defenses can be organized according to a developmental continuum beginning with less differentiated projective/introjective and broad splitting or dissociative mechanisms, to higher-level increasingly differentiated defenses.

(8) **Attachment and Separation-Individuation Issues**: although densely woven through the deep tissue of character defenses, due to their biological implications especially during early development, the *actual* history of attachment and separation experiences play a key role in personality structuring and unconscious motivation, as does the recapitulation of these issues during the adolescent passage. Both, in my opinion, ought to be imperative investigative and interpretive dimensions of any analysis.

(9) **Cognition and Thought** processes also operate unconsciously and are highly influenced by defenses; 'reasoning' may actually be 'rationalizing', feelings intellectualized, and perceptions and understanding, heavily conditioned by primitive needs, beliefs, or self-esteem preserving strategies. Cognitive style, also, varies immensely from person to person. There may also be professional areas of functioning and mastery that remain uncontaminated by conflictual areas of the personality: thought processes and the way a person is reasoning are always important dimensions of any analysis.

These, in addition to the contextual scrutiny of here-and-now interactions, I believe, are the nine most prominent referential perspectives from which contemporary psychoanalysts derive their knowledge and interpretive understanding of the unconscious. That there are numerous aspects of the psychical that are descriptively unconscious was very familiar to Freud: as early as 1915 (p.172) he made a clear distinction between the System Ucs. and the secondarily repressed; and again, in 1917, distinguishing between the infantile unconscious of the 'wish' and that of the day residue to which it attaches in dream-formation, he wrote, "People consider a single unconscious as something fantastic. What will they say when we confess that we cannot make shift without two of them?" (p 227)—or indeed, nine of them?

Where language is the only currency words acquire quite formidable powers, taking on or substituting for many of those expressive functions ordinarily discharged through actions and behaviors. Language in this setting must transcend its own limitations and become a medium for mutuality: as in poetry it must capture, depict and give shape to eruptions of unconscious experience by transforming the hidden, amorphous, and transient, into the symbolically represented. Only language offers the breadth and scope of denotive reference capable not merely of expressing but of *transforming* what is felt into what is known; only language lifts experience out of the senses crystallizing it into symbolic form. The transformative features of the talking cure mirror the symbolic functioning of the human mind; many cerebral functions converge in symbolic activity contributing to elements producing language "...so that perception and fantasy and memory, intuition and even dreaming take their special human form under its continual and increasing influence" (Langer, 1972, p. 345). Higher, and certainly conscious, organization is infused by linguistic mediation that seeps through all levels of experience reaching beyond cognitive to deeply emotional spheres.

This is why the exploratory process has to be contextual, flexible, exhaustive, detailed, encompassing, stretching from nonverbal to ideational content: We are interested in understanding *how* an experience is revived, relived, remembered and retold; to what degree it is still organically vital and to what extent it has been revisited and narratized with a sense of the pastness of the past. "Working through" is the crucial referential activity of this semantic. Operating in tandem with the observing ego it renders the process of analysis personally transforming while laying the foundations for continuing to exercise the central mediating activity of this interpretive framework. Like all creative thinking, working-through tends to suspend all other actions, requires a capacity for delay and considerable tolerance for the disagreeable tensions associated with feeling emotionally charged experiences while trying to channel them through words. "The German verb can, in fact, be used either transitively, in which case it means 'to finish or perfect something,' or reflexively for 'making ones way'" (p. 340), writes Gedo (1995). It is a particularly apt term because its ambiguity encompasses both interpersonal and intrapsychic dimensions of therapeutic activity. According to Gedo (1995) the metaphor was coined to cover a "disjunction between our theory of therapy and our theory of mind," the real focus of treatment being to identify areas of primitive thinking and "promote the maturation of the relevant cognitive functions" (p. 345). Yet working-through results in broader, deeper, more momentous psychic modifications than the cognitive learning of new communicational skills: we experience an impressive amplification of awareness at each new plateau of conscious gain, a palpable sense of growth, control and mastery through self-understanding, which sharpens and enlarges the spheres of what can be spoken about, leading to more general powers of conception. And this amplification of intellect goes beyond the idea of more adept cognition or improved interpersonal skills. Becoming 'conscious' appears to generate its own maturational momentum and spread, carrying in its tide toward higher functional organization a number of closely related differentiating and individuating processes that promote autonomy of thought while expanding the capacity for symbolic abstraction in other areas. As with any new learning or creative formulation, the task, necessarily slow and demanding, is experienced as mentally taxing. We understand this better when we realize that symbolic formulation is not simply a passive process of becoming aware but a laborious mental activity in various self-propelled stages that identifies, formulates, organizes and transforms unconscious material.

My intention in the above was to place the multiplicity of theoretical and referential perspectives of our interpretive semantic within the compass and vocabulary of human communication. Grounded in contemporary knowledge of the mediating roles of language and dialogue this approach yields operative principles that unify theory and practice by correlating psychological integration and maturation with semiotic and dialogical processes. It is not enough, in my opinion, to vaguely claim that psychoanalytic therapy entails "putting feelings into words" but that the whole contextual interplay of textured layers engaging the participants involved in analytic work partakes of this complex, laborious, new symbolic articulation. Only from within the hub of a significant human meeting can the mediating function of language serve as a bridge between minds becoming an instrument of insight and transformation.

The search for common ground ends when we understand this common ground to be the methodological unity of an interpretive semantic that engenders particular and uniquely revealing psychical processes in its discourse fields, a semantic that by its multidimensional, biopsychological sweep of reference and broad range of investigative goals, continues to expand our understanding of the human unconscious.

* * * *

In these four essays on the theme of human-interactions I have tried to lay down the conceptual underpinnings for a basic, metatheoretical reorientation that views communicative phenomena, whether projections, transmissions, evocations, enactments or verbalizations, as a direct window into the organizations and nature of the human psyche. It may not have escaped the reader that woven through are represented all five metapsychological dimensions requisite for a full psychoanalytic presentation, each theoretically accounted for through the prism of observable communicative process. The task of tracing the developmental transformations of communicative modes as language becomes our primary medium and dominant channel, and the ways in which earlier, more primitive and less mediated forms continue to inform, as interpreted in psychoanalytic situations, is tackled in the following movement.

THIRD MOVEMENT
THE MORPHOLOGY OF HUMAN COMMUNICATION

"…treat of the network and not of what the network describes."

Wittgenstein, 1922/1961

INTRODUCTION

What follows is a developmental model of communication delineating how human interactions are transformed by sign- and symbolic-mediation and how semantic and discourse reference determine the nature and meaning of what is spoken about. The purpose of this model is to identify and differentiate various projective, enactive, inductive and narrative forms, to trace their evolution ontogenetically and then as they reappear in analytic dialogues. The model ought to assist in pinpointing similarities and differences between primary developmental processes and their recapitulative forms in analytic situations, while locating certain internally consistent laws of semiotic progression.

The fundamental premise underlying this study is that communication is reciprocally constructed between a communicant and an interpreter; by definition, this implies a dialectic. The unit of study, therefore, must include the reciprocal interplay and respective contributions to the communicative process, of both parties. From this perspective we cannot logically separate interactions and relationship. I am, therefore, proposing an interactive model of communicative forms for the continued study of the *individual* mind with a primary focus on the psychoanalytic clinical and supervisory situations.

The growing recognition of the intrinsically interpenetrative, bi-directional character of communicative processes, as well as the widening scope of psychoanalytic therapy, have required analysts to become aware of the importance of examining the quality of minute-to-minute contextual exchanges. Current trends toward increasingly detailed investigation of sub-verbal interactions necessitate the recognition of a new range of unconscious communicative modes. In order to be able to resonate with these unconscious transmissions and be in a "position to make use of everything he is told for the purpose of interpretation," (Freud, 1912, p. 115) the analyst's attunement has to be sensitized toward a spectrum of unconscious derivatives.

Our focus has gradually shifted from a primary interest in what is known to *how* it is known: from content to an awareness of the *functions* of form. Despite having long recognized the technical importance of monitoring ones own responses in both a counter-transference and non-counter-transference sense, we still lack a theoretical framework that can logically exhibit the differences between these two classes of response – reactions that are contaminated by the personal, versus those that are activated by the *forms* of the communications themselves. It has been customary, thus far, to lump an excessively broad range of these responses into typologies of "countertransference" without making a theoretical distinction between counter-transference proper and inductions due to resonance to the *forms* of the communication themselves. It seems to me that this difference is important and needs to be stressed if analysts are to differentiate between attunement and countertransference. Thus far we have no clearly conceptualized internal working model to turn to when experiencing, addressing or teaching these differences. This is one of the lacunae this model attempts to fills.

Nowhere is this lack more apparent or acutely felt than in the supervisory situation where didactic requirements call out for clearly defined concepts and terms for these phenomena, and where manifestations of these very inductive currents and replications are dramatically played out. Here the dialogical character of these often powerful experiences are palpable, observable and accessible to both supervisor and supervisee, providing opportunities to grapple hands-on with phenomena that in many ways echo those of clinical process. Familiarity with all levels and forms of communication and their differential impact becomes a technical necessity. The benefits of studying these phenomena through the supervisory encounter cannot be overestimated since their *in vivo* reactivation provides a veritable research arena into the dynamisms of discourse processes. The model proposed begins to discern, name and systematize the principles of their organization.

One of our primary methodological requirements is that the observer's contextual experience and theoretical vantage-point be taken into account, not only because these are sources of analytic inference but because both are fundamental to the inquiry. My observations were informed by the developmental principles of symbolization which grounded my understanding of different communicative forms in this multi-directional semantic field. As mentioned in the introduction, the context for my observations of the supervisory process was a weekly study group in a two-year supervisory training program, which met for discussion immediately after the observed sessions. Under the expert eye of an "instructor," our group meetings were to serve as feedback for the supervisor-in-training. In addition, they proved extremely informative by providing rich and ample opportunities to experience the rippling reverberations of dynamic patterns reenacted among group members as well as the recapitulation of thematic overtones and undertones from the content of observed session. It became apparent that until these dynamisms had been thoroughly identified and thrashed out verbally between us they did indeed continue to be reenacted unconsciously in the group-process. The fact that the overarching purpose and goal of psychoanalytic discourse is to arrive at greater awareness and understanding of unconscious process, and of the phenomena that make up the process, I believe, not only added to the hall of mirrors effect but also accentuated the need for a vocabulary to refer to these diverse communicative forms.

In this sense, the distance afforded by an observational stance once or twice removed from the clinical process itself, while still privy to its dynamic patterns, was of inestimable value because it provided the requisite space for objectifying phenomena that are otherwise very difficult to identify when one is immersed in them. The advantage of an observatory stance from the supervisory process heightened both visibility and awareness of the phenomena in question. Collusions, blind spots, parallelisms, various word dances and postural mimicry, were brought vividly to light on these occasions.

What I observed was a spectrum of transmissive, replicative and narrative modes of recounting along a continuum from unconscious to conscious form-varieties. Pre-symbolic expressions shadow symbolic articulation and residues of earlier stages infiltrate and fuse into the higher forms. Each of these contributes to the whole account so that differentially assimilated and mediated elements of information interweave throughout the supervisee's report. A careful process-analysis of supervisory discourse reveals a dynamic display of alternating verbal and replicative forms of recounting and different modes of recall some of which are partially familiar from the clinical situation. Analytic understanding takes this unevenly projected, presented and represented report as a seamless continuity through which the unconscious account of a clinical process unfolds. Through the interplay of projective and transmissive tellings and showings, objectifying and exemplifying, a whole picture appears: the narrative-account contains what occurred, how it was experienced, what of this the supervisee has metabolized and understood, and what cannot yet be put into words.

It is important to recognize that the account itself *contains* and *embodies* the clinical process as it was experienced, as well as disclosing the different modes in which verbal information, interactive pattern and unconscious dynamics, are assimilated, recalled and transmitted. The only reliable "data" of psychoanalytic situations, I believe, are elements and features of the discourse process itself; and the only objectifiable phenomena are its forms and transformations. As Schaefer (1981) has pointed out, "one of the first things that would make a psychoanalytic theory of discourse just that would be its providing some internally consistent set of rules for retelling in one way events that have already been told or are being told at that moment in another way" (p. 20).

This model categorizes these stratifications and systematizes their forms: it begins to lay bare certain organizing principles of semiotic mediation and lays down a preliminary vocabulary through which to identify and refer to their different forms. Unconscious communications and meanings emerge in the interrelationships between form and content; 'content' is often a metaphorical reflection of process, just as process often reiterates and echoes content.

Psychoanalytic situations reveal how different kinds of experiences and information are assimilated, accommodated and semiotically mediated. Just as the analysis of transference provides a window into those formative experiences that created both psychic structure and psychic reality, the analysis of the supervisory report and parallel process disclose the unconscious nature of the clinical interaction and to what degree it has been understood. The unconscious transfer of experience, occurring in both, from one context to another, suggests that both situations provide opportunities for observing universal patterns of internalization.

The direct observation of supervisory sessions through a one-way mirror proved to be ideal, quasi-experimental conditions for naturalistic research. Once I became familiar with the setting, over the course of the two years, I took the opportunity to test two loose hypotheses: the first focused on a sequence of phases in verbal symbolization marked by body and eye movements; the second had to do to with the multi-directional inductive power of unconscious transmissions within our semantic fields. With respect to the first: the evolution in stages of symbolization appears quite clearly during supervisory discourse because both interlocutors share semantic and referential perspectives and, presumably, collaborative goals. Their joint striving toward understanding and verbal articulation of their subject is clearly observable as are their moments of collusive inattention, blind spots or derailment, when dwelling on content or management issues at the expense of unconscious process.

With respect to the second: as I experienced the ripple effect from the triadic supervisory field and observed it impacting on those participating in the group discussions (an effect that sometimes lingered for days or even weeks) it became apparent that the parallel process is not a unitary phenomenon but is made up of many types. There are different kinds of parallel process, often operating simultaneously, mirroring multiple levels or patterns associated with affects, images, dynamic interactions, words, stories, etc. Singular aspects of these patterns were 'held' and distributed between different group members each of who contained and reflected, and often enacted, these facets. Configurations from each aspect of parallel processes seemed to infiltrate the minds, interactions and discourse of those who entered their transmissive spheres or became involved in their semantic fields of influence. This relates directly to Person's (1989) penetrating observations on relationships between plagiarism and the parallel process in her attempt to tap the conditions for these inter-mental phenomena. I agree with Person (1989) that the parallel process needs to be considered in a broader context because it offers a window "through which to explore aspects of inter-subjectivity, affect transmission, and the investigation of a dyadic object relationship" (p. 61). The second section of the model is devoted to an examination of this kind of unconscious transmission.

In order to carve out a manageable unit of analysis for my chosen preoccupation with form, I developed the idea of the "communicative event," a slice of process, consisting of a sequence of four or five utterances examined vertically and horizontally. Ideally, this sort of micro-analysis benefits from video taping that enables one to still each frame and identify, in detail, what was being said in relation to what was being done, and how, and in what ways, ones' impressions coincide or differ with others. The idea of studying a slice of process cross-sectionally as well as sequentially, embodies an organismic approach to communication in which the primacy of the verbal component is relative and fluctuates according to the particular function language is serving at any given moment: verbal content may be carrying or obfuscating some facet of a much broader and deeper exchange.

The thesis expounded throughout this work is that the psycho-analysis of communication must encompass dynamic interrelationships between linguistic and non-linguistic forms: words cannot be divorced from actions as mirrors of mind; what was said cannot be decontextualized or fully understood without knowing how and in what way, in which sequence, in what tone and in which sense...and all of this will still not reveal much without knowing what was being done at the same time, how this was felt and experienced. Psychoanalytic dialogues are *not* texts but dynamic human interactions. In a semantic of *unconscious* meanings the supremacy of the spoken or written word is doubtful. There is no valid "verbatim" clinical or supervisory "text' outside of, or separate from, the analysand's associations and the supervisee's report. This is why observation of supervisory sessions *in vivo*, which contain the clinical *within* their current process, is such an exceptional research tool.

Psychoanalytic domains are unique in establishing rules of discourse for the purpose of exploring and understanding many levels of meaning. Multidetermination makes of every utterance a condensation of many diverse streams; consequently the interpretive potential in any slice of process is very broad indeed. This leads to another important implication for the observational inquiry of the supervisory process, namely, that psychoanalytic discourse is amenable not merely to one or two dimensions of study but to many and, certainly always several, simultaneously. The chosen vector of investigation will determine what is seen, heard and understood, and each of these foci of observation can be studied in brief micro-process segments or over the span of several months in broad macro-process phases. It is virtually impossible to adequately harness the complex, multifaceted simultaneity of psychoanalytic phenomena sequentially, or do justice to the subtle gradations and hues of so rich and refined an experience as that of psychoanalytic listening.

The advantage of studying human modes of interaction through the morphology of their communicative forms is that this conceptual lens eliminates the inside/outside dichotomy, neither reifying nor distorting direct manifestations of "mind." Most importantly, because the processes in question are observable phenomena, and the observer's experience is included as part of the interpretive understanding, principles of theory and practice are brought together and anchored in 'data' which can yield empirical hypotheses.

Many interdisciplinary streams converge in the holistic paradigm of which the following model is an expression. And while I cannot refer to the vast literature that underlies this conceptualization, I am particularly indebted to the works of Vygotsky, Bahktin, Piaget, Bateson, Langer, Bruner, Goodman, great thinkers in psychology, philosophy and epistemology whose ideas are woven into this integration. This is a *psychoanalytic* model, however, derived from informal observations of the psychoanalytic and supervisory processes, and is especially influenced by the orientation of psychoanalysts such as H. Loewald, N. Freedman, H. Searles, G. F. Basch, S. Greenspan, and T. Shapiro, to name the central few.

A word about the diagram; as the title implies — morphe; form: genesis; coming into being: The developmental model is arranged in terms of forms and transformations of communicative means along a continuum from natural signals to symbolic modes as these first appear in ontogenesis and are recapitulated (*not* replicated) in psychoanalytic contexts. The model is layered to convey the epigenetic quality of a hierarchy of communicative forms evolving one out of the other. However, these ought not be viewed as fixed stages so much as transforming organizations of experience and knowledge, along a fluidly mediating continuum. The first three stages build toward language, the last three build upon it. It is important to keep in mind, however, that *all levels continue to operate all the time*: the contrapuntal appearance and multidimensional quality of our material, so much a part of the phenomenology of psychoanalytic discourse, is thereby taken into account.

Psychological defenses tend to split components of experience and elements of communication. This obliges us to conceptualize psychoanalytic models that can account for disguised and disjointed or distorted communicative pathways in terms of an elaborate hierarchy of defensive strata. Higher level defenses are often layered over earlier, more primitive defenses and so on, all of which seep into and permeate communications and communicative style. Differentiating between transmissive, enactive and inductive, versus expressive and verbal, elements of a complete communication provides conceptual distinctions that are necessary to explain phenomena such as when language is the primary carrier of explicit information but not of its implicit meanings; or when verbalization of what ought to be affectively charged material is delivered in an emotionally flattened, meaningless way. In part this reiterates an idea with which communication studies have long been familiar, namely, that there are two (probably many more) facets to all communications, one that is content based and linguistically structured; the other that is nonverbal, analogical, transmitting interpersonal or sense-information through subtle signals. In most human interchange both aspects co-determine the whole message.

But a psychoanalytic study of communicative processes has to yield deeper insights into the minds of those in clinical and supervisory dyads, particularly with reference to the nature of what flows between them. The broad formal distinctions between transmissive-contagions and communication proper, initially proposed by Escolona (1953), seemed a good place to begin. Accordingly, the broadest distinction in the diagram is that dividing morphic (or signaling) from lexical (signifying) sentience.

This study begins at the experiential hub of the supervisory process to which I will return often for illustrative purposes. This is to try to render as vividly as possible the phenomenology of the supervisory encounter and to illustrate how each of the formal modes, arranged developmentally in the model, reappear and rise to ascendance at different junctures and with different consequences for the supervisory process. I would like to state at the outset, that this group of simultaneously occurring phenomena that are prominent in supervisory situations, it may be safe to say, probably constitute normal, universal forms of assimilation, affect- and interaction-transmission, and phases of accommodation, symbolization and narrative construction.

In view of the educative function of supervision and the implicit evaluative position in which supervisors are placed by training institutions, a number of extrinsic factors, from both sides, also impact on the already unconsciously edited report of the supervisee. Dynamisms involved in the desire to both reveal and conceal, express confidence and vulnerability, knowledge and insecurity, all at the same time, further complicate the communicative forms revealed in this situation. Nevertheless, when all is said and done, transactions arising in this particular discourse arena provide invaluable, palpable interactive sources from which to observe the interplay of diverse conscious and unconscious forms of communication.

ILLUSTRATIVE VIGNETTE

For several weeks, a supervisee with whom I enjoyed a good working relationship had been expressing increasing discomfort with a particular patient and growing misgivings regarding her competence to treat this case.

The patient in question, a young man, presented a dramatic history of neglect in a well-to-do family, with a suicide attempt during his college years and a lifelong coercive struggle to obtain some care and attention from an unreachable, surgeon father and an inaccessible, alcoholic mother. The last of several children who had witnessed bitter parental fights, he had found some support in an older sister on whom he was still very dependent. The opening phase of treatment had been marked by considerable ambivalence, devaluation and reservations regarding the usefulness of the treatment process, his ability to pay for it, the therapist's competence, and in general, the hopelessness of his plight. His precarious self-esteem vacillated from day to day. Alternately he bombarded the therapist with violent, sadistic fantasies or questioned the purpose and value of anything, particularly in the therapist's ability to effectuate any change. He felt isolated and worthless—unable to form friendships, unable to be alone. There had been frequent phone calls in between sessions and frequent scheduling changes. Despite noting the urgency behind these attempts for more contact and special consideration, the therapist rationalized that they were merely scheduling calls due to the nature of her patient's freelance work.

Similarly my supervisee had called me on several occasions, at odd times, regarding what seemed to be trivial decisions on management and policy issues. Given her novice status I had responded, but when next we met I questioned what prompted these uncharacteristic calls for advice. She saw nothing in it, focusing instead on other cases where things were going smoothly. Reticently, and at the very end of our time, she brought up the patient in question. She had been uncomfortable the whole week, unable to gauge the depth of his depression or get a handle on the material and then the patient had reported a violent dream. The supervisee then began shuffling nervously through pages of notes (I do *not* encourage written reports) mentioning the patient's having questioned her ability to keep all his information in mind. I asked what she recalled of the dream. Looking at her wrist watch she blurted out that it was something about him having taken a gun and shooting randomly at everyone in sight at work and an image of a splattered brain on a white screen. . .at which point she hurriedly gathered her notes and got up to leave, remarking "it's hard to tell what are his fantasies and what could potentially be real with this patient. Thank you, see you next week."

Left hanging, I puzzled at the palpable change in my supervisee. I had noted her defensive avoidance of this case and evasiveness but was struck by the last comment, so clearly did it appear to be induced by the mounting anxiety she was experiencing with this patient. Moreover what he had reported was clearly a dream not a fantasy; the patient had not confused the two; what was it about this patient and their interactions that caused my supervisee to lose her bearings and confuse the two? As she recounted the dream she seemed petulant, dismissive, avoidant, anxious, already half way out the door. In my mind the dream had immediately called up an image referring to one of this patient's very early memories, as reported by the therapist, early in the treatment. The little boy had been awakened at night by his parents fighting. He had gone to his father's drawer and come down stairs carrying a gun threatening to shoot. It wasn't clear if or who he intended to shoot. His later suicidal threats and depressive symptomatology apparently covered a deeper, more frantic, rage or panic filled fear of loss of impulse control and disintegration. His surface adaptation masked and disguised a heavily defended "splattered" core. The unspeakable anxiety around this potentially fragmenting center, and its underlying terror and rage, had to be discharged in projective forms onto any potential caregiver. My supervisee had fled in a hurry leaving us no time to reflect upon or understand this material or to mitigate its countertransferential and inductive effects.

At our following meeting the therapist was openly despondent about this case. She felt inadequate, unhelpful, found herself dreading the sessions and had now been put "on the spot," as the patient had announced that following his sister's advice he had asked his father for a prescription for Prozac and was already taking it. Caught off guard, the therapist told him that she would have to report this to the clinic psychiatrist, but realized that this had been an uncalled for retaliation for the patient having gone behind her back and then telling her this as a *fait accompli*. In the same breath she asked me what she should do. I responded with several practical recommendations centered primarily on further exploration of what this action meant in the context of their interactions. But mostly I questioned her feelings of incompetence, despondency, avoidance and dread, and focused on the degree of anxiety this case seemed to be inducing. No, she answered, this was not so, it was just that she found it harder to work with better-defended, neurotic patients than with severely disturbed or overtly psychotic patients. She left seemingly reassured but in agreement with the need for further exploration and discussion of what was going on.

In the following supervisory meeting she recounted two sessions with this patient. In each, her patient had begun with a taunting "well, have you told your supervisors yet?" Torn between my recommendations that she analyze everything and a fear of institutional regulations she experienced this provocation as a challenge and coercion. In the same breath, she turned to me and again asked me what I thought she should do, knowing quite well where I stood on this, and that I was unlikely to give directives or answers. Again, I laid less emphasis on the content but reflected back my opinion that it seemed worthwhile to explore in depth the coercive quality and challenging nature of her patient's opening, provocative confrontations and their interactions around this issue, what they were inducing in her and how she could understand this. Again she agreed. Maybe her patient's aggression was emerging via this taunting and "putting her on the spot...." Further exploration might open an inroad to begin to interpret her patient's warded off, coercive aggression which masked a desperate plea to be adequately taken care of while preempting this by destructively devaluing any potential caregiver. Yet, she added, she felt uncomfortable and put on the spot by institutional rules; what did I think. I asked her if she had followed through on my recommendation that she check to be sure what the institutional rules really were. Had she ascertained that the effects of the medication were being monitored by the prescribing physician? No, she answered, she had not. I noted this paradoxical neglect, but did not immediately make any remark. At this point I again emphasized that given the dynamics it was important that these transactions continue to be analyzed in the treatment process with her patient. Truthfully, she answered, she was torn, worn out and drained and wished the "whole thing" would go away, but again left reassured and prepared to continue her analytic task.

Next I heard from her in a hurried and awkward phone call. Offhandedly she informed me that since our last meeting she had sought advice in the institution group supervision where it had been categorically decided that she should report the patient to the clinic director right away. This she had already done, she just wanted to let me know. Caught off guard, put on the spot and struck by my supervisee's acerbic tone I wondered why she had called, and said we would talk further at our next meeting. As I hung up I became aware of a mounting annoyance stirred by this abrupt and confrontative call. Clearly, she had succeeded in finding someone who *would* tell her what to do, she had disburdened herself of the tensions involved in the responsibility of analyzing her patient and of understanding the process rather than "managing" the case, and she had gone behind my back, reporting this to me offhandedly over the phone as a *fait accompli*. She was recreating the coercive and provocative tensions she experienced with her patient in our relationship to a T, and enacting a very similar triadic pattern of events. I noticed how I too, uncharacteristically, wished I could wash my hands of the whole thing.

As we sat down for the following supervisory session a deep rift had descended between us. The tenor of the exchange was to be set by my supervisee who, visibly upset and agitated and avoiding eye contact, began telling me how things had proceeded to get even worse. She had told the patient she had reported him but then subsequently discovered there had been no need to do so, there was no such policy; she had been misinformed. She then had to tell him <u>that</u> as well, so that she felt foolish and appeared incompetent as he had anticipated. Sitting nervously on the edge of the chair, my shaken supervisee then proceeded to pour out a flood of rebukes; I had not given her sufficient guidance; I had not told her what to do; I answered questions with questions; it wasn't fair, she shouldn't have to take this much responsibility, etc. Moreover, I was not fulfilling my duty as a supervisor; while she understood my analytic approach she was frustrated and anxious by the whole process and by not being told explicitly how to proceed. Now she felt it was my fault that she had been made to "look bad," because of incongruent information. Seizing a pause in the deluge I tried to understand her distress in the context of the analytic process with this patient, but to little avail. I then resorted to the observation that apparently, like her patient, she too felt she had not received either adequate or appropriate care.

We then carefully went over the sequence of events and their systemic reverberations, as these had rebounded dyadically, triadically and even at group and institutional levels. This seemed to help. She could reflect on these more removed processes. Moreover from this vantage point the parallelisms stood out in vivid relief. Together we could now trace and begin to process some understanding of the echoing phenomena at hand.

A powerful parallel process had been underway inducing the therapist to reproduce those unspeakable aspects of her patient's fragmenting anxiety in an enactment with me, which conveyed the desperate cry for help and containment this patient's unconscious coercions were really about. She was enacting and inducing what she *felt* but did not *know* of this patient's desperate pleas for safety and care underlying the depression and had recreated a credible scenario where she could include all the coercive, mistrustful and rebuking nuances that characterized her patient's conscious and unconscious communications to her.

Given the solid learning alliance established prior to this derailment and my unswerving commitment to understanding this enactment in terms of a triadic dynamic, we were able to isolate its inductive impact from her own countertransference issues and the patterns of replication in our relationship. I would not have been able to do this had my stance not been sufficiently guided by a disciplined capacity to observe my own induced responses. We regained our moorings as my supervisee began observing the events and the various decisive *actions* she had taken to mitigate her mounting anxiety, for which she had then tried to blame me. Over the next several weeks and months, aided by the fact that her patient continued in treatment and by the occurrence of a similar but more muted version of the same dynamic, with sufficient distance and time for 'reflection' we were able to sift out induced from countertransference aspects of what had transpired. Haltingly my supervisee became cognizant of parallelisms and of the immense power of unconscious inductions and transmissions, continuing our work with heightened awareness and an increased, deepened understanding of the meaning of analytic neutrality as a therapeutic stance.

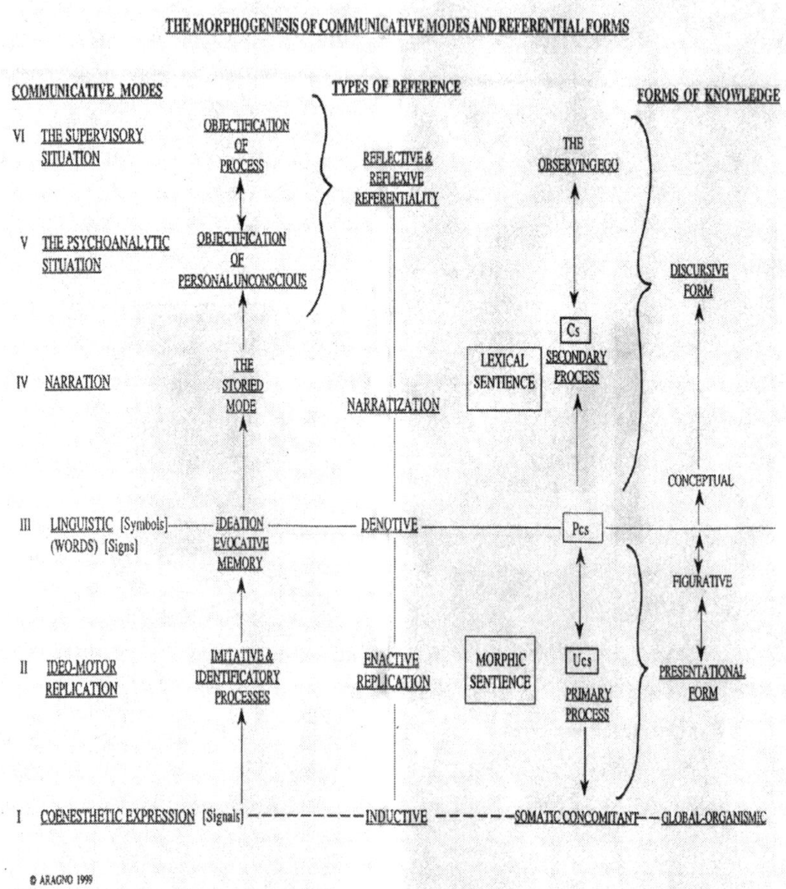

THE MORPHOGENESIS OF COMMUNICATIVE MODES AND REFERENTIAL FORMS

I
COENESTHETIC EXPRESSION

The Sensory-affective Anlage

> The movements of expression in the face and body, whatever their origin may have been, are in themselves of much importance for our welfare. They serve as the first means of communication between the mother and her infant;...she smiles approval, and thus encourages her child on the right path, or frowns disapproval. We readily perceive sympathy in others by their expression; our sufferings are thus mitigated and our pleasures increased, and mutual good feeling is thus strengthened. The movements of expression give vividness and energy to our spoken words. They reveal the thoughts and intentions of others more truly than do words, which may be falsified....To understand, as far as possible, the source or origin of the various expressions which may be hourly seen on the faces of the men around us, not to mention our domesticated animals, ought to possess much interest for us.
>
> Darwin, 1872, pp. 364-365

Disadvantaged by prolonged dependency, the human infant is amply compensated by the biological endowment of a highly effective communicative system consisting of eight primary affect-signals associated with widespread glandular, muscular and behavioral manifestations. The ability to activate and recognize this basic repertoire of human expressions is phylogenetically inherited through subcortical centers and mediated by the autonomic nervous system. Facial expressions are the immediate, observable indications of organismic states or dispositions, each of which is accompanied by broad physiological responses generating sensory feedback. Tomkins (1962-1963), who considered affects to be our primary motivating system, listed and described the features of eight universal expressions: surprise/startle; interest/excitement; enjoyment/joy; distress/anguish; anger/rage; fear/terror; and shame/humiliation (Vol.1 p.337). Human infants are equipped from birth to communicate their inner states via these facial and bodily expressions.

Because facial and vocal patterns can automatically arouse similar responses in others, affects are highly contagious. It is important to differentiate between primary affect-forms — present at birth — from their later, modulated elaborations into subtly nuanced complex emotions. Initially, infantile affects are contentless; the expressive behavior means only itself and functions like a signal, designed to elicit a satisfactory reaction. Their expression and intensity is intimately tied to innate temperamental disposition and the nature of responses with which their expression meets. Very quickly primary affects are shaped through interactions that mediate their expression and modulate intensity. Signaling turns fast into *signifying* gestures and expressions that indicate wish or intent more effectively. Depending on whether care-giving responses are understanding and timely or frustrating and delayed, affect displays will change qualitatively, decreasing or increasing in intensity, the latter an automatic mechanism associated with "density of neural firing" (Tomkins (1992 p. 56). The manner in which infantile signals are responded to, therefore, is most consequential insofar as early conditioning interactions lay lasting neurophysiological traces predisposing toward particular interactive expectations.

Whereas in animals innate responses are tied to survival behaviors with little other communicative value, in humans the opposite is true (Basch, 1996a). The human infant's survival is completely dependent on establishing and maintaining effective attachments: hence the repertoire of innate human behaviors is predominantly made up of various expressions with high communicative value. Communication, learning, and adaptation, are all so interwoven as to be virtually inseparable in the development of the human psyche or 'mind'. Basch (1976a) expresses the same idea:

> How significant an infant's messages are in bringing about whatever takes place within him and to him must play an important part in determining the eventual sense of confidence and "basic trust" in his transaction with the environment. That is, the substrate or *anlage* for a future conviction that he can create meaningful order from experience and that a temporary disorganization does not herald unmanageable trauma, or threaten chaos, depends on the efficacy of the system of communication between mother and infant. The language of mother and infant consists of the signals and cues produced by the autonomic, involuntary nervous system in both parties. These transactions generate an experiential pattern that influences later character development. The baby's observable behavior is therefore not simply a discharge phenomenon, an affective release which is only incidentally informative for the mother, but a form of communication whose significance is either understood or misunderstood with similar consequences that adequate or inadequate communication has for conflict and adaptation in later life. (pp. 766-767)

As a communicative means, affect-signals function by transmitting feeling-patterns that are immediately recognized by any member of the species. The efficacy of the signal is contingent on the others' willingness to read, react, or resonate with that signals expression. A continuum of response-patterns within the signaling-form can, therefore, be traced, all of which begin with the same inductive process. At the earliest, most undifferentiated, level facial and vocal patterns spontaneously activate organismic like-responses, a morphic echo. Contagion operates through *contamination,* by infecting with an affect, automatically. More evolved and differentiated responses function by eliciting an abbreviated version of the affect-pattern, accompanied by some awareness of the activated feeling. In the most mature response, 'empathy', only a transient, internal reactivation of the affect is induced and awareness of that fleeting feeling engendered is used informatively, to *understand* the other's state; "...the perception of emotional expression leads the observer to an unconscious, merely incipient imitation of the fleeting act, and the resulting faint tensions involve an equally faint feeling by which he understands what is passing in the other person," (Langer, 1967, p. 176). Maturation along this continuum is contingent on a decrease in egocentrism and a correlate capacity to tolerate and recognize a whole range of emotional states. Again, it is important to remember that this mode continues to operate via the same inductive means; the transmission of feelings, images, thoughts, ideas, etc. — no matter how abstractly they are represented — may engender correlate responses that repeat the contagion-awareness-empathy sequence.

Both Piaget (1962) and Vygotsky (1934) addressed the phenomenon of contagion but from different perspectives. Piaget's biological orientation emphasized the functional continuity between sensorimotor and representational form, an approach which, when applied to communication, stresses the persisting impact of early modes on subsequent forms. Vygotsky (1934), on the other hand, who was interested in semiotic processes, focused primarily on interrelationships between sign use in social interactions and their formative impact, when internalized, on the development of higher mental processes. In Piaget's framework, what I refer to as coenesthetic expression, our primary signaling *mode*, forms part and parcel of the foundation out of which all successive stratifications of thought and communication build. For Vygotsky, the sign function, and the generalized categories language enables, must be distinguished from primitive automatic, biological stimulus-patterns. This primary unmediated signaling mode of transmission, devoid of anything that can properly be called *signified* content or meaning, does not qualify as genuine social interchange. In fact for Vygotsky even signs serving merely an *indicative* function do not meet the criterion for genuine social interchange, which must be based on the use of generalized signs for communicative purposes; "In essence, such social interaction that uses expressive movements does not even merit the name social interaction: it should instead be called *contagion*. The frightened gander that recognizes danger and spreads alarm to the whole flock is not really communicating to it what it saw but is rather contaminating the flock with fear" (Vygotsky, 1934, p. 11, in Wertsch, 1985, p. 96).

For Piaget (1962) on the other hand, the appearance of contagion marks the developmental point at which the simple reflex has given way to a stimulus response by reproductive assimilation, a shift that corresponds with the beginning of six stages of imitative assimilation considered to be the very manifestations of sensorimotor intelligence. As early as the second month Piaget observed a clear form of contagion whereby the voice of others stimulated the baby's own voice. In order for this to occur the baby had to have already become familiar with their sounds and intonations since contagion is a circular reaction, triggered automatically only in the case of crying because of the strong affect that accompanies this sound. Vocal contagion is viewed as the beginning of phonic imitation; and microstages in imitative assimilation are understood, in a Piagetian scheme, as the continuation of efforts at sensorimotor accommodation.

Both these great psychologists identified this phenomenon of pre-signification, each interpreting its functioning from their particular framework. Piaget considered the functional mode or organization to which any experience is assimilated and accommodated; Vygotsky looked at the function the semiotic form is serving, dismissing signals as pre-social. From the psychoanalyst's perspective, however, the very aspect of contagion that is most important in the interpretation of the deep unconscious is ignored by both. Whereas it is true that signals incite stereotypical action-patterns in animals, in humans, affect-signals induce feelings: and feelings shape experiences, generating signified forms (images) and meanings, which also *inform*. The centrality of the affective dimension in the development of mind and communication, both phylo- and ontogenetically, fairly leaps to the eye. It must have been as fundamental in human evolution and adaptation as it is in individual psychological development. Certainly it is fundamental in understanding unconscious transmissions as records of our earliest interactive experiences; Basch (1976a) comments, "we tend to overlook the fact that in terms of total communication, especially in terms of motivating communication, purely discursive speech plays a relatively small and belated role in our human lives" (p. 764). From the beginning, basic survival patterns — approach/avoidance, fight/flight, the whole panoply of attachment behaviors — are titrated and patterned through affectively charged interactions forming a core interactive matrix through which all future messages are filtered.

As analysts, we are interested in signals emanating from this pre-representational mode, not only because their expression is wordless but because they persist, diminished and partially subsumed by higher forms, yet still reflecting broad character traits that eventually permeate the analytic dialogue. It is this primary matrix, patterned during the first two years of life, which is remobilized at the heart of the archaic transference. The transmission and projection of qualities of interaction pertaining to this deeply conditioning primary encounter can be elusive, deeply disturbing yet highly informative, insofar as we are able to become aware of them. As Basch (1976a) put it, "Once affect is identified as an adaptive behavior, a form of communication mediated by the autonomic nervous system and relying primarily on chemical transmissions of messages,…it ceases to be a mysterious event and takes its proper place among physiologic processes and their psychological manifestations"(p.771). These modes are subcortically conditioned and recorded, deeply entrenched, and have enormous impact on basic life-enhancing or self-defeating attitudes that, because they are so pervasive, are also extremely difficult to change.

From a developmental perspective, and to inform genetic reconstructions, it is important to make a clear distinction between infantile affects and the semiotically mediated meanings underlying more complex emotions. Their apparent equation is highly misleading. It is as much a mistake to adultomorphize a baby's spontaneous expressions and survival behaviors, as it is to minimize the impact of failures to respond adequately to these first attempts at engaging the human milieu. The fact that infants produce facial expressions corresponding with emotional states to which we attribute meanings does not justify our assigning to these basic signal-patterns the significance of differentiated emotions. In fact, "We may claim only that facial patterns seem to be expressive *reactions* and then go on to deduce what might be the nature of these reactions" (Basch, 1976a, p. 769).

Affective expressions are the behavioral correlates of feelings, they speak directly from the human soul; and feelings rapidly acquire forms in a species driven to organize, recognize, signify and ultimately symbolize stimuli. 'Emotions,' on the other hand, imply the capacity for differentiated, nuanced and signified responses, greater proprioception, and levels of awareness that cannot exist prior to linguistic mediation: "The shame-humiliation reaction in infancy of hanging the head and averting the eyes does not mean the child is conscious of rejection, but indicates that effective contact with another person has been broken," writes Basch (1976a, p. 765). The reappearance in analysis of even minute traces of these reactions needs to be noted and explored in detail. Genetic reconstructions are based on inferences regarding the nature of our earliest adaptive responses to interactive experience, therefore "by conceptualizing affective behavior as a system of communication, antedating and independent of verbal language, it become possible to explain systematically how it is that the paradigmatic patterns for later adaptation as well as for later psychic conflict are already laid down in infancy, long before language and the kind of reasoning it makes possible can be brought to bear on experience" (Basch,1976a p. 768).

A psychoanalytic model of human communication must begin with a reintegration of this primary communicative mode in terms of what its signals and survival reactions imply for the nuclei of self-experience and self-organization, and subsequent psychological development. In order to assist in this task, Basch (1976a) provides a reading of Tomkins' (1962-1963) eight basic expressive modalities that incorporates a translation of their communicative significance. Following, is my own abbreviated version:

> **Surprise/Startle:** a reaction which readies the organism to attend to stimuli in order for these to be integrated as messages preparing for adaptation to a new situation.
>
> **Interest/Excitement:** a reaction indicating the pursuit of the significance of a message.
>
> **Enjoyment/Joy:** a reaction indicating stimuli have been successfully integrated into sensorimotor matrix, manifesting when adequate pattern-matching or pattern-making occurs.

> **Distress/Anguish:** a signal-call indicating need and an expression of the inability to organize stimuli into recognizable patterns.
>
> **Contempt/Disgust:** a reaction to stimuli that are noxious or become so through association (withdrawing, rejecting or spitting out).
>
> **Anger/Rage:** a reaction to immutable, intense frustration — with active attempt to impact on situation or ward off frustrating stimuli.
>
> **Fear/Terror:** a reaction to non-fitting or threatening stimuli with readiness for flight. Message is organized but threatens integration of coping capacities.
>
> **Shame/Humiliation:** a reaction to rupture or failure of contact function with significant others accompanied by a collapse of self-integration and initiative.
>
> (from Basch, 1976a, pp. 762-763)

One of the most eloquent of the early psychoanalytic baby watchers, S. Escalona (1953) considered "The network of patterns which constitute the totality of the baby's social world, and especially the process of communication between baby and mother," to be "the most mysterious and fascinating part of infancy research" (p. 33). Presiding over a panel discussion on "Emotional Development in the First Year," addressing forms of transmission and interaction between mother and infant, Escalona suggested making a distinction between contagion and communication. The former she defined as "those processes whereby a feeling state transmits itself from mother to baby, as when an infant cries when held by an acutely tense and anxious person but seems quite content when held by one who is relaxed;" (p. 314). The term communication, on the other hand, would be reserved for the "conscious and purposive sending and receiving of information" (p. 35) She speculated that contagion is never fully under "voluntary control" (p. 34), and that "currents of feeling" (p. 35) emanating from contagional processes probably continue to play a significant role throughout life. Contemporary baby-watchers have drawn our attention to the intense mirroring of the mother/infant dyad in face-to-face interactions. Behind these subliminally choreographed expressive duets are the seeds of wholesale introjections, identifications, and the internalization of patterns of interaction. One wonders how much of the underlying *unconscious* attitudes are also assimilated and adopted.

Mothers can and do use contagion intentionally to exert a soothing or calming effect on their infants, with excellent results. I can personally vouch for its success from first hand experience, as when my infant daughter underwent the removal of eight stitches from an eyelid without so much as a blink or a whimper, with only my own soothing arms, intense eye contact and reassuring murmurs to calm her. Describing her own attempts to understand precisely what goes on in her when approaching a baby with an intent to sooth, Escalona (1953) determined that in preparation she deliberately altered her feeling-state toward calmness banishing all else but her interaction with the baby from her mind. In order for reassuring contagion to be effective, then, the *quality* of the adult's disposition is important; and this implies unconscious as well as conscious attitudes and feelings. There is now much well-documented research regarding the impact of maternal states even prior to birth, during the intrauterine phase. Apparently whatever the adult is really feeling is what is transmitted. However we conceive of 'truth' in this ambiguous world, human affects, particularly if unconsciously felt, not only do not lie, they wield considerable power.

Escalona's (1953) panel drew a distinct line between contagion and communication proper. In the attempt to pin point what flows between people without the aid of words, and by what pathways, I believe there is more to be gained by placing contagional processes within a unified framework and examining the kind of information that is transmitted by each of the interactive modes. What is transmitted directly via these expressive and inductive pathways are dispositions and emotional attitudes and qualities of inner states; signals, eliciting agonistic or antagonistic responses that alert the organism to react in a number of ways. The least differentiated, most primitive of these responses, contagion, is a mechanism ensuring maximum and immediate responsiveness to vital messages. It functions like social glue, contaminating the whole group to move in unison, ensuring a primal form of social bonding that probably originates in limbic circuitry, bypassing cortical functions altogether. If we think of human interactions in terms of a continuum of increasingly differentiated modes with contagion at one end and intentional verbal communication at the other, as did Kris in Escalona's (1953) panel, we might say that at the contagion extreme there is automatic reaction to stimuli that at more advanced developmental stages are either not perceived or are rapidly mediated. Barring extreme danger situations, 'selection' favors 'higher' forms of communication allowing sensory-emotional cues to sink and merge into the background at subliminal levels. Different modes of attention, however, can orient toward different *kinds* of stimuli eliciting conscious responses fitted to different types of information.

One of the primary conditions for effective maternal induction is a complete focus of attention, which predisposes toward the second, a loosening of the boundaries created by linguistic mediation and thought. A third prerequisite, however, cannot be prescribed; it requires a genuine and fully felt intention to sooth. In infancy the entire sensorium is vulnerable to inductive input. Babies are notoriously sensitive to "attention and intention" two central qualities in shaping an interactive matrix where the first bond of trust is potentially forged. One of the most important of mothering functions is to be able to 'contain' and modulate the infant's affects. She cannot do this if she is agitated, depressed, anxious, resentful, or harboring intolerable ambivalence and in need of affect-containment herself. She can exert a calming effect on her infant only if she is able to engage in a totally invested form of attention that conveys unconditional *involvement*, saying, in essence, "I see you, I'm here for you, everything is all right." This is why the *quality* of the maternal gaze is of such fundamental and lasting importance: even more than a mirror of the soul, it is statement of relatedness, conditioning the infant's core state and experience of self. To the degree that a mother's gaze is merely a reflection of herself projected into her baby's eyes, the infants embryonic self is negated. To be truly nurturing, the maternal gaze has to see the 'Other' in her infant and, in their subverbal vocabulary, has to convey what is best described as a form of 'devotion'. This beneficent disposition toward her infant, to the degree that it is accessible to her, creates an inter-influential nexus whereby the inducer's conscious and unconscious emotional states and intentions are directly transmitted.

This is the soil of basic trust, a mold from which all future intimate ties are cast. Luckily empathic tendencies are heightened and cultivated in mothers during the early phases of mothering, "The language of mother and infant consists of signals and cues produced by the autonomic, involuntary nervous systems of both parties" (Basch, 1976a, p. 776). If we conceptualize the major developmental task of the neonate to be that of regulating and coordinating basic physiological systems, the mother's primary function is to maintain stimuli within a tolerable range. Paradoxically the mother's own regulatory capacities — which echo *her* own mother's — her attitude toward her baby's affects and the quality of handling, holding, feeding and care-giving this generates, is introjected wholesale by her infant. In this way mothering and interactive styles are transmitted intergenerationally.

The skin is the dominant sensory organ in the neonate and early in life we receive significant impressions largely through direct physical contact. Threshold and reflex studies reveal that touch, taste, temperature, pain, and probably kinesthetic sensations, lead to relatively specific responses, whereas (barring extremes which elicit startle responses) vision and audition are less developed and do not, initially, evoke differentiated responses. This creates a narrow orbit for the mother/infant dyad. As perception and audition achieve prominence, however, visual contact comes to replace the regulatory functions obtained through direct physical contact. Breathing rhythms, heartbeat, muscular tensions, holding patterns and facial expressions, i.e., the whole sensory-kinetic underlay that formed the basis of this first encounter, once introjected, is gradually supplanted by visual cues. These primal adaptive patterns resurface in analysis where they appear in the subtlest reenactments of broad interactive rhythms of engagement and withdrawal, relatedness and disconnection, in the dynamic tensions of micro-sequences that recapitulate the pulse of this earliest bond.

Subliminal currents emanating from this sensory-affective anlage leave lasting impressions to which subsequent perceptual input will orient. The dim records of this uneven encounter are emblazoned in our stance toward the world, in the faintest pulse of breathing patterns, how we hold our bodies, look, touch, move, and read environmental cues; they color our tendencies to become involved or to retreat, toward expectation of benevolence or fear, affecting how we attune and respond to others. Primary interactive schemas are grafted into the innermost self-experience. These underlying neurophysiological channels are obscured but not eliminated by more mediated, symbolic organization and continue to play a part in our apperceptions, which means that they remain amenable to therapeutic modification (see Schore, 1996, 1997a). Taking a neurobiological approach to communication in the psychoanalytic treatment of schizophrenics Spotnitz (1985) prescribed units of verbal contact that were to be carefully administered, like optimal "dosages of appropriate humanizing communication" (p. 111). He was appealing to this earliest, deepest and most vulnerable of human cores. Drawing attention to the enormity of the therapeutic demand made on the patient, he wrote "it entails the reorganization and reintegration of the nervous system, with the multiplicity of physiochemical changes that, as we now recognize, accompany that transformation" (p. 111).

The point this entire work stresses is that affect is not an antonym to reason and cognition but its complement, the inner face of outer information: "affect, so-called, is in fact an onto- and phylogenetically early form of communication" writes Basch (1976a). "It seems that affective communication does not represent a unique class of activity, as has always been assumed, but is basic for cognition and, by exercising a guiding function on later cognitive developments, provides the motive power for both maturation and pathologic adaptation" (p. 776).

We turn now to examine the ways in which these modes of transmission and forms of interaction manifest in psychoanalytic and supervisory situations.

For analysts at work, this is the deepest, often the most disturbing, amorphous and least differentiated of experiential levels: it is also the most difficult to identify and resistant to shaping by words. For some these are uncomfortable regions of interchange since they require a receptivity and openness to inductive input of primal, raw feelings that may arouse tensions threatening the stability of even the most solid psychic composure. Frequently no adequate words can be found to transpose what flows between people interacting along these transmissive channels. And characteristically, the unutterable seeks a direct projective outlet, a milieu or an encounter, on which to displace and play out what presses from an inner proscenium. Analytic situations provide just such a space, their semantic focus and discourse functions designed to elicit a reawakening and spontaneous replay of even these dim regions of unconscious mental life.

Yet focused interest in differentiating between distinct forms or types of un-verbal transmissions, thus far, has been scant and theoretical progress in this area lags far behind all others. Part of the problem, according to Jacobs (1994) stems from the very nature of this realm: "It is the earliest and most primitive form of expression, and for many, if not most, people it evokes a world best forgotten —....for some analysts, to put themselves in close touch with the nonverbal world is unconsciously experienced as a threat that must be warded off (p. 746). One of the best ways of doing this, writes Jacobs, is to ignore its existence. But to ignore these profound levels of human interchange is to eclipse precisely what is, today, of most relevance. The psychoanalyst's spheres of observation and reference are now deeper and broader than ever, virtually demanding investigation and theoretical integration of these forms of interpersonal connection. As Reik (1948) noted, "It is the unconscious mind of the subject that is of decisive importance, and the analyst meets that with his own unconscious mind as the instrument of perception" (p. 132).

Unconscious perceptions remain attuned to the subtle accompaniments to linguistic communication of "speaking gestures" (Reik, 1948, p.132). These emanate from an interplay of facial and bodily expressions, movements, gestures and looks that supply "psychical data" in the form of "neurodynamic stimuli" (p.135) that are absorbed and synthesized unconsciously. Exchanges taking place at these subliminal levels do not "proceed in a vacuum," (Reik 1948, p. 139) but play a major role in forming unconscious impressions: "The minutest movements accompany every process of thought; muscular twitchings in face and hands and movements of the eyes speak to us as well as words. No small power of communication is contained in a glance, a persons bearing, a bodily movement, a special way of breathing" (p.135) The sum-total of these fragments of sensory information yields a pattern conveying a sense of the others inner state. Reik (1948) advocated sharpening acuity to these "subsensuous phenomena" (p.

142). His famous "third ear," sprouts from just such exercise and is dependent on heightened proprioception for optimal functioning; "the only way of penetrating into the secret of this language is by looking into oneself, understanding ones own reactions to it" (p.147).

These "subterranean" signals do not, however, transmit clear information. The ability to register and trust their tiny, transient impressions, and use them informatively, is not possessed by everyone in equal measure. Psychoanalysts must aim at bringing into their spheres of semantic reference many such transmissive stimuli that would otherwise remain completely outside of the range of awareness precisely because their only mode of access is via emotional attunement. Reik (1948) believed that many of these rudimentary senses, traceable to the prehistory of our species, are still significant at unconscious levels (p.138). He hypothesized that the earliest organ to reflect what was going on within was originally the skin (p.143).

These early observations are today amply confirmed in the contemporary research of neurobiologists such as Schore (1996) who examine the impact of early attachment patterns on the brain. In wondering what these neurohormonal pathways of transmission actually transmit, and looking to the source of their vocabulary in the primordial unit of mother/infant exchanges, we might speculate that from this communion originates the human experience of a transcendent-self, the soul. Are we to assume that a dialogical process that reactivates early affect-states and potentially reopens vestigial channels of interpersonal connection can thereby restore, regenerate, and even *create* connections where none existed, or heal those that were severely malformed?

Gaining accessibility to these porous, undifferentiated levels is to expose oneself to projective/introjective processes, becoming vulnerable to inductive influences of the most disturbing kind. The closer we approach these deep layers, the more is verbal content and lexical form overshadowed by evocations of broad interpersonal patterns and archetypal constellations. To reenter this interpenetrative realm consciously and contain what streams from its powerful unconscious dynamisms, can be disorganizing and give rise to exceedingly disagreeable tension-states. It is one of the analyst's most taxing technical obligations, a task made all the more difficult by the requirement that what transpires unconsciously be held until processed verbally. This requires rapid referencing of induced or transmitted feelings by using words to express senses.

In the most extreme cases of induction or projection, the experience is of being forcibly cast into a role or of being taken over by dynamisms that invade the analytic space. Any hope of reflection or symbolic communication, at these times, is temporarily lost, and the only way to disembroil the entanglement is to try to identify and anchor the experience in words. Paradoxicallly, the degree to which one can identify the distinct qualities of such induced feelings, images or moods, is also the degree to which these evocations can be used informatively. For the beginner this potentially destabilizing experience is the most alarming and difficult to metabolize analytically, yet one that can only be learned hands-on, through practice. In order to use it optimally, one has to have become conversant with these deep layers of experience within oneself.

My own first encounter with the potentially noxious power of these interpenetrative modes is grafted in my memory: These were my first weeks at a state hospital, as a naive intern who still believed in the effectiveness of good intentions. I can vividly recall a brief brush with a tall, deeply detached schizophrenic man I had stealthily attempted to engage. Towering above me as he strode stiffly by, apparently sensing I was easy prey, he threw me an acidic glare so piercing and pregnant with devaluing disgust it well nigh pulverized me and my good intentions. Having heard I was "psychoanalytically" inclined, he murmured through clenched teeth, "Why don't you go psychoanalyze yourself," effectively nipping our first contact and any attempt at communication in the bud.

More commonly analysts can and do maintain contact with their analysands, even through silence. The psychoanalytic literature on silence in the analytic hour is replete with descriptions of its many paradoxical, resistive yet "communing" effects, its meanings, functions and messages. In a context where the only requirement is to speak, and everything is grist for the analytic mill, silence is anything but empty. Through it are delivered richly textured overdetermined moods, distinct images and subtle mental states that impact bi-directionally. Once these communicative channels have been established they persist in their *modus operandi* transmitting along unconscious frequencies, even without words. Both patients and analysts become highly attuned to the emotions, preoccupations and thoughts underlying varieties of silence and when this does not occur it may be a signal of narcissistic defense. Silent messages are received not only through the usual "basic configurations" (Zelig, 1961, p. 15) of facial and postural expressions — shiftings, twitchings, sighings, and the typical repertoire of nonverbal noises — but through 'vibratory' cues, a condition of intense resonance to each other. It is difficult to conceptualize so intense a form of mental attunement other than in terms of interactive frequencies to which both 'tune in,' as it were.

The ambiguity of silence, however, enables its space to be endowed with any number of contradictory qualities and meanings. Zelig (1961) and Arlow (1961) refer to varieties of silence as serving functions of discharge, defense and complex unconscious communications, or a gratifying confluence of all three. Analysands may betray both the motive and content of resistance through nonverbal means. As Greenson (1961) points out, the absence of verbal exchange "may itself be the content which the patient is trying to convey" (p.80), a sound can "become the auditory representation of a mood — an affect equivalent" (p.81), "Great emotions are wordless but not soundless" (p. 80). Resistive, enactive or coercive as a silence might be, these transmissions may be a way of communicating the deepest most primal interactive experiences, what Greenacre (1954) considered to be the *basic* transference.

I know of no psychoanalyst whose sensibilities are more acutely attuned to these profound affective processes or whose observations more vividly illuminate them than H. Searles (1965). It is fitting then that, in a seminal 1955 paper identifying the Informational Value of the Supervisor's Emotional Experiences, Searles would be the first to draw attention to the informative power of inductive processes, moving in both directions, that occur in psychoanalytic supervision. He wrote:

> The emotions experienced by a supervisor — including even his private, 'subjective' fantasy experiences and his personal feelings about the supervisee — often provide valuable clarifications of processes currently characterizing the relationship between the supervisee and the patient. In

> addition, these processes are often the very ones which have been causing difficulty in the therapeutic relationship and, because heretofore unrecognized by the supervisee, have not been consciously, verbally reported by him to the supervisor. (p.157)

With these bold, opening lines Searles alerts us to a phenomenon he will refer to as "*the reflection process*" (p.159) an emotional response to a supervisee which is less an aspect of the therapist's own personality than a "transitory unconscious identification occurring as a function of his relationship with the patient" (p. 161). In this paper Searles unveiled his awareness of the arousal in himself of an emotional signal that functioned as a reflection of some aspect of the therapist/patient interaction or of some problem area in the analytic process. This reflection process, he emphasized, ought not be thought of as "holding center stage" throughout the entire supervisory hour but as pertaining to a small portion of the events occurring in the supervisory situation, but added, "…its part is a vital one, for it may offer clues to obscure difficulties besetting the patient-therapist relationship" (p.159).

The parallel process phenomenon will be discussed in depth, in terms of its developmental underpinnings, in the next section. Here, however, I would like to propose the idea that parallelisms occur along a continuum of transmitted patterns, from gross contagional processes emanating from sensory-affective strata to the reenactment of interactive, behavioral and verbal, or even narrative, patterns. What is common to them all is that they are unconsciously transferred, their content and essential dynamic *pattern* reproduced unawares, through replicative enactments. Searles (1955) identified the former affective version, while Arlow (1963), in an equally seminal paper on "The Supervisory Situation" described the latter behavioral variety; "At the point where the therapist should have introduced an interpretation, he responded with an identification" (p. 581). Searles (1955), and most psychoanalysts since, have not gone further than suggest that 'transitory unconscious identification' is central to the "reflection" or, parallel process.

Due to the ubiquity of these recapitulative phenomena it would seem that they are fundamental forms of pre-representational internalization or universal ways of exhibiting unmediated interpersonal experiences. Understanding the function and form of parallelisms in the supervisory encounter, no matter how subtle, is as central to 'learning' in the supervisory process as is the key role of transference/resistance in the analytic process. Infact so central to the interpretation of unconscious dynamisms are these processes that a supervisor who is unable to identify or use the parallel process informatively in this situation is as useless as an analyst who is oblivious of transference and resistance, both of which may be extremely subtle and difficult to detect. On the other hand they may also be exaggerated. In supervision where the purpose is to recount a clinical process the supervisee's unconscious dramatization may accentuate the dynamisms and take on an illustrative, evocative function that becomes an index of reference.

In my experience, parallellisms are not limited to emotional or interpersonal patterns but take many different forms — behavioral, gestural, figurative, ideational, even musical — from the most subtle and understated to the most shaking of contagional inductions. The point is that these unconscious modes continue to operate bi-directionally, throughout life. In an effort to understand the origins of such transmissive phenomena, Person (1989) similarly, stated; "Emotional contagion may play a greater role in early development than psychoanalysts have previously acknowledged, and it may have an ongoing role in adult life" (p.54). Within the conceptual model of a continuum, what began as affect-contagion at the undifferentiated primal end evolves into receptivity to more differentiated, symbolic forms, at the other. *All* modes, however, continue to be subject to *contagional* influence. As an unconscious transmissive *modality*, contagion continues to be operative throughout life but the *contents* of what is *contaged* change according to semiotic form and semantic field.

More than any other discourse situations psychoanalytic contexts revive these archaic, vestigial sensibilities that must be honed and put to interpretive use as part of our technical instrumentation. One is struck in Searles' (1955) paper by his extraordinary attention to nonverbal cues — facial and tonal expressions, mode of relatedness, subtle interpersonal indicators exhibited repeatedly over time, a general attitude or mood that remains invariant regardless of verbal content, all are noted and used informatively to show "the kind of behavior...the patient was exhibiting concerning which he, the therapist, was most in need of assistance from me" (p.166). Searles made several other important points; he emphasized form, the *manner* in which the therapist reports despite differences in verbal content; he noted the *condensed* nature of the reporting, in which an interplay of several psyches appeared compressed into one dramatization; he observed a relationship between depth of emotional involvement and degree of affect-transmission, and lastly he pointed to the rehearsal-like nature of the supervisory presentation as it displays the therapeutic problem in "miniature scale" (p.173), as he put it, to enable the therapist to carry back this understanding in working with the patient.

It is very important to make a distinction between this source of emotional information and countertransference-proper, "...these emotions...do not represent foreign bodies, classical countertransference phenomena, but are highly informative reflections of the relationship between therapist and patient" (Searles, 1955 p.158). I would stress, in addition, that this kind of emotional knowledge is not arrived at through empathy which is more intimate, more emotionally complex, and requires a kind of engagement with the inner experience of the other. Given the purpose of the supervisory context, the receptive supervisor is attuned to these transmissive frequencies through a heightened resonance to patterns and condensations that exhibit affects, interactive dynamisms, behavioral or narrative-actions that directly transmit via inductive means. The task is to process this subsensory information, assess its dynamic significance in the therapeutic process, and gauge the degree of the supervisee's awareness, while modeling the use of such attunement through verbal inquiry and discussion.

To illustrate the nature of the phenomena he was calling attention to Searles (1955) offered rich and plentiful clinical examples of which seven occurred in dyadic settings and three in groups. It is striking how pronounced and predictable is the occurrence of contagion in group dynamics. Searles described, and I experienced, the "strikingly tangled interrelatedness" (p.172) of group discussions after the supervisory presentations. It is helpful to think of these phenomena in terms of psychical or morphic fields — dyadic, triadic, or small and large groups. Boundaries in these situations are created by affiliative intent and are reinforced by participation, involvement and, where discourse is prominent, by semantic fields that cement ideological cohesion. These boundaries can be loosened or sealed, expanded or constricted, they can include and contain or reject and expel. Whether we are speaking of two, three, ten or fifty people, these modes and forms of connectedness are rooted in a primal sensory-affective underlay that provides the genetic social blue print priming us for attachment and affiliation, even before birth.

At this juncture I would like to refer back to the illustrative vignette for a vivid example of this kind of contagional phenomena. As my supervisee had correctly intuited, her patient's functioning belied a highly precarious defensive structure that was beginning to show vulnerability to dissolution and breakdown. He could not have been in touch with the profound, disintegrative layers of anxiety, panic and rage underlying the depressive symptomatology which ostensibly had brought him into treatment. Nevertheless, it had erupted very early on emerging through elaborate externalizations and projective maneuvers which coerced the therapist in various ways but also induced in her a profound sense of inadequacy, hopelessness and incompetence. Needless to say, my inexperienced supervisee was extremely vulnerable to this anxiety overload and very soon the tensions and generalized insecurity this generated began rippling systemically through the various hierarchies of the teaching institution. The way this patient could discharge the degree of anxiety he felt and evoke the chaotic nature of the family dynamisms which had precipitated it, was to engender its replication within another psychical field. This he did, very effectively, by involving a lot of people and eliciting the appearance of a sort of general, institutional "incompetence" paralleling his disordered, dysfunctional family. An implicit cry for care and containment in this patient's coercive behaviors and toxic transmissions were the means by which he could induce and reproduce, and thereby *transmit,* the affective quality of his traumatic experience and the only way he could "take control" or claim attention. Only by these unconscious inductive means could he recreate the kinds of systemic tensions which might approximate those causing the magnitude of the traumatic anxiety he experienced and had reacted to, originally, with a panic-stricken threatening gesture.

Grinberg (1990, 1991, 1995) refers to the therapist's response to a patient's transmitted affects as a "projective counteridentification reaction." In fact throughout the psychoanalytic literature affect-induction is viewed as an "identificatory" response. In my opinion, the transmission and induction of anxiety and other broad affect-states originates in undifferentiated contagional strata rooted in modes ontogenetically more primitive than, and antecedent to, "identificatory" processes which correspond to more advanced and differentiated levels of perception and internalization. Had my supervisee been able to contain even some of her patient's intense inductions she would not have confused the dream image with reality. In fact, her confusing the two belied the parallelism itself, in the overwhelming, disintegrative quality of the anxiety. The idea of affect-echoing as a mode of resonating with induced emotional information, implicit in Searles' 1955 title, has greater significance when we are able to isolate discrete forms from within the broad vocabulary of the deep "Ucs." By relating these micro-morphic differences to developmental roots, we can begin to decipher different orders of unconsciously communicated meanings.

In this case the feelings emerged not only because the feelings were primary but also because they were so intense and so unacknowledged. In all fairness to the patient, he did try to convey the nature and dimensions of his anxiety through the dream. But my supervisee was too engulfed by her own anxieties and the induced sense of incompetence, and defenses against this, to explore either the dream or the case. She avoided both. Instead she enacted the whole thing through the institutional group supervision which provided her with an avenue for acting out rather than analyzing and understanding the process. Affect-signals, it must not be forgotten, are by their nature an inducement to *re-act*; they exert quite formidable and unmediated responsiveness.

In order for these feelings to move from a somatic to a semantic universe, they have to be recognized, identified and named. In the supervisory situation, what the supervisee has been unable to metabolize or explore in the clinical process will be brought in and handed over *in toto* for the supervisor to figure out. In the case of deep affects and particularly traumatic anxiety, the supervisory field provides an ideal provisional or liminal space—betwixt and between — for replication, which is exactly what occurred in the case of my supervisee. She experienced, enacted and duplicated with me the entire unconscious emotional scenario between herself and her patient, taking on all roles and recreating all facets; the kind of chaotic situation her patient most feared yet provoked and engendered; the nature of the anxiety itself, as well as her defensive attempts to deal with it and her patient's defeating of her, were all evocatively paralleled.

The important question of what to do with these deep forms of affect transmission in supervision and how to respond instructively to different kinds of parallelisms has yet to be addressed. Suffice it to say that recognizing such inductions as being informative and modeling for the supervisee the capacity to tolerate the elicited tensions, while exploring their meanings, is a big help in the difficult task of transforming amorphous feelings into psychological understanding. Ultimately the narrative will cohere and the telling will replace replication; words will appear to give form to unspeakable experiences that could only be conveyed through enaction and induction.

We have focused too little on this primal mode of human intercourse. I would give preeminence to the interactive soil of this sensory-affective anlage that shapes the nucleus of self-experience (not to mention central and autonomic nervous system activity) laying seeds from which all subsequent communicative acts build. To avoid a systematic exploration of these preverbal modes is to perpetuate dualisms separating a body/mind continuum that treats the biological as though it were not part of the psychological. This entrenched philosophical split is misleading, conceptually, theoretically and clinically, and continues to impede the proper theoretical integration of emotion with cognition, the organic with the symbolic, a unity which psychoanalytic methodology insistently practices. Body, mind and communication cannot be separated in a semantic of unconscious meanings that exhibits the interwoven nature of all three. Language is itself embedded in sensory-affective experience, emanating from strata that, like a basso continuo, provide a perpetual subtone of latent meanings accompanying surface higher-clef manifest variations. The functional continuity of the organismic developmental model of symbolization, on which this model of communication is founded, provides a unifying framework subsuming these quasi-biological, pre-semiotic modes and their symbolic mediation.

In the foreword to Ekstein and Wallerstein's (1972) classic text on the teaching and learning of psychotherapy, B. Lewin commented, "Finally, after having viewed the learning situation and its supervisory variety *sub specie aeternitatis*, there remain the factors of a universal nature — indicated but not explained by the remark that they 'come from the unconscious'" (p. viii). It is too simplistic today to sweep different forms of unconscious phenomena under the general rubric "the unconscious." The broad categories designated one hundred years ago — unconscious, preconscious, conscious — have become *too* broad to accommodate the microgenetic shifts in mediated progressions along a continuum toward consciousness. If Freud (1915) had to "assume the existence...not only of a second consciousness, but a third, fourth, perhaps of an unlimited number of states of consciousness, all unknown to us and to one another" (p.170) the time may have come to systematize these form-variants. In 1948, Reik wrote: "I should like to draw a distinction between these data and certain other data, also unconscious, helping the former to shape our impressions, but such that their precise nature can only be surmised. That is to say, we receive impressions through senses that are in themselves beyond the reach of our consciousness" (p.137). From the standpoint of communication, I would draw a similar distinction between this primal mode of affect-pattern transmission, the essence of which may never be fully verbalizable, and the next mode, also unconscious but more organized and integrated with perception, through which some explanation of more differentiated parallel process phenomena may be derived.

II
IDEO-MOTOR REPLICATION

> Perhaps we shall do well to draw a distinction between this part of our psychical data and another, even though the distinction may prove at a later stage to be purely descriptive. It is true that the facts with which we have just been dealing are unconscious, but they do undoubtedly fall within the group of sense-perceptions of which we have knowledge.
>
> T. Reik, 1948, p.137

The principal distinction to be made between this and the previous interactive mode is a functional advance in form, namely, a shift from signal to sign. The former mode can only incite an automatic reaction through contagion whereas 'ideo-motor replication' is so named because it evokes a detectable pattern of information through an enacted behavioral duplication. By taking these nonverbal forms as communicative means and studying their morphological transformations we also observe the progressive course of representational or symbolic functioning. Examining the ontogenesis of these pre-representational modes we note that functional/form determines what kind of information can be transmitted by each of these increasingly differentiated organizations. We also note that when unconsciously replicated dynamic patterns of behavior are taken as signs, their inductive power diminishes as our awareness of them increases.

The difference in informative potential then between signaling and signifying behaviors, in ontogenesis, is both functional and formal: signifying behaviors are indicative of more discrete and differentiated perceptions, higher organizations of meaning, greater specificity of intent. The capacity to single out and identify something is evidence of a perceptual gestalt, a formal abstraction of information that already implies some learning and transactionality. Signifying gestures presuppose the establishment of joint attention and the expression of several possible meanings including intentional indication, request or denotation. An act of signification is therefore perceptually and kinetically differentiated reflecting a clear, albeit primitive, referential *purpose*, precursor to what will subsequently take shape linguistically. Purposeful actions and behaviors in interaction are the foundations of reference and meaning, "Language will serve to specify, amplify and expand distinctions the child has already about the world. But these abstract distinctions are already present, even without language" writes Bruner (1983, p. 30).

An expanding spectrum of unconscious meanings comes into view when we adopt our interpretive lens and referential perspectives to identify and specify distinctions between different microstages in transmissive and communicative forms. Ontogenetic development provides a template for the normal evolution of representational and symbolic capacities which assists in identifying these discrete forms, much as fluency in any given language is contingent on the mastery of its grammar and knowledge of its vocabulary. However, I must stress again, that while these communicative strata are here presented sequentially, their development is epigenetic; each successive mode incorporates, abbreviates and finally transforms the formal features of the previous ones while retaining meanings that are subsumed and condensed within subsequent signs or symbols, much like a layer cake which is created by stratification but consumed all of a piece! The unpacking of these richly textured manifestations is the laborious work of inquiry in psychoanalysis.

Our understanding of the underlying operative features of the parallel process, its multiple forms, multidirectionality, and the contextual factors that bring it into sharp relief, is enhanced by taking a developmental perspective toward the origins of assimilation and internalization, and how these manifest in supervisory discourse.

Of the many papers written since the sixties exploring the complexities of the parallel process, none relates it systematically to its developmental roots or identifies its diversely manifesting forms and functions as they appear in supervisory contexts. In the following I will posit some explanatory conceptualizations considering these three dimensions—the functional-developmental, the formal-semiotic and the deictic (contextual). By examining this phenomenon for its wider implications, I am suggesting that parallel processes are ubiquitous and normal unconscious reiterations of patterns of information as diverse as a tune, an image, an interaction, or a story, that are transmitted and received unconsciously by others who are 'tuned-in' to similar semiotic or dynamic spheres. Viewing the parallelism phenomenon as a general class or mode of unconscious transmission means recognizing that the specific content or nature of what is transmitted may vary depending on the context, its referential focus and semiotic features.

Psychoanalytic dialogues set up multidirectional, interpsychical regions of influence or, morphic fields, creating optimal conditions to identify the transmission of emotions and the psycho-dynamisms of unconsciously internalized interactions. In order to sharpen our theoretical clarity we are obliged to make several new definitional distinctions that inherently reveal the complexity of these processes; the first, already mentioned, is between signaling and signifying transmissions; the second, between *acting out*, and *enactive replication*, i.e., the difference between unconscious repetition of the infantile, historical past and the evocative duplication of more contemporary, unmediated assimilations; the third is the difference between *unrepresented* and *dynamically* repressed or *suppressed* material; the fourth, is between the supervisee's *presentational* and *representational* account of the clinical process; and lastly, we need more precise definitions pointing to the functional differences between internalization, identification (transient or otherwise) and empathy, terms used loosely, sometimes even interchangeably, with overlapping meanings in the literature.

The developmental perspective leads to an understanding of parallelism phenomena as recapitulations of sensory-affective and sensory-motor, imitative modes of assimilation in the attempt to accommodate *representationally* what was experienced and observed but not mediated linguistically. Both its ubiquity and specificity in supervisory contexts are accounted for by these universal origins and the logical differences between presentational and *re*presentational forms of reference. The following analysis of the operative factors and situational features of the parallel process will encompass three dimensions — the functional-developmental, the formal-semiotic and the deictic — all central to its understanding and, it goes without saying, all intimately intertwined.

Two questions orient the ideas that follow: What is the parallel process? Why does it emerge in supervision?

What we observe in psychoanalytic situations is the ubiquitous unconscious importation of experiences transferred from one context into another. In the clinical situation the sources of transfer are early internalizations, entrenched identifications and dynamically repressed material originating in the biographical past now structured intrapsychically. In the supervisory situation what is projectively replicated are unconsciously assimilated affective and behavioral dynamic-patterns from a contemporary situation, reflecting how these were experienced in the clinical process. The clinical transference replays the past in the present, the supervisory parallel process duplicates entire interactional segments from the clinical scenario. What they have in common is their unconscious nature and enactive, projective form. Person (1989) puts it very well:

> In transference, we see how the past profoundly influences the present and how significant memories and predispositions are enacted in the present...the emphasis is on what the monadic mind (already structuralized) brings to an interpersonal encounter in the present.
>
> In contrast, parallel process illuminates the contemporaneous change that occurs in one mind upon exposure to another mind. Parallel process, as described in the literature on supervision, appears to have the potential for "demonstrating" if not "explaining" emotional contagion. (p. 65)

In order to understand the parallel process, Person (1989) later comments, "one must try to grasp the conditions prerequisite to its occurrence" (p 65).

Certainly, as with transference, we are astonished by the regularity of its appearance, by its inductive and evocative strength, its figurative precision, its "amazing mimicry" (Person, 1989, p. 61), by the piercing power of its intromission into the feelings and reactions of even the most attentive and seasoned of supervisors, by its capacity to infiltrate the dynamics of virtually any dialogue or discussion of a supervisory account and by its forceful interpenetrative, multidirectional impact on all those involved. While most of what analysts experience during analytic sessions can in some way be identified as relating to the patient, and most transference patterns can be objectified and observed as being projections of the analysand's inner world, the parallel process has a way of taking over and of gripping ones senses in ways that are both more insistent and alarming, as though it held the key to that eternal blind spot in each of us that can never reach consciousness without the help of a reflective mirroring of an observing other.

Both transference and parallel process are evocative, presentational phenomena that projectively reproduce what was unconsciously assimilated and internalized. Both are brought to light, identified as being psychologically informative and referred to verbally, only in psychoanalytic contexts. What is most striking to me about these phenomena is the nature of the semantic that brings them into sharp relief. For here we have different sources and situations from which originate particular kinds of narrative modes pointing to different types of information which, in the recounting, converge in the unevenness of their reportorial forms. Characteristically different aspects of content (and different kinds of information) are alternately recounted, enacted, induced, evoked, and occasionally abstracted, implicating mnemonic, transmissive, communicative, and referential processes all in one. Greater theoretical clarity might result from distinguishing between the specific formal properties of each of these modes and examining how this relates to differences between the clinical transference and supervisory parallel process.

To ask what makes the parallel process work, however, in my opinion, is to approach the inquiry from the wrong angle. It's not so much what makes it *work,* as what makes it stand out. As Person (1989) and others have noted, like transference, this spontaneously arising phenomenon is probably a normal manifestation of the unwitting *illustration* of unconsciously assimilated experiences. Our viewing of this duplication as informative comes into focus only in specific discourse situations where it is identified, given a name, and utilized interpretively. In order to grasp the conditions prerequisite to its occurrence we need only recognize that these conditions are provided for, indeed created, by the special semantic domain, the referential features, educative purpose and technical protocol of the supervisory situation. The psychoanalytic semantic not only expands the spheres of what is interpretable and therefore knowable to encompass unconscious-meaning forms, but provides the methodological lens, the dialogical protocol, or *the conditions for* observing how the distant and more recent past, typically, are transferred and replayed in current situations. This, as previously mentioned, puts semantics, semiotics and deixis at center stage. These interpenetrative processes do indeed arise in our dialogic settings; but they arise as a function of discourse and semantic referentiality; because we identify them, use them, and assign them mnemonic significance.

I maintain that transference and parallelism phenomena emerge visibly in psychoanalytic situations as a result of the features, functions, purposes and referential perspectives of psychoanalytic discourse. We are able to identify these universal, unconscious narrative modes, because our interpretive semantic and referential focus is geared toward their observation and use. The only analogy I can think of is that of blood analysis: blood courses through the veins of each living one of us, but blood *work* can only be done under lab conditions with a microscope by a skilled technician who is trained to isolate and analyze the chemical properties of each blood sample. Similarly, the psychoanalytic phenomena that enter into the purview of our interpretive domain may well be universal aspects of human experience, but only under the "lab" conditions of psychoanalytic situations, that enable us to study the nature of their occurrences in process, are we able to undertake a careful analysis of their various *forms*. Careful differentiations and scrutiny of our phenomena may begin to reveal the kinds of regularities from which theoretical principles can be derived.

Among various reasons why the underlying mechanisms operating in the parallel process have been elusive the most obvious is that there has been little attempt to deepen our understanding of enactive phenomena beyond Freud's (1914) initial observation that what is not remembered is repeated in action (p.150). Despite Searles' (1955) clearly identifying the "reflective process" as an emotional induction containing important information about the clinical dyad (specifically pointing to problem areas in the unconscious dynamics of their interaction) neither the transmissive nor the contagional nature of this bi- and multi-directional phenomenon has been investigated in its own right. Today, Freud's (1914) general observation regarding repetition as remembrance appears too broad to account for all the features of the parallel process. At first glance it does not even distinguish between the inductive quality of the *nonrepresentable*; the dyadic projective reenactments of the *unrepresented* and the *dynamically repressed* or *suppressed;* and the multidirectional dynamic spread of the parallel process —all 'unconscious' reiterations, but infecting by different means. Each of these forms appears, in some way, in the transference, for instance, but not all appear in the parallel process.

D. M. Sachs and S. H. Shapiro (1976) did notice several different kinds of enactive forms of remembering in their supervisory group settling on the term "identificatory reproduction" for the most prominent in the parallel process, a term previously coined by Loewald (1973 unpublished) to denote a transference enactment of a figure identified with from the past. As Person (1989) comments, by linking "identificatory reproduction" to parallel process they faithfully describe what seems to occur but leave unexplained the mechanism and motive for the appearance of this form of enactment in the supervisory context (p.64). Yet parallel process reproductions are contemporary transfers, not from the past, and the term "identification" in psychoanalysis usually refers specifically to an intrapsychically structured internalization of traits and behaviors belonging to important figures from the developmental years. We cannot correctly say that parallelisms reflect "identifications," in this sense of the word. The temporal factor would appear to be significant in pinpointing the difference between enactive repetitions in the clinical dyad versus inductive reproductions appearing in the supervisory situation.

The same term is used again in reference to parallel process, but with a different meaning, by Arlow (1963) who, rather, stressed certain similarities between the clinical and supervisory situations. His understanding of the parallel process focused on the supervisee's shifts between verbal reporting and "experiencing empathetically" (p.581) viewing these as a recapitulation of oscillations between observing and experiencing which characterize psychoanalytic listening. Presumably, what the supervisee is aware of having observed can be reported verbally whereas lapses into "transient identifications" produce enactive parallelisms: "What he had failed to report in words, he had transmitted in action." writes Arlow (1963). "The phenomenon of transient identification with the patient, which is so important in the conduct of analysis, it struck me, is also important in the supervisory experience" (p.580). While focusing primarily on the formal shifts between verbal and enactive reporting, Arlow's understanding of the parallel process, however, includes a decidedly dynamic factor, "At the point where the therapist should have introduced an interpretation, he responded with an identification" (p.581).

But why identification? The notion that transient identification adequately explains the underlying imitative mechanism of parallel process has been taken more or less for granted. Yet neither its reportorial quality, its multidirectionality or its interpenetrative, inductive force, are accounted for by the concept of "identification," therefore, in agreement with Bromberg (1982) "…I see no reason to call it an identification" (p.110). The term "identification" only obfuscates the reciprocal, interactive nature and communicative, even informative function, of the parallel process. In stressing the reciprocal oscillations between enactment and verbalization, empathic identification and observation, Arlow (1963) pointed in the direction I would like to go, namely, toward identifying different unconscious modes of communicating different kinds of information correlated with reciprocal modes of reception.

Caligor (1984), whose voice seems to be representative of the interpersonalists approach to the parallel process, invokes the concept of participatory-observation, equating it with empathy "— the noncognitive process of emotional learning and emotional communication —"(p.25) in accounting for the inductive and interpenetrative power of the parallel process: "We are speaking of *participant* as an empathic function and *observer* as a cognitive function" (p. 25). But to thus split empathy in two defining half of it as "noncognitive" because it involves emotion is, I believe, gravely misleading. No part of mature empathy is "noncognitive." Moreover the requisite oscillations of the analytic stance impel self monitoring, and hence self-awareness, as part of the process of understanding, both of which involve reference and cognition, at the very least. Today we need conceptions that do not fall into the error of splitting cognition from emotion, particularly where psychoanalytic understanding is involved.

Purposeful "transient identification" *is*, however, an accurate description of an aspect of mature empathy which, by definition, implies a conscient, differentiated act of re-cognition — we empathize with someone else's feelings, state, experience or situation, someone from whom we are fully differentiated and perceive as separate and distinct. But the 'transient identification' of empathic re-cognition can only be understood developmentally, in terms of a continuum along which less differentiated, precursor contagional forms lie at the primitive, opposite end from fully differentiated, cognizant forms of mature empathy as used in psychoanalytic understanding. We cannot correctly say that empathy is operative in the inductive and indicative transmissions of the parallel process or that the supervisee is necessarily empathic when enactively reproducing a clinical interaction. Rather, these point to unmediated forms of assimilation and reproduction taking place when lapses in the requisite distance provided by the observing ego occur and mediational activities that go with it are unavailable: in other words where supervisory supplementation is needed. In this case the 'motive' for the appearance of parallel process in supervision would implicitly carry a request for assistance accompanied by a demonstration, just as the replay of transference enacts what is not remembered.

Interestingly, unconscious "patterns" or "content" that is passed on in parallel processes, exhibits all the characteristic features of 'presentational' form: it is dynamically multidetermined, condensed and subject to displacement and projection; its polyvalence simultaneously encompasses many voices and elements from the whole scenario. The supervisee evokes the nature of the interactions through a replication of their feel and form, from multiple angles often simultaneously, in a plastic imitation — like a rough sketch — that duplicates various emotional and behavioral interactive dynamisms from the clinical situation. What is assimilated is an interactive *pattern*, and the pattern consists of a condensation subsuming what came from the patient, how it was played out in the session, how it was experienced by the supervisee, and what was observed; a polypsychical blend or hybrid echoing the undercurrents of what transpired unconsciously.

Out of a general class of unconscious communications we distinguish between the inductive and the indicative modes for which Searles' (1955) and Arlow's (1963) landmark papers provide perfect illustration. From their different orientations and focus, each offered superb examples of the informative potential of induced emotion (Searles, 1955) and the dynamic condensations indicated by replicative behaviors (Arlow, 1963). Both these modes contribute to the parallel process which directly projects, induces and presents, *in vivo,* what cannot yet be put into words. These uneven accounts, lacking representational articulation, are saying: "This is how it went, this is how it felt" and, given the deictic factor, "Tell me what is going on." The supervisee's presentational replay is *implicitly* a request for representational clarification.

The relationship between representation and reference is an important one and both memory and verbalization are contingent on both. Recalling and reporting are *re*presentational constructions. The parallel process accomplishes a number of expository feats, including vividly recreating the dynamic impact of interactions, from both sides simultaneously, by means that are more direct and immediate than words could ever be. It relays emotions and behavior, or *experiential* information, which was noted but not denoted, registered but not represented. We can thus correctly say that the parallel process in supervision is a presentational account of the unconscious, dynamic and unrepresented dimensions of the clinical report. But for unconscious experiences to be reported along psychoanalytic lines, they have to have been identified, processed and further understood within a particular frame of reference that must capture the complexity of feeling, behavior and dynamics, all in one. The difficulties of supervisory reporting are not only due to insufficient self monitoring or blind spots and inexperience; they are also due to the nonlexical nature of much that has to be included in a polished account.

I would suggest avoiding the term "identification," which fuels ambiguity and conceptual confusion when referring to the parallel process and substituting it with "imitative reproduction," a more precise term connoting the mimicry it employs that distinguishes between supervisory replications and transferential repetitions. Both are unconscious, presentational forms of telling, but they tell different tales. The transference externalizes the intrapsychically structured "inner world" replaying the biographical past; the parallel process transmits unconscious dynamisms from contemporary interactions, relaying assimilations from the present. Different mnemonic tracks and motives are involved due to the different referential focus and purpose of the two situations. Herein lie the dangers of loosely transposing terms from one phenomenon to another: parallel process does not repeat what has been forgotten and repressed; it exemplifies what is striving to be represented. If we isolate the central operative mechanism underlying the parallel process we find that it is a recapitulation of sensorimotor modes of assimilation and introjection, manifestations of stages in the re-presentational process itself. Person (1989) came close when she wrote "... it is as though we are witness to some form of internalization taking place before our very eyes" (p. 64).

In order to understand the origins of this form of internalization, we have to know that its ontogenetic course begins in imitation and is directly linked with representation and the growth of symbolic functioning. The persistence of a sensorimotor core throughout life means that pre-representational modes of registration and assimilation continue to be active subliminally, especially during social intercourse, and that the gap between registration and mediated assimilation will be most pronounced in learning situations where attempts are being made to grasp and retain new information. This gap will be most evident in a context where unconscious, dynamic aspects of interactive experiences must be articulated in psychoanalytically insightful ways. The recapitulation and dramatic externalization of this sensorimotor form of deferred imitative accommodation, to which we bear witness in supervision, is a reflection of this gap. The parallel process then is a *way* of recounting, and a *phase* of representation.

No one has left more detailed or sophisticated accounts of the initial stages of pre-representational imitation than Piaget (1962) who observed and enumerated no less than six discrete stages of sensorimotor imitation paralleling the progress of representation and the genesis of cognition. Repeatedly Piaget (1962) stressed that imitation is a "continuation of the effort at accommodation" (p.5) that it is "always a continuation of understanding" (p.73). He wrote, "Although it is outstripped,...by conceptual intelligence, which develops the initial schemas into rational operations, sensory-motor intelligence nevertheless remains, all through life, and in a form very similar to its characteristic structure in stages V and VI (from ten to eighteen months), the essential tool for perceptive activity and the indispensable intermediary between the perceptions and conceptual intelligence" (p.75).

In his observations of children at the early stages, Piaget (1962) focused on the function of imitation "...it was as though she felt the need to mime what she saw in order to grasp it" (p. 63) and further on, referring to a little boy, "he was merely adding a kind of plastic representation which would help him to understand what he was perceiving" (p. 71). Emphasizing the functional continuity in development, Piaget's (1962) studies traced gradations in a succession of six sensorimotor imitative stages moving toward increasingly interiorized and deferred forms of reproductive assimilation until both assimilation and accommodation are internalized and executed on the mental or representational plane. This progression does not, however, automatically imply a shift in consciousness, since "mental" or cognitive operations characteristically take place unconsciously. However, the fact that parallel processes recapitulate these early stages with, what Piaget (1962) would call, a "vertical lag," confirms the idea that representational activity (and semiotic mediation) is again in its early forms and involves the same efforts to differentiate or distinguish between what is internal and what external. It is important to realize that imitative reproduction continues to be an indicator of both a lack of differentiation and the attempt at representational accommodation.

In order to appreciate the dynamic, multidetermined and idiosyncratic nature of internal representations, we have to keep in mind that they are a complex amalgam of affective, motoric and perceptual elements. Ideomotor-replication is a phenomenon between gross sensorimotor imitation and the fully 'mental' representation (it is precisely not 'mental' as long as it is enacted). As Piaget (1962) noted, "on the one hand imitation is merely the continuation of the accommodation of sensory-motor intelligence, and on the other the first mental images are interiorized imitation" (p.75).

Piaget (1962) concluded that even at the highest levels of representation the image is not a copy of perception but the result of imitative accommodation, the construction of an activity "above perception and action but below reflective thought" (p.75). He wrote: "The image is therefore not the continuation of perception as such, but of perceptive activity which is an elementary form of intelligence deriving from the sensory-motor intelligence characteristic of the fist eighteen months of life" (p.77). (This explains the phenomenalistic creations of dreams!) By the last of the six stages, with the advent of two developmental achievements, evocative memory and the semiotic function, experience is sufficiently differentiated for its assimilation and imitative accommodation to occur "internally" or on the mental plane where, in the words of Gal'perin (1969) "the abbreviated operations are only presumed, not executed" (p. 257 in Wertsch, 1985, p. 66).

This implies that internalization and signification coincide; it also explains why the parallel process, like the dream and other presentational projections, functions as a *signifier* (not a symbol) for what it displays, pointing to its multidetermined elements and retaining the intensely emotional undercurrents of little-differentiated experiences. In the supervisory situation we observe a recapitulation of this pre-ideational accommodation in the attempt to understand—a figuring *in,* in order to figure it *out*, as it were! In this sense the parallel process is not so much a reflection process as a replicative process in search of its reflection. In order for it to become fully conscious, an additional referential step has to occur: the felt-representation, as the signifier of the experience that evokes it, has to be identified, processed, interpreted and understood, along psychoanalytic lines. This is the referential step that is *specific* to this discourse situation. In this way, its understanding can be communicated as well as conceptualized. Given that the overall purpose of psychoanalytic situations is to uncover unconscious phenomena, particularly in supervision, we have the opportunity of observing the stages of evocative presentation and of increasingly linguistic symbolic referencing unfold before our very eyes.

Context, purpose and reference are therefore inextricably intertwined because entrance into a referential perspective, the establishment of joint attention, and a grasp of the 'things' or subjects that are referred to in any given semantic field, is situational and specific, a dialogic enterprise. As Bruner (1983) has pointed out, referential acts are basically a form of social interaction involving two people negotiating, they are "highly context sensitive, or deictic" (p. 69): a communication means something in a specific circumstance. Learning a new language or a new vocabulary entails learning to identify, indicate, denote, and refer to those kinds of things that are spoken about in that semantic field. More than that, it entails knowing how to interact with the help of these verbal signs according to the discourse protocol, adhering to the purpose, customs and implicit codes of that situation. The functional parallelism between language acquisition in childhood and any learning situation lies in the recapitulation of this elementary struggle to enter into and become familiar and conversant with the world of the referent, because that world holds the key to making ones way within that social milieu. We cannot logically separate 'relationship' from dialogue, from this perspective, since the substance and form of communication is the woof and warp through which both are woven.

Consideration of the deictic factor is, therefore, extremely important to understanding what transpires in psychoanalytic situations. We do things with words that are done nowhere else — we use them, insistently, consistently, persistently, to identify and refer to what is unconscious. Words in our dialogues are acts — acts that are both organic and symbolic. Psychoanalytic contexts establish semantic fields that expand the ordinary functions of language and narrow range of referents to include unspoken, transmissive modes as well — induction, evocation and indicative enactments become themselves *forms of reference* in contexts where nonverbal, projective and enactive forms are recognized and taken as indices of meaning.

The psychoanalytic semantic encompasses within its referential orbit those transmissive forms that can only be accessed through a combination of observation, listening and introspective awareness. Sensory input and symbolic meanings infuse contextual experiences with information that is referred to and interpreted in this discourse alone. When we say that psychoanalytic learning is "experiential," this is what we mean: what is being taught through the supervisory dialogue is how to adopt and sustain an attentional stance and referential focus that looks inward and outward at the same time, one that attends to content while experiencing process and considers both as reflections of each other. The supervisory process is the establishment of an ongoing dialogue between an uneven pair, in which the supervisor models the kind of observing, experiencing and thinking that produces the kind of questioning and exploration of conscious and unconscious contributions to the supervisory report. In this sense, there is an analogy between the clinical and supervisory situations, as Arlow (1963) noted: the supervisee learns how to analyze the clinical process through the *experience* of having those affective projections and behavioral exemplifications identified and reflectively fed back into the dialogue. Learning takes place in the dialectic of a reflexive discourse in which the interpreter is always identifying and verbally pointing to those presentational, unconscious aspects of the report, while the supervisee is always striving to represent them, refer to them and articulate them verbally. Unconscious transmissions take many forms; affective, imagistic, ideational, auditory. It takes time and much experience to begin to isolate and identify the full impact of these often subtle resonances. The referential acts of noting and denoting these unconsciously enacted and projective elements of the report focuse attention inward in such a way as to encourage the supervisee's constant self-monitoring and questioning of his/her personal reactions, thereby reinforcing the reflective referential eye that is essential for the introspective vigilance that accompanies the analytic task.

It seem to me that Piaget's (1962) approach, with its insistence on the functional continuity of sensorimotor and representational intelligence and its attempt to encompass the complexity of different forms of early representation and semiotic activity, is most relevant for understanding this trajectory of psychoanalytic discourse. Piaget (1962) believed, and I concur, that only when the study of the symbolic function covers all the initial forms of representation "will the functional unity of the development which leads from sensory-motor to operative intelligence be seen through successive individual and social structures" (p 4). The supervisory dialogue gives us the opportunity to observe phase-transitions in the microgenetic stages of pre-semiotic internalization which, at the very outset, include a plastic, ideo-motor replication of what was seen and experienced.

It was again Piaget (1962) who recommended that psychological study not invoke "social life" as a whole, but that its scrutiny should enter into the particulars of "a series of relationships established in all possible combinations between individuals of distinct levels of mental development, and as a consequence of various types of interaction (coercion, co-operation, imitation, discussion, etc.)" (p.4). It is precisely the deictic factor, the overall purpose of the supervisory meetings and the complementary roles, intents and uneven preparedness of the two interlocutors, that governs the discourse-dynamisms and sets the stage for the semiotic events that will transpire within it. Bruner (1983) emphasized; "Parties to a referring act infer its referent from an *utterance in a context*. Any account of the ontogenesis of reference must take this deictic feature into account" (pp. 69-70). The study of the development of reference could, according to Bruner (1983) be restated as "the problem of how people manage and direct each other's attention by linguistic means. We may properly ask how *linguistic* attention-management is superimposed on prelinguistic means and inquire as to how the first extends and modifies the second" (p. 68). The supervisory context has much to teach us about this very transition.

To summarize: the parallel process emerges in supervision as a function of the features and purpose of the supervisee's report and the supervisory task, in a discourse context where it is identified and denoted as a consequence of the psychoanalytic semantic and its referential perspectives. Whether it becomes informative or infective will depend on the supervisor's stance and skill. In my opinion, the parallel process is to be understood as a normal and ubiquitous manifestation of unconscious assimilations striving towards symbolic accommodation; as such, the imitative replications of the supervisory report exhibit phases of signification and semiotic mediation through projective and presentational modes of referencing. The supervisee's report, in its entirety, is in the service of learning how to understand what transpired in the clinical process: and it is precisely the unevenness of referential accessibility to the unconscious aspects of this material that brings the parallel process so sharply into view. The gap between the reporter's and the interpreter's symbolic organization (vis-à-vis unconscious material) recreates a functional parallelism between this learning situation and early development.

Characteristically it is the analysands and supervisees who are susceptible to developing the most intense feelings toward the influence of their analyst and supervisor. As Doerhman (1976) suggested; "An extension of this idea is that every teaching or helping relationship is subject to exactly the same forces" (p. 74). Given their dynamic conditions and dialogical nature, examining the genesis and evolution of referencing in early development—the prototype for all linguistically based learning—ought to provide some insight. In early dialogues, the child, is operating and using language at less advanced stages of symbolic organization than the adult who, typically, encourages and fosters linguistic articulation. This creates an ongoing, functional gap between the child's grasp of things and what he/she perceives the adult to know. The parallel seems obvious. In psychoanalytic dialogues, similarly, the listener or interpreter always seems to hear and know more than what is actually said. A comprehensive account of the factors co-contributing to the emergence of the parallel process requires an analysis that takes the three perspectives mentioned at the outset—the developmental (semiotic), the semantic-referential, and the deictic—into consideration. Each of these perspectives may be associated with the works of Piaget, Vygotsky and Bruner, respectively, three great psychologists, a synthesis of whose ideas is woven through the above.

I believe this discussion adequately responds to what seemed to me to be important points raised, in particular, by Person (1989), who emphasized the need to better understand the "mechanism and motive for identificatory reproduction in parallel process (and in life)" (p. 64), and Caligor (1984), who proposed that the emergence of parallel process in supervision is "in the service of emotional learning and supervision" (p. 23).

Out of a host of papers on the parallel process addressing its specificity within a complex, multi-directional network (Gediman and Wolkenfeld, 1980); its multiplicity of forms (Doerhman, 1976); its use as a vehicle in a process-centered approach (Ekstein and Wallerstein, 1958); its relationship to a general class of modes of remembering by enacting (Sachs and S. H. Shapiro, 1976); its intersystemic nature and informational value (Searles, 1955; Baudry, 1993); its structural and dynamic properties (Arlow, 1963; Gediman and Wolkenfeld, 1980); and even regarding the impact of the supervisor on the analysand's transference (Luber, 1991), only Person (1989), Caligor (1984) and Bromberg (1982) posed truly pointed questions that challenged finding explanatory answers, and none related the parallel process systematically to developmental or semiotic factors.

To return for a moment to my illustrative vignette (p.125), I feel sure that aspects of my supervisee's behavioral attitudes — the abrupt change in her demeanor, her loss of composure, her mood, and the surprising urgency in her coercive phone calls; the particular tense way she sat at the edge of her seat, her accusatory, rebuking, sulking tone and disconnection from me — all uncharacteristic of her—reflected and expressed the reproduction of dynamisms and behavior patterns which typified her patient's unconscious attitudes and inductive transmissions to her. In particular, her accusations and coercive rebukes, which seemed designed to shake my confidence and rattle my professional stance, and stood in sharp contrast to all that had come before, alerted me to the inductive power and presence of a parallel process. While the flare up of the emotionally charged crisis itself reflected a contagious induction, the overall behavioral patterns and attitudes she replicated in interactions with me gave me the opportunity to *experience* what she was experiencing with her patient, an ideo-motor duplication which, in turn, exhibited by evocation what she was unable to reflect upon or communicate verbally.

How words will come to re-present these interchanges conceptually, when and in what ways they will be used as signals, signs or symbols, as principal means and vehicles for referring to them, describing them and, eventually, understanding them along psychoanalytic lines, will be explored in the following stage.

III
VERBAL FORM

> The importance of symbol-using, once admitted, soon becomes paramount in the study of intelligence. It has lent a new orientation especially to genetic psychology, which traces the growth of the mind: for this growth is paralleled, in large measure, by the observable uses of language, from the first words in infancy to the complete self-expression of maturity,....There is an increasing *rapprochement* between philology and psychology — between the science of language and the science of what we do with language.
> Langer, 1942, pp. 26-27

> Words provoke affects and are in general the means of mutual influence among men. Thus we shall not depreciate the use of words in psychotherapy and we shall be pleased if we can listen to the words that pass between the analyst and his patient.
> S. Freud, 1917, p. 17

Nowhere is the efficiency and power, the decisive impact on intellect and consequence for behavior of the symbolic function more dramatically epitomized than in the use of words. The advent of language in early development, its rapid spread through communication and momentous influence on mentation is the most striking evidence of the modulating, regulatory effect on human experience of semiotic mediation. As a vehicle of communication a tool for thinking, it is unsurpassed, a precision instrument of infinite plasticity. Used initially in its simplest, indicative form, language is able to grow to meet the conceptual needs of its user: "Not higher sensitivity, not longer memory or even quicker association sets man so far above other animals...; no, it is the power of using symbols — the power of *speech* — that makes him lord of the earth" (Langer, 1942, p. 26).

The cornerstone of a model of communication that correlates transformations in communicative means with shifts in mental (semiotic) organization, rests on the premise that adopting a system of verbal signs — the grammatical edifice of language — and the increase in symbolic activity this engenders, alters the very nature of experience, knowledge and awareness. Even more, it opens the door thereafter to a reality which becomes both structured and defined by its use. In its representational capacity language detaches thought from action, fortifying evocative memory and enabling conceptualization and abstraction. In its communicative capacity language anchors interactive experience in social conventions, habits and dynamics that lay their stamp on internalizations that will become structured into the 'inner world'.

The difference between the ideo-motor indications of the previous presentational mode and the advent of speech marks a momentous event in human communication and mentation; a shift from signifying *actions* and behaviors to the use of a *symbolic medium*, so that "Between the clearest animal call of love or warning or anger, and man's least, trivial *word*, there lies a whole day of Creation — or in modern phrase, a whole chapter of evolution" (Langer, 1942, p. 103).

The relationship between outer semiotic process and inner representational means is an intimate one. Our perceptions, knowledge and experience are shaped by the semiotic medium we are currently adopting and by the semantic attributes and vehicular means this symbol system is able to carry. In the case of words, we enter into a linguistic universe essentially by learning to pair a verbal signifier with its referent. The indicative or sign-function of words precedes their fully symbolic, conceptual use. At the beginning words wedge their way between immediate sense-impressions in a world of action, impression, sensation and impulse, and the delay imposed by their selection and articulation leaves the genesis of thought in its wake.

Just as language emerges through use in daily interactions and further expands through a variety of discourse situations, so too the germinal potential of the symbolic function blossoms and proliferates through dialogue and exposure to other symbol systems. We come to know as we learn to speak and we learn to perceive and conceive of those things to which language has drawn our attention. Denotation is the distinctive referential characteristic of language, nourishing communication and intellect alike, for "as soon as an object is denoted, it can be *held*" (Langer, 1942, p.135). A word first uttered and then taken inward, or decontextualized, becomes the mind's possession, a means of recollection and contemplation carrying both object and context within: "A word fixes something in experience and makes it the nucleus of memory, an available conception" (Langer, 1942, p. 135). Precisely because of the denotive quality of verbal reference — its capacity to single out and re-present — it stimulates evocative memory, thought, imagination, while it's purposeful disciplined use reinforces symbolic conceptualization. In language, wrote Langer (1942) "we have the free, accomplished use of symbolism, the record of articulate conceptual thinking; without language there seems to be nothing like explicit thought whatever"(p.103).

In its initial communicative function, speech serves as a bridge, mediating between natural signals and cultural signs, so that the transmission of family custom and national culture go hand in hand with the internalization of semiotic process and form. Language acquisition implies learning to *interact* verbally; knowing when and how to speak, what to say, with what intonation, and how to negotiate things with words. From the outset, therefore, speech not only modulates expressive signals, transmuting the indicative and denotive gestural signs of sensorimotor intelligence, it also comes to incorporate and subsume the referential world along with the dynamic patterns of those in whose company it was first used. The nature of compromise and its entrenched contribution to character formation is virtually indistinguishable from linguistic habit and form and the ways in which verbal interchange will be used, later on.

At its most essential, language is a semiotic tool, an instrument of immense plasticity which can be used at different levels of functional organization and can be made to serve different expressive, cognitive and dynamic purposes. Vygotsky (1934), and the Russian formalists pointed out that language "is not a single form of speech activity, but an aggregate of diverse speech functions…" (p.297 in Wertsch, 1985, p.85). Even at the very outset, speech combines three or perhaps four distinct primary functions: that of social intercourse, and of indicative and denotive reference which, when internalized, lead to thought, the cognitive function of language. In connection with a discussion regarding speech functions from a Vygotskian perspective, Wertsch (1985) presented Vygotsky's various types, categorizing them in terms of four sets of oppositional pairs:

> The signalling versus the significative function.
> The social versus the individual function.
> The communicative versus the intellectual function.
> The indicative versus the symbolic. (p. 89)

From early in ontogenesis and out of the pre-intellectual or sensorimotor stage of development, come Vygotsky's (1934) *emotional release* and *social contact* forms of speech-action, out of which evolve the *communicative* and *intellectual* functions of language (Wertsch, 1985, p. 93). These latter, writes Wertsch (1985), can be understood as further specifications of the broader Vygotskian division drawn between the **social** and **individual** functions of language, the different formal differences of which can be traced to distinctions between dialogic and monologic forms of speech.

Given the central role of free-associative, monologic speech as a means of accessing the inner world in the clinical situation, it might be helpful here to take a glance at the ontogenetic roots and developmental course of monologue, through the eyes of Piaget and Vygotsky. Although both studied the egocentric speech of children's early monologues, they differed considerably in their conclusions as to its function and fate. For Vygotsky the origins of egocentric speech lie in social speech, which, once internalized becomes an intrapsychical form of self-regulation, a permanent personal accompaniment, as it were, reflecting both the qualities and functional properties of its interpersonal precursor. Its egocentric nature is viewed not merely as a reflection of the child's egocentric attitude, but as an important factor in the planning and regulation of action, in thinking itself, its ultimate fate to be silenced and internalized as inner speech. For Piaget, on the other hand, egocentric and monologic forms of speech are accounted for by the child's joy in word usage, their functional assimilation occurring through practice in play as a form of wish fulfillment and an expression of the still minimal differentiation between actions and words. Piaget observed the gradual decline in egocentric speech paralleling a general decrease in egocentrism, coupled with an increase in explicit, social communication.

The developmental vector for Vygotsky moves from social, to egocentric, to inner speech, while Piaget's account, based on a general decrease in egocentrism, moves in the inverse direction, from egocentric forms of individual monologue, to social, dialogic communication. I think it worthwhile for psychoanalysts to be informed of these views. The origins and course of early speech forms must have considerable impact on intrapsychic structuring; its re-externalization in the free associative stream might become even more informative once we are aware of just how much the early environment is still present in the regulation of thought and behavior.

There is nothing particularly new, then, in approaching words by re-emphasizing the functional diversity of speech, or in joining the pragmatist's position vis-à-vis context and language use. Only that the logical consequence of pursuing the concept of "function" in speech is that it leads to a comprehensive view of the complexities of meaning, particularly in our extraordinary communicative fields in which verbal analysis and interpretation has to encompass so many dimensions

For a field embedded in the linguistic medium, soaked through and through with evidence of the mysterious, transformative alchemy of verbal exchange, it is astonishing to what degree psychoanalysis has turned a blind eye to the complexities of language and to the different kinds of meanings that are introduced and subsumed by verbal form. At first glance there are the denotive, connotive, signific and symbolic use of words. Then there are the differences implied by conventional word-meanings, their contextual and idiosyncratic sense, their current dynamic function and purpose, their genetic soil and associative threads, whether they are to be taken literally or metaphorically, as informative or expressive, a mask for deceit or a means of disclosure, their tone of deliverance sardonic, sweet, sarcastic or sincere.... In no other dialogue, contrived as it might be, are the organic, multi-determined, dynamic roots of language and meanings made and conveyed, more clearly marked than in psychoanalytic situations where the interplay of experience and word, of action, reaction and interaction, converge to revive, replay and retrace an unconsciously woven subjective account. Upon closer examination, 'meaning' is a topic vast, complex and as intricately dense as the Milky Way. With this in mind, to say verbal or nonverbal, is to say nothing at all

Many things can be done with words; I am interested in examining not only what *is* done, but what *only* psychoanalysts do with them. This means that I am interested in exploring the enwebments of linguistic, para-linguistic and pre-linguistic forms, the signific, symbolic and proto-symbolic meanings that spread around, beneath, and through the fabric and forms of our dialogical situations. In particular I am interested in considering the consequence of such semantic spread in a communicative field that pushes the potential for language to function as a reflexive vehicle for self-expression, self-understanding and, above all, an instrument of integration and transformation.

However we elect to approach the study of the many ways verbal meanings are made, we will have to explore the complexities of language also in terms of its malleability of form and function. As psychoanalysts, we are in the singularly privileged position of working in a living laboratory where the intermingling of these multiple forms and different functional organizations pervade the space, permeate its interactions, and parade before us hourly. This is why in the analysis of unconscious meanings a combination of process and content — and the interrelationships between the two — represents the full semantic scope of interpretability, and why such an analysis should proceed by paying careful attention to the semiotic organization and primary function of the locutions in question. Words and linguistic meanings are *servants* of this dynamic *contextual process*, constrained, yet also created, by it and not the other way around. The way language is currently being *used* beyond mere verbalization is relevant to psychoanalysts since an interpretive semantic that includes unconscious presentational forms must logically be based on an understanding of the ways different kinds of meanings are made, from the ground up as it were.

Take the simplest of these functional distinctions, between the **signific** and **symbolic** use of words, as Langer (1942) put it; "In an ordinary sign-function, there are three essential terms: subject, sign, and object. In denotation, which is the commonest kind of symbol-function, there have to be four: subject, symbol, conception, and object" (p. 64). The 'idea' is the added factor. As previously mentioned, these subtle but important differences can be identified by the mental *experience* they evoke in the listener. To reflect on an experience or a situation is not the same as reacting to it impulsively; "In talking *about* things we have conceptions of them, not the things themselves; and *it is the conceptions, not the things, that symbols directly 'mean'*" (Langer, 1942, p. 61). The principal distinction between signific (indicative) and symbolic referencing, then, lies in the cognitive consequences of their diverse semiotic forms. Signs point to their objects; symbols induce us to conceive of them. The same referent may assume entirely different functions, in a psychical sense. This important distinction has significant implications not only for the meaning of a communication but for the degree to which its subject is accessible to consciousness. In ordinary discourse sign and symbol interweave seamlessly so that any "nameable item of reality may stem from a signific experience and enter into the role of a symbol..." or "may act momentarily as a sign," In the psychoanalytic clinical process this seemingly minor detail proves to be a distinction of major consequence: words may persist as servants of unconscious dynamic, developmental or restitutional needs, they may serve as labels to indicate, or they can serve a truly symbolic function by becoming instruments of *higher* aims to *transmute*, even *transcend,* experiences by transposing them to conceptual planes. In this last capacity words arrive at their higher destination by an additional act of *symbolic* referencing, a further abstraction that lifts language to ideational, conceptual levels.

Vygotsky applied this semiotic distinction in penetrating the manifold expressions of "meaning" and "sense." Wertsch (1985) explains:

> On the one hand, language has the potential to be used in abstract, decontextualized reflection. This premise underlies his analysis of concept development, categorization, and syllogistic and scientific reasoning. In...this aspect of his research he focused on the potential for decontextualization in language, especially the decontextualization of "meaning"

> (*zrachenie*). On the other hand, there is a side of linguistic organization that is rooted in contextualization. In this connection Vygotsky introduced the indicative function of speech, and he studied the ways in which the structure and interpretation of linguistic signs depends on their relationship with the context in which they appear. This aspect of his semiotic analysis provides the foundation for his account of inner speech and relies on his notion of "sense" (*smysl*) (p. 95).

In my experience, and particularly in psychoanalytic contexts, these two tendencies intermingle, operating simultaneously to determine the structure and interpretation of speech. Insofar as language is primarily pointing, it is functioning only as a preliminary to conceptualization and abstract thought; and it is this *conceptual, contemplative, abstractive* function of language that gives evidence of a genuine analytic attitude, a truly *symbolic* di-stance vis-à-vis its subject matter.

Awareness of these functional distinctions ought to be part of any analyst's listening and interpretive skills. How we hear what is being said and how we respond to what we think it "means," in our semantic, ought to include an informed awareness of the operative level at which the speaker is speaking. Words may be functioning primarily as signal-equivalents or affect-substitutes; for anxiety discharge, as presentational signs, or symbolically, as the bearers of ideas. In fact, as our discourse would indicate, the pathway toward consciousness goes from nebulous feeling, to presentational or figurative form, to label, to symbol. Speech begins as an accompaniment to gesture and action, participating in the expression of feeling, intent and request. To name a 'thing' is to give it objective status. The functional advance that language promotes is grounded in this denotational specificity. Once securely paired with a referent, the word serves as a "nominal specifier" (Bruner, 1983, p. 76) conjuring an envisagement of the absent object in the mind's eye. Langer (1942) believed this "*naming, fixating and conceiving of objects*" (p. 132) to be the primary function of language even beyond its communicative purpose, "the practical application of something that has already developed at a deeper psychological level" (p.132). Nonetheless, words spring from interactions: they are social signs before they are conceptual symbols. For Vygotsky, similarly, the word is initially an indicator; the *indicatory* function, the original function of speech. But the word is also a 'thing,' an audible phonic sound-pattern, publicly recognized, privately held, its meanings nourished by denotational and connotational tributaries, its sense colored by context and convention. Only gradually, with continued use and decontextualization, will the word-as-symbol, multidetermined, complex, and fully formed, with its denotive specificity and connotive underbelly, rise to the inner eye in its full blown "meaning" for the individual.

The use of verbal signifiers *as symbols*, then, is a stepwise process, promised but not guaranteed by the advent of speech. It is contingent on sufficient differentiation, objectification, the ability to generalize and abstract, as well as participate in the symbolic space of make-believe and play, to enter the realms of metaphor, imagination, allegory, story, myth and meanings. Lacking both the referential specificity and the multidetermined richness of meaning that typifies the symbolic use of words, both signals and signs are an invitation to misinterpretation. The word-as-symbol, by contrast, is both more abstract and more complex, possessing an inner and an outer face that adds new dimensions to its functional use. As a result, a word that 'indicates' and a word that '*means*' are in two different referential hemispheres: they are two strictly different functional forms.

Consider the three most evident ways in which 'meaning' is made: signification, denotation and connotation, each quite distinct and in no way interchangeable. Their functional differences hinge on the diversity of their referential forms. Once language becomes the dominant vehicle of communication meaning is generated by the syntactical, grammatical, tonal and referential arrangements that most closely express the 'sense' of what we currently "mean" by what we say. Most spontaneous acts of signification originate and continue to spring from deep within the bowels of organic experience, consequently their expression and forms will be tied to functional organization and dynamic intent.

Psychoanalysis is in a uniquely privileged position to study these dynamic underpinnings of communication. Ours is the first semantic and only discourse in which a fourth legitimate dimension of meaning—unconscious, organic *expressiveness*—is explicitly brought into the referential field. By virtue of its semantic and methodological mandate psychoanalysis expands the range of interpretable meaning-elements to encompass all modes and dimensions of human expressiveness. In so doing, I believe, it pushes its interpretive charge to join the ranks of art. And as with any interpretive art, those who enter its practice ought to acquire a thorough understanding and mastery of their medium, as well as the technique to use it in highly skillful, professional ways. Ours is the *only* linguistic semantic required, through genuine *symbolic* articulation, to transpose ambiguous presentational, enacted patterns of meaning that, heretofore, have erupted via symptomatic or sublimatory expressive channels. This makes it all the more important to thoroughly investigate the functions and forms of the semiotic instrument through which its dialogues materialize. Verbal form may be used at various levels of semiotic organization and serve many different dynamic, extra-linguistic functions. Only its *symbolic* use and articulation, through the working-through process, yields genuine psychoanalytic insight. I say this emphatically in order to dispel a commonly held misconception that verbalization is automatically also symbolization.

A peculiar paradox of psychoanalytic discourse is that despite it being a verbal "method" *par excellence* its interpretive charter does not coincide with what would commonly be considered a truly linguistic enterprise. Psychoanalysts use words to perform many nonverbal feats. A situation in which words will substitute for various vital developmental needs, where many communications will aim at promoting integrative and transformative functions, by adding non-indexical forms to the fray of interpretable elements, expands 'dialogue' well beyond the verbal plane while still adopting only words as instruments.

Language, discourse-context, and sense, are interrelated in complex ways; 'meaning' is in great part merely a *potential* realized and co-constructed through dialogue, determined by the semantic field, agendas, and interpretive perspectives of the discourse participants. Schole (1980) explains:

> The interpretant is generated by the interpreter through a process of selection from and perhaps modification of the

> semantic field which the interpreter has developed for the particular sign in terms of its previous appearances in other utterances. A dictionary or lexicon of any language is simply an attempt to codify the results of this process. (p.203)

Yet words are also fairly malleable, their particular sense and significance subject to the speaker's conscious and unconscious intent, the function and semiotic organization that currently molds them. A word, in psychoanalytic discourse, is understood by everything that clusters around it; by the tone and timing of its utterance, by identifying the voice in which it is spoken, its pivotal sense, and double meaning in the current moment, its dynamic relationship to the past. What is the utterance *doing*, the analyst wonders, directly, indirectly or obliquely, as the speaker's unconscious intent reveals itself at the interstice between the form of the communication and its content. Is it depicting, describing, evoking, coercing, transmitting? Why these words and why now? When and how have they come up before? What ideas, images, and memories do they conjure, refer to, or express, the analyst questions, as the exploration burrows to sublinguistic roots buried deeply in unconscious soil entangled in a web of associative ramifications. And it is here, in this muddy, subterranean gravel that psychoanalytic meanings are unraveled, spun out and transmuted into a new, jointly created psychoanalytic co-construction.

In general, then, 'meaning' and sense are not fixed or inherent properties of words. They issue, rather, from a semantic attitude toward communications *within a particular context*, the result of a meaningfully negotiated or created 'sense' that emerges when we consider an utterance in its *total* relation to everything that surrounds it. Citing Austin's (1962) use-based theory of language, Bruner (1983) reiterates "...an utterance cannot be analyzed out of the context of its use and its use must include the intention of the speaker and interpretation of that intention by the addressee in the light of communications conventions" (p. 36).

According to philosophers of language and the logic of discursive thought, only that which language can define can be known; verbal symbolism supplies literal meanings and produces logical conceptions, everything else that falls outside the bounds of this semantic, that pervades everyday speech and life, is to be considered expressive of desire, feelings and emotion,"… not symbols for thought, but symptoms of the inner life, like tears and laughter, crooning, or profanity" (Langer 1942, p.83). It hardly bears repeating that it is precisely such "symptoms" of the inner life that psychoanalysts are most interested in deciphering in the belief that outer expression reflects inner landscape. Our focus is on filling in the gaps, piecing together what is not told but shown; much of what we attend to bursts through in these behavioral or "symptomatic" forms. We understand human expressiveness to be rooted in the body, the emotions, whether conscious or unconscious. Our task is, by increments, to give form to the inchoate, to shape the unshapen, name it, explore it, interpret it, to reconnect body and mind. From the obverse direction, our attention is peaked by those linguistic forms — synecdoche, metonymy, tropes and metaphors — symbolic connectives, depictives, descriptives and explicatives that infiltrate the verbal mass spinning their magic, shedding colored hues on the grey march of words as do the subtle shadings of a master's palette surreptitiously guide our gaze: "Only a mind which can appreciate *both* a literal and a 'poetic' formulation of an idea is in a position to distinguish the figure from its meaning," writes Langer (1942, p. 149).

Language, in psychoanalytic situations, must stretch to meet the referential demands of the discourse. What was unknowable, unthinkable even, out of an inducement to take shape, will slowly rise to representation, often through the pathway of imagistic metaphor, an envisagement spun to bridge the unconscious with the conceivable. Interpretation and insight are both characterized by a search for the right words in which to capture fleeting, richly nuanced yet ineffable experiences through semiotic vehicles that by their constitution do not lend themselves either to their polyvalence or to the soaring *qualities* of feeling they must describe. When a term is sought to express something new, we call first on metaphor: straddling two realms of experience, in one instantaneous iconic flash, metaphor fuses word and image, welding two modes of cognition. A figurative evocation in verbal form succeeds both in *presenting* and *re*-presenting a novel idea; while literal and non-literal meanings are determined by context and the speaker's intent, metaphor strikes both chords simultaneously.

'Novelty' according to Langer (1942), and 'oddity' according to

Goodman (1984), are the marks of metaphor: "The novelty is what the speaker is trying to point out or to express"(Langer, 1942, p.139) "The oddity is that metaphorical truth is compatible with literal falsity" (Goodman, 1984, p.71). In a context where only *psychic* truth is relevant we note that metaphor is more than both; it is a fundamental *law* of ideation, a principle of the processes of symbolization. Metaphor effectuates that semantic transformation which is the hallmark and goal of psychoanalytic interpretation. Its presence, so strikingly a part of psychoanalytic discourse, is due to the feat it accomplishes: it is the simplest and most effective transitional device the mind can conjure between no form and a signifying formulation. Insofar as it works partly by evocation it is not strictly *referential* at all; metaphor is "our most striking evidence of *abstractive seeing*," (Langer, 1942, p.141).Whenever new and "unexploited possibilities of thought crowd in upon the human mind, the poverty of everyday language becomes acute" (Langer, 1942, p. 149). This is why metaphor—half image, half idea—with its implicative multi-dimensionality and descriptive depth, is often the closest approximation in words that can be found for unconscious meanings

A strange thing occurs when patterns or processes are fitted into verbal form; sensations, impressions and intuitions that spontaneously and simultaneously rushed through the mind, must now be unwound and strung along sequentially. Words stand discrete, separate from one another; the only picture that language can paint is of "things," its "facts" objectified in the very act of their pronouncement. Words reify fluid, iconic, multidetermined and interactive processes. What language does not "picture" well, is the polymorphous, ambiguous, richly nuanced, experiential *quality* of inner life. "One name stands for one thing, and another for another thing, and they are connected together. And so the whole, like a living picture, presents the atomic fact" wrote Wittgenstein (1922, 4.0311) By reason of its linearity only thoughts that can adapt to this stringent ordering are communicable by words. What is lost in verbal form are vast amounts of sensory cues and subliminal features that resist the proscribed arrangements of this sort of semantic. The musical analogy is drawn to underscore the fact that much of what is transmitted unconsciously is precisely what is most elegantly and eloquently evoked through the suggestive compositional-patterns of musical rather than verbal phrase. On the other hand unconscious meanings are slippery, ephemeral, elusive, woven on gossamer threads that come and go and quickly disappear, on which we have tenuous hold were we not able to seize and harness them through the fixity of words.

Throughout development language participates in the gradual blanching and objectifying of experience; speech grows increasingly conventional and bland as language proceeds to spell out distinct meanings that earlier were merely implied by the vibrant use of a single, vital word.

Not so at the beginning, when the toddler's summary one word sentence subsumes within its unadorned, undifferentiated content the atmosphere of an entire scenario and all that is associated with it! From its early anchoring in action and sensory-affective experience, the word will undergo increasing generalization and abstraction, until its meaning is torn from highly personal or idiosyncratic associations and tied to its conventional use and sense. In its most elementary form, a word contains the whole process-storied situation implied by its evocation. "All gone" is put to all kinds of compelling uses when called on to refer to experiences of disappearance, conclusion, completion, consumption, ending, elimination, separation, absence and loss —to name just a few. But such idiosyncratic and arbitrary application of its sense proves excessively vague and ambiguous so more and more words are added to modify the original expression; "grammatical structure evolves by emendation of an ambiguous expression, and naturally follows quite closely the relational pattern of the situation that evokes it. In this way, the context of the primitive word-sentence is more and more adequately expressed in verbal terms" (Langer, 1942 p.137).

It is important to keep in mind that learning to use words goes hand in hand with context, interaction and quality of relationship. The genetic roots of language as *interaction*, Bruner (1983) emphasized, are embedded in the prelinguistic, early relational milieu from which it sprung:

> Language does not "grow" out of prior protophonological, protosyntactic, protosemantic, or protopragmatic knowledge. It requires a unique sensitivity to a patterned sound system, to grammatical constraints, to referential requirements, to communicative intentions, etc. Such sensitivity

> grow in the process of fulfilling certain general, nonlinguistic functions — predicting the environment, interacting transactionally, getting to goals with the aid of another, and the like. These functions are first fulfilled primitively if abstractly by prelinguistic communicative means. (p31)

Whether interactions were wrought with anxiety or filled with joy, whether they engendered curiosity or fear, encouraged to conform or confide; whether the will was served or made subservient to acts of speech; whether communications were clear or confusing, direct or indirect, personal or formal; whether interchanges served narcissistic needs or referred to ideas; whether their predominant tone was instructional or transactional, playful or stern, dismissive or respectful, their sense, metaphorical or literal, abstract or concrete, *all* impact on subsequent habits of speech, influencing the manner in which language is used. Dynamic factors and identificatory features are woven through lexicon and communicative style: the superego, in particular, is predominantly an auditory, linguistic internalization.

Whatever is being done with words, language is always context and subject sensitive: as simple a verbal act as 'naming' already implies reference to story, situation, and relationship. In a context which invites us to follow each associative trace to wherever it leads, we are constantly surprised to find just how much there is in a name. We are in a position to trace it backward, as it were, to that place where affect, imago and meaning — always tightly knit — make their appearance in one striking metaphor. Words can become triggers, like the flick of a switch, suddenly casting light on an entire scenario of untrammeled history; the means for summoning a presence, rekindling dormant feelings, recapturing an event, a place, a sound, a smell, a situation. Through their dynamisms words can convey an atmosphere, conjure emotions, transport us, transfix us, transform us; words transcend limitations of space/time, freeing experience from the eternal present into future projection or past recollection by the grammatical turn of a tense. The recapitulative, reconstructive aspects of psychoanalytic exploration draw attention to the dual dynamic vectors that converge in verbal form: words are products, emblems and expressions of unconscious imagination, as well as pointers, indicators, definers, the creators of conscious exegesis and narration. Verbalization is not a simple unitary phenomenon: at times it is a means, at others an exemplification, at others still it becomes an end. Citing studies by Lorenz and Cobb (1953), Rycroft (1958) pointed out that "many of our so-called intuitive judgments of others are in fact based on our unconscious perception and evaluation of their linguistic and syntactical habits…and that disturbances in object-relations, self-awareness, affectivity, etc., are reflected in habits of speech" (p. 414).

Internalizations need neither originate in the distant past nor be so deeply entrenched in order to reemerge in the course of a spontaneous account. Aside from the impressive impact of the parallel process in supervision, a less dramatic phenomenon occurs at the mere mention of a patient's name, which may bring with it an entire tonal and expressive shift, the coloring and nature of which discloses information regarding the qualities and undercurrents of the clinical encounter that are completely absent in the verbal report. Some of the subtle inflectional cues and even kinetic tensions that creep into the supervisee's spontaneous account may be less apparent than the insistent or repetitive use of a particular word—which upon questioning usually turns out to have been used by the patient—the dynamic unconscious significance of which the supervisee will reveal, even if unaware of doing so. This is yet another instance supporting a view that spontaneous reporting of clinical process in supervision is superior to verbatim accounts and yields the *kinds* of unconsciously transmitted, contagional information that is most relevant to psychoanalytic discourse.

I am reminded of another interesting example of this taken from the supervisory process of the supervisee/patient pair from my illustrative vignette. As part of the training protocol, we were required to work with a few taped sessions in order to get an *in vivo* sampling of my supervisee's interactions with her patient. Leaving aside all the practical and technical difficulties which seemed to arise around these recordings (the tape recorder became dysfunctional, batteries were dead, the volume had not been turned up sufficiently, the replay was inaudible, etc.) and the initial, distracting impact on the patient, as the sessions finally got underway and the patient was entering into a meaningful and, for him, painful realization, he punctuated his words with loud bursts of nervous laughter. These had the effect of dissipating the impact of his insights but also of minimizing them. Had I not heard the defensive quality of these explosive, jarring self-interruptions I would not have grasped the full implications of the way he was communicating his new found awareness. The laughter was the only reliable indicator of what he was *still doing*, behaviorally, namely recreating a habitual trivialization and devaluation of his capabilities and accomplishments. In other words, the laughter carried his repetitive pattern of self-denigration and embarrassed belittlement vis-à-vis a transference figure, despite the content wherein he was, ostensibly, gaining insight into the very dynamic he was still repeating. This illustrates quite vividly how I could not have relied on a textual report which would have given a very skewed rendition of his new awareness. Rather, it highlighted the transferential underpinnings maintained through the manner in which he was communicating. The supervisee had responded counter-transferentially with a rather indifferent silence, missing the expressive message of her patient's self-defeating submissiveness as it continued to trip him up by inducing depreciation through the very form of his self-disclosure. This stresses that the full sense and deeper significance of an utterance is always subject to the emphasis given it by the expressive qualifiers that surround it.

Psychoanalytic dialogues are not, or not merely, textual but *contextual*. Much paralinguistic information, which is "data" in our interpretive semantic, is simply not packaged in linguistic form but appears in spontaneous asides departing from verbatim process reading. Consider if the impact of an abrupt shift in tone, a fleeting expression of pain or fear or disgust, a burst of hilarity, a sudden gush of tears or swell of compassion, can adequately be rendered in a verbatim reading; or if the subtle impact on the listener of a sudden break in a word, a spell of verbosity, a wistful silence or pensive stare, can reliably be documented in a written text. I think not. Yet many unconscious meanings are found in the qualifying folds of such fleeting expressive moments.

This points to a mixture of speech functions and communicative processes the complexities of which are astonishing: words are not only put to multiple uses while retaining at surface their most conventional, literal meanings, they can simultaneously be operating from different points along a continuum of symbolization, from a spectrum of dynamic, developmental and narcissistic needs, as well as serving immediate interpersonal goals. Listening from the psychoanalyst's chair, one is struck by the fluid alternation of informative and expressive channels, the relative place and weight of words in their contributions to the full meaning-function of any utterance. It is remarkable how effectively and creatively word arrangements and tonal modulations combine to reflect unconscious attitude and sense as well as transferential meanings. "Thus," Shapiro (1991) writes "we watch and listen for dissonance, consonance, and sequential shifts in the vehicles of expression for clues to understanding how emotions hide in communicational sequences…" (p.337). Commenting on the relationship between words and feelings in psychoanalytic dialogues from a sophisticated bifocal lens straddling linguistics and psychodynamics, Shapiro (1991) continues:

> We read how the patient feels about us at that point of the analysis by how she addresses us in the dyad. A sudden lapse into baby talk, lisping shyness, the aggressive tone, silence and obsequiousness, all have meaning in the transference. This ought to be looked at from the standpoint of *what do these behaviors stand for* and what do they add to our knowledge of the significance of her utterance in the traditional semantic way. We ask: what is being said that cannot be read from the grammar or the semantics of the words themselves, but must be a composite derived from context, tone, and elocutionary force as well. (p.341)

Psychoanalysts are trained to withstand multiple contradictory streams of information; to seize an image, feel a silence, tolerate ambiguity, forego judgment, to curb the tendency to reach hasty conclusions, while allowing all sensory input to incubate and ripen, as it were. We are primed to conceptualize communication as a multidetermined, multidimensional, dynamic inter-activity, and to remain attuned to different informative codes, implicit and explicit. Ours is therefore a complex and peculiar relationship with words; our listening extends along multiple dimensions simultaneously attending to manifest meanings and their metathematic, metaphoric shadings, their particular sense in the current context and their idiosyncratic associative underpinnings. We listen for their current dynamic and transferential implications, exploring the internalized attitudes the voice of the current moment is echoing, and how it relates to other genetic factors. And we are interested in identifying at what level of semiotic organization these words are being used, whether they are scripts for enacted exemplifications, functioning as symbols for reflective thought, or whether they are serving as substitutes for signaling cries. Given this unique and peculiar methodological immersion in the verbal medium, psychoanalysis has a particular responsibility to conceptualize the yields of its observations in ways that maximize the uniqueness of its specialized semantic. Distinguishing between speaking that is serving restitutional or substitutive functions from speech that is functioning symbolically, however, is just the beginning for an interpretive agenda that recognizes phase-transitions in symbolization that may begin at biological levels and move only gradually to elaborate symbolic ideation and thought.

In fact, rather than being used for this abstractive function, at different times words serve to hold, touch, to cling to or push away; they are used to shock and surprise, disgust and delight, to commune and merge, or attack and detach. Words may be used to do and undo, convince and cajole, to adulate or demean, destroy or repair, bully or bless. Words can evoke, convey, conjure, or replay and recall, articulate and remember; they may illuminate or obfuscate, disclose or disavow, and serve equally well to conceal as to reveal, to show off, turn off, cut off. Words can be played as instruments or toys, wielded as weapons, offered as gifts; they can be used to beautify, soil, to fill space or pass time: they are used in concrete, literal, onomatopoeic, analogical, and metaphorical ways, to signal, signify or symbolize, and they can substitute for a plethora of physiological discharge purposes. When words are operating as "psychical discharge," as E. Sharpe (1940) referred to this, their functional equivalency takes precedence over any genuine "linguistic" *meaning*. Content, in this case, is of little relevance; "Only when the analyst can find that these discourses serve the same purpose as a stream of urine, a smoke screen, flatus, bleating, is he able to get behind the words to the unrecognized, unfelt anxiety" (Sharpe, 1940, pp. 158-159).

Psychoanalysts practice a profession suffused by language, awash in a world where words are the means, the medium, the medicine, and cure. For the better part of their days analysts are surrounded, smothered, submerged, and sometimes baffled, bewildered, touched and awed, by the power of the currents of words that swirl around them. Denied habitual channels of casual exchange, where expression can freely escape by alternate route, all things that pass between our patients and ourselves must ultimately be funneled through the forms we've give them in speech. Verbalization permeates the relationship, the space, the process, the situation; it governs the transformations which occur along multiple vectors, at multiple levels and in multiple ways, in our dialogues. Words structure the method, mold our understanding and modulate our minds; and words alone are the instruments we may carry into our practice. No wonder, then, that in these contexts language acquires quite formidable powers.

Not only are analysts acutely aware of nuance and tone, the motives, sources and functions of words spoken to them; they are *super* conscious of those uttered by them. If in most colloquial exchanges words can be flung nonchalantly this way and that, analysts, rather, must thoughtfully select, dose and time what they say. The primacy of our therapeutic intent dictates that every communication have a deliberate aim, words delicately picked and deliberately planted as seeds for their potential to promote growth. In the supervisory situation words used by the supervisee during the report may or may not be the same as those spoken by the patient, their sequence and sense having certainly been unconsciously edited by the dynamic filter of the supervisee's own "secondary revision." It is, nevertheless, very important to be aware of the very words that are used, at times to inquire and determine whose they are, to observe how they are spoken, what they evoke, note which expressive, gestural or tonal embellishments fill in the gaps that qualify the verbal account. In many ways these details will duplicate the unconscious dynamisms of the clinical process that is partly transmitted and partly recapitulated through the report. In this way we become directly privy to the *experience* of the clinical process and bear witness to spontaneous narration as an organic, living activity that reflects the internalization of multileveled interactive processes.

In this regard, I would like to return for a moment to my illustrative vignette (p. 124): At the height of the crisis, recall, my supervisee had come in very upset, full of rebukes, blaming me for her own actions in an uncharacteristic outburst in which she blurted out that I had not offered sufficient directives and that I had failed her by not telling her explicitly what to do. Her vociferous complaints about me belied several threads of anxiety: on one level her scene reproduced and paralleled her patient's transferential coercions. It mimicked his provocative style designed to test her tolerance and ability to adequately care for his emotional needs, while implicitly reproaching her for not "being enough." On another, deeper level, his demanding and panicky pleas for containment resonated with and triggered her own fears that she would be confronted with a situation she would not be able to handle. A third exacerbating element was her conflicted desire to do the "right" thing institutionally, while feeling that these requirements were not in the best interest of the patient or of safeguarding the therapeutic alliance and process. The conflictual tensions and anxiety thus aroused precipitated an enactment that was in part induced and in part countertransferential — she too needed containment. Most striking to me was not only her replication of her patient's overt and covert communications to her, but the tone, demeanor and linguistic bent she adopted that session which, in style and attitude, stood out as being quite unlike her. Not only was she duplicating the unconscious scenario of the clinical situation but this replication echoed the very speech patterns even the words in which her patient's plaintive and provocative dynamics were played out. This suggests that in unconscious assimilations words, interactions and behavioral dynamics are internalized together.

In a similar vein as Rycroft (1958), Sharpe (1940), and Vygotsky's (1934) I would like to outline ten broad categories of language-use that stand out in the psychoanalytic situation. This is not an exhaustive list, yet when approaching communication from an organismic-developmental orientation it becomes clear that neither is all speech communicative, in the full sense of the word, nor is verbalization always truly *linguistic*. To the extent that speaking is serving discharge, contact, self-stabilizing, posturing, exhibitionistic or boundary-titrating purposes, it is not truly functioning as an instrument of communication or as a tool of thought. By treating speech activity as *significant behavior* we note that language is often used to serve several different functions simultaneously. The following ten speech-functions are dynamically distinct from one another although they may mix and overlap; identifying them, I believe, is helpful when conceptualizing verbalization as an organismic activity serving substitutional, restitutional, creative, communicative, and cognitive functions — or an admixture of these.

The first speech-function serves to establishand sustain ***contact***; here the vocal line functions primarily like a thread, as a means for making and maintaining a social connection. There are, of course, numerous variants along this dimension and gradations in the intensity with which it is pursued depending on whether it is motivated by a need for attachment, attention, social interaction, emotional containment and support, or intellectual conversation. Regardless, the desired response implies a reciprocal, complementary investment in the interaction.

The second is that of ***discharge***; here the vocal channel functions like an exhaust valve, to release various types of emotional and/or psychological tensions. Words are used to eject, project, reject, ventilate, and eliminate undesirable bodily contents or unmanageable mental states. As Sharpe (1940) put it, "…words themselves become the very substitutes for the bodily substances" (p. 157), or as Rycroft (1958) commented, a patient "will use speech as a symbolic substitute for infantile sexual activities. At such times he will not only use his own speech to discharge oral, anal, or phallic drives, or to gain exhibitionistic or narcissistic pleasure, but will also endow the analyst's speech with identical or complementary meanings" (p. 413). When speech is serving such quasi-organic functions responsiveness spans the gamut of container and holding purposes; from garbage pail to gilded mirror, from toilet bowl to cherished vessel, from impartial listener to soothing, comforting organizer and holder.

The third is that of ***thought***; originating in the inner speech of childhood, this monologic stream of verbalization gradually turns inward, persisting partly as that familiar stream of consciousness that accompanies our waking experiences but also becoming an available internal referential activity which can be deliberately activated as in planning, reasoning, considering or contemplating.

The fourth is that of ***play***; here words, and speech itself, are used as an instrument of hilarity. From babies babble and childhood word games to adult punning, rhyming, joking and verbal sparring, people love to play and have fun with language. Teasing, flirtation, humor and humoring are all done with words as indispensable accoutrements of sensibilities which seem to rise out of and flower through speech, so that language and laughter — a highly infectious pair — often intermingle and are tied together.

The fifth is the ***communicative, informative*** function of speech, and were it not for our pervasive search for unconscious meanings, might be as straight forward as it appears to be; a means for imparting information. Yet no piece of information, however simple, is devoid of surrounding qualifiers and contextual implications — the reason for it coming up now, what came before and follows after, what is being done simultaneously, or how it is communicated, its transferential shadings, etc.…so that a psychoanalytic inquiry is incomplete without attempting to grasp this whole array of meanings…and a cigar is rarely, if ever, just a cigar…

The sixth is that of ***metabolizing*** (as in working-through); here speech is serving a cathartic function by providing specific content while processing toxic or intensely charged memories. Language helps to organize, contain and express traumatic thoughts and feelings, to give shape and meaning to subjective states and reactions. Words are fundamental in formulating, describing, sharing and articulating symbolically the quality of profoundly stirring or disturbing experiences, defusing their hold through the verbalization of their impact and significance. The metabolizing function of speech can also subsume the contact, discharge, expressive, integrative and transformative functions.

The seventh is that of ***conceptualizing***, when speech is serving a strictly symbolic and intellectual function, that of formulating, articulating, elaborating, reasoning through, abstracting, and deliberating on ideas. As an extension or continuation of thinking, conceptualizing is the deliberate gestation and manipulation of ideas at high levels of abstraction. When listening to this kind of speaking we are, similarly, induced to 'thought' and the articulation of ideas.

The eighth function, I call the ***artistic*** or ***poetic*** use of speech. It is the most expressive, inspired, evocative, and deeply personal articulation of language, springing from imaginative sources and creative sensibilities that mold and combine words to generate a novel, aesthetic verbal envisagement. This kind of speech 'touches' us, evoking a participatory response, even a transcendent experience.

The ninth and tenth, the ***integrative*** and ***transformative*** functions of speech, apply specifically to the reflective expression of personal insight in clinical psychoanalysis and to the analyst's therapeutic intent when identifying, naming and bringing into the linguistic orbit what becomes manifest unconsciously. The *integrative* function serves to bring together disparate facets and differentially organized aspects of experience, i.e., linking affects and ideas with words, image with meaning, past with present, primary with secondary process. In the *transformative* function the analyst's intent is catalytic, designed to effectuate a complete transmutation in the nature of an experience and how it is known, accompanied by a transposition in form through which it can be communicated. The two functions work synergistically through the recursive dialectic of psychoanalytic dialogues; the former paves the way, or makes possible, the high degree of self-awareness and higher levels of synthetic and symbolic organization expressed through the latter.

The *integrative* function brings together, unifies and consolidates the personality: by its linguistic articulation and insightful content, when uttered by the patient, the *transformative* function reflects profound psychological change in progress. Both the integrative and transformative functions of speech arise out of the analyst's thinking, understanding and interpretive activities, as an expression of authentic, contextual responsiveness to unconscious manifestations and meanings. Both functions imply the activity of a steadily working observing ego which, in turn, is part of the requisite referential equipment of the analytic attitude; "Insight gained in such interaction is an integrative experience" wrote Loewald (1960, p. 240). It is an indication of the analyst's ability to move freely between unconscious apperceptions and the symbolic verbalization of there possible meanings, so that "The analyst, in his communication through language, mediates higher organization of material hitherto less highly organized, to the patient" (Loewald, 1960, p. 241). The referential activities of the psychoanalytic interpretive semantic are implemented through the dialectic of its discourse processes and specific use of verbal form.

MODULATION

> A musical modulation is a smooth transition from one key into another. The seamless quality of this tonal change is achieved by an intermediary passage through a perfect cadence with a "pivot" chord that has several notes common to both keys so that the shift is continuous, occurring within and through the structure of the musical line
> (Collins Musical Encyclopedia, 1959 ed.).

The analogy is chosen for its specific fit: from an examination of the transition from natural to verbally mediated modes of communication, we are now moving to an analysis of forms of knowledge for which words and discourse are indispensable. The transition effected by this brief bridge, then, represents a shift from documenting the developmental progression of natural expressions and the advent of speech, to a study of ways of knowing that are shaped by language through dialogue. This marks the midway point along an increasingly complex continuum through which we are tracing morphogenetic transformations in communicative means, and will now study the impact of semantic and discourse reference on knowledge and awareness.

Once we are functioning predominantly within the realm of language and linguistic interchange, mechanisms of interaction become subject to the infiltration of semiotic activities that may dramatically impact on all systems. The mind truly becomes master when conscious choices are deliberated by means of thought, by articulating ideas that override biologically-based motivations. This is less about a sharp divide than it is that new and different processes take over the executive governance of the organism's actions producing a cascade of effects influencing all neurobiological systems. The importance of understanding dialogue is not only for its semiotic processes but for its widespread impact throughout the organism.

Scholes (1980) has emphasized that words ought to be thought of in terms of a sign/semantic field of "potential meanings" that are "partly governed by social code and partly individualized by the unique features of whoever utters or interprets them." When a verbal sign is used in a speech act, he writes, "each interpreter (including the speaker) narrows the field down and so isolates an interpretant for the sign in this particular utterance, discourse, context and situation" (p. 203). The Saussurian distinction between *langue* (language) and *parole* (utterance) might here be used to illustrate how language supplies the referents while discourse implements their meanings.

While this general principle also applies to psychoanalytic situations, insofar as our overarching interpretive semantic orients to what is 'unconscious', our referential scope works somewhat in the opposite direction: rather than narrowing the field it expands it considerably, slanting interpretive understanding toward everything that emerges unconsciously. This vastly expanded referential sphere calls on unusual emotive/cognitive faculties requiring a special attentional stance. Psychoanalytic knowledge and understanding continue to originate from an experiential matrix involving "more than the usually listed perceptual and communicative modalities" (Loewald, 1970 p.286).

The overriding impetus to move everything toward conscious awareness that orients psychoanalytic methodology makes of its discourse situations ideal windows to; (a) identify the developmental building blocks that organize communicable forms of experience; and (b) to trace the mediational exchanges and stages in verbal referencing that lead to becoming consciously aware. It will be impossible, therefore, in the ensuing exploration, to avoid the issue of consciousness, particularly if consciousness is understood to be a phase or stage in the process of verbal symbolization achieved through the confluence of dialogical and referential activities. Our analysis will turn to the *specific* semantic, semiotic and discourse features that create the kinds of phenomena and forms of awareness that are generated by the situational purpose. The clinical situation is designed to make conscious the analysand's inner world; the supervisory to increase the supervisee's conscious grasp of the clinical process. Both situations function by way of a dialectical exploration of contextual emergent phenomena contingent on the establishment of a special introspective and reflective referential attitude.

Conscious awareness and referential factors, therefore, are closely interrelated and always context- and subject-specific. The discourse parameters established by the particular "situational definition" (to use Vygotsky's term) or "format" (to use Bruner's) determine the conditions for emergent phenomena and the interpretation of meaning within them. This is relevant not only for psychoanalytic dialogues but as a general principle of discourse. Most importantly, it has relevance here for a systematic understanding of the regular appearance of transference/resistance and parallel processes, and the reasons for their coming into sharp relief in these situations. My goal in the following analysis of the psychoanalytic and supervisory situations will be to identify among a multiplicity of influential factors those that are specific to communications leading to; a) the kind of psychological integration and change resulting from insight in the clinical process, and; b) the enhanced grasp of clinical process that is learned through supervisory interchange.

This analysis will be guided by three key Vygotskian concepts that are central and indispensable to a semiotically informed approach to discourse analysis. In order to do justice to Vygotsky's sophisticated thinking, and because his terminology is intrinsically tied to semiotic ideas, I am careful to define these terms through Wertsch's (1985) authoritative presentation. The fundamental assumption underlying Vygotsky's general laws of cultural development is that "all higher mental functions appear first on the interpsychological plane and then on the intrapsychological plane" hence "interpsychological functioning," or social discourse, is inextricably linked with intrapsychical functioning. Consequently, any change in the former will produce corresponding changes in the latter (Wertsch, 1985 p.158). Understanding the semiotic activities and discourse processes mediating this transition from external dialogue to intrapsychical structuring, particularly in the establishment of higher, more complex, forms of ideation, was Vygotsky's primary interest. To this end he advocated a type of analysis that considers the specific *situational definition* and identifies the various ways in which different types and levels of *intersubjectivity* are engendered within that discourse context. The *"situational definition"* refers to "the way in which objects and events in a situation are represented or defined" (Wertsch, 1985, p. 159). It is necessary in the analysis of communicative exchanges and contexts functioning "interpsychologically," because "it allows us to characterize the fact that interlocutors may differ and may change their representations of the same set of objects and events" (Wertsch, 1985 p.159) as a result of dialogue. This difference may be especially pronounced in the kinds of communications taking place in the *"zone of proximal development,"* between individuals at disparate levels of development or with dissimilar frames of reference and representational means. Children, for example, are not ordinarily able to grasp word-definitions or the full significance of behaviors, events and actions, in the way that adults may assume. Similarly, anyone entering a new discourse field or situation will require some time to become familiar with its semantic range, categories of reference, and speech conventions. Individuals interacting in this *zone of proximal development* approach their communications from different referential perspectives, with different expectations, often representing aspects of the situation in very different ways. Given such inherent difficulties, it is a wonder anyone can engage in effective communications at all!

In order to analyze these problems of language and discourse, Vygotsky invoked the notion of *"intersubjectivity,"* a term defining the joint establishment of a mutually understood referential and representational vocabulary through which communications can transcend the different personal, subjective worlds of the participants by having successfully generated a temporarily shared world view: "Intersubjectivity exists when interlocutors share some aspect of their situation definitions. Typically this overlap may occur at several levels and hence several levels of intersubjectivity may exist" (Wertsch, 1985 p.159).

Clearly, the term "intersubjectivity," thus defined, was never intended to convey the concept of a permanent state or fixed condition but, rather, that of fluctuating speech activities, the function of verbal negotiations through which different kinds, and greater or lesser degrees, of intersubjectivity are established, maintained, lost, and recemented through continued verbal exchange. These semiotically mediated transactions come to define the special sense of a set of primary referents in a given context and, out of a large pool of meaning-potentials, what kinds of meaning are attributed to particular, events, words and utterances, within that situation. At those points of contact within the dialogue in which a basis of mutual understanding has been attained, interlocutors will have succeeded in establishing some level or form of "intersubjectivity" that is specific to that situation. However many dynamic factors contribute in complicating how interlocutors understand each other. Issues can range from basic trust, or apprehension about a person's intentions and capabilities, to the way a particular meaning or referent has been understood. On the other hand, even a minimal degree of intersubjectivity may suffice in providing a basis for the internalization of the semantic and referential activities of an interpsychological dialogue

Vygotsky derived these ideas from his studies of learning and development in school age children, particularly from his investigation of relationships between instruction, learning a specialized skill and the more general impact on overall development of formal studies in the academic disciplines. He was aware that similar learning dynamics may continue to operate even at later stages of life (Wertsch, 1985). Because of the semiotic grounding of such Vygotskian concepts as "intersubjectivity" and the "zone of proximal development," we can surmise that similar dynamics of disparity, whether due to unfamiliarity with vocabulary or of the regulatory codes of a discourse, are reiterated, more or less, throughout life whenever an implicit unevenness between interlocutors is re-encountered.

The Vygotskian ideas here presented point to the need in psychoanalysis of studying our discourse contexts in terms of their "situational definition" and unique semantic and referential features in order to identify in what ways these factors are influential in engendering those events we have labeled the clinical and supervisory "processes," beginning with the therapeutic and learning alliances. Vygotsky's semiotically oriented concepts and terms help characterize many of these discourse-engendered processes as arising out of a *type* of discourse situation, embedded in a special semantic, and as a function of a number of dynamically interrelated speech and referential factors that bring certain phenomena into sharp relief. Although distanced from psychoanalysis both historically and conceptually in this citation Vygotsky (1978) might just as well have been referring to its methodology:

> Any psychological process, whether the development of thought or voluntary behavior, is a process undergoing change right before our eyes. The development in question can be limited to only a few seconds, or even fractions of seconds (as is the case in normal perception. It can also (as in the case of complex mental processes) last many days and even weeks. Under certain conditions it becomes possible to trace this development.... Using such an approach one can, under laboratory conditions, provoke development. (p. 61)

For psychoanalysts, our method is our "laboratory." In order to understand how our dialogues operate and how their semiotic and referential activities are internalized, a process-analysis of discourse events arising in the clinical and supervisory situations, from within the hub of their contextual interactions, is necessary. This transformation, involving the internalization of dialogic processes, takes place slowly over time. Changes occurring in the shift inward involving voluntary attention, memory, concept-formation and most semiotically-mediated higher functions, entail alterations in their interfunctional relationships, a result of extensive engagement and internalization. In psychoanalytic dialogues, similarly, these interfunctional shifts occur slowly, over time, creating the typical phase structure of our processes.

The ensuing examination of two psychoanalytic discourse situations is prefaced by an exploration of narrative form, or, rather, of modes of narrative-action that tell of psychical tales: a concept of enactment as the unwitting exposition of deeply structured voices and interactions, of conflicts, compromise and belief, the metathemes and metacodes that constitute the experiential hi-story of the internalized past and of how these becomes narrativized as *psychoanalytic* tales.

IV
NARRATIVE MODES: NARRATIVE FORM.

> The study of narrative is no longer the province of literary specialists or folklorists borrowing their terms from psychology and linguistics but has now become a positive source of insight for all the branches of human and natural science. The idea of narrative seems...to be repossessing its archaic sense as *gnãrus* and *gnosis*, a mode of knowledge emerging from action, a knowledge which is embedded not just in the stories we tell our children or to while away our leisure but in the orders by which we live our lives.
>
> W. J. T. Mitchell, 1980, pp. ix-x

Language and life, both, proceed linearly, in time, obliging us to put one word and one foot after another. The consequence of temporality is sequence, in action and thought. And where we find sequence, causation follows close behind. We organize experience, generate belief, endow events with meaning by looking backward, retrospectively, and the stories thus created are the stories that guide out lives.

All people, everywhere, at any time, have a story to tell. Narration is a human universal—transcultural, transhistorical, transgenerational. Narrative is one of the clearest expressions of the symbolizing and synthesizing tendencies of the human mind. People make moral judgments, think, remember, anticipate and believe, from the confidence of narrative. Stories provide paradigms for how to think about phases in life crises' and stages in natural events: the ordinary is transformed into the extraordinary by means of a storied account. Each of us is constantly carving out structures of value, morals and meaning, out of daily occurrences that make up the fabric of human experience.

What is not narratized remains uncontoured, inconclusive, unsynthesized by the kind of coherence that encapsulates a string of happenings in narrative form; narration promotes the storied structure, sequencing and ordering its subject matter in ways that endow it with meaning, value and coherence. Even at first glance we can see that the urge to recount subsumes at least two important psycho-social functions: that of communicating, or sharing, and making sense of experiences. At certain times these dual functions appear to become a psychical necessity. The seeds of psychoanalysis were in fact sewn in Anna O's evening narratives, her story-tellings to Breuer, an activity she found to be so calming that she called the 'talking cure.'

Not every telling, however, is a narrative; and not every narrative tells a story. We distinguish between a recitation, a confession, a sermon, a speech, a report, an account, a free-associative stream! Even a brief foray into narratology reveals that there are very specific formal and structural requirements for a telling to qualify as story proper, criteria which, on close scrutiny, are not particularly representative of the subjectively propelled, partly enacted, partly depicted and partly remembered, uneven accounts of psychoanalytic tellings. Despite the fact that, as Schafer (1980) says, "We are forever telling stories about ourselves" (p. 31), it strikes me that we have been tossing around the idea of "story" and "narrative" in psychoanalysis far to loosely without sufficiently paying "minute attention" to form. (Reed, 1995, p.718)

Disciplines set their own boundaries and insofar as they adopt terms associated with other specialized fields are under some obligation to carefully redefine their use in order to avert misunderstandings. Fudgy transpositions lead to theoretical and conceptual confusion. Different discourse interests and conventions yield different types of narratives; every situation will beget its own story and its own version of stories that are engendered by its particular setting. This, as I understand it, is the source and nature of *genre*; and, as Derrida (1980) emphatically cautions "Genre's are not to be mixed" (p.51)

We cannot assume that what a psychoanalyst means by narrative and story necessarily coincides with what a narratologist or literary theorist intends by the same. Even within these disciplines opinions vary according to schools. The point is I do not think it fruitful for a discipline grounded in unique methodological goals and so specialized an interpretive semantic to rest satisfied with the simple notion that psychoanalytic tellings and retellings yield stories and story lines only. To the extent that we are content with such a simplistic conclusion we foreclose on the possibility of undertaking a detailed process-analysis of those very narrative and storying *processes* that render our discourse features so unique. A genuine commitment to the investigation of form leads to a closer examination of the specific *kinds* of narrative voices, narrative actions, storied meanings and narratizing interactions that emerge and are pieced together in psychoanalytic dialogues. This line of inquiry points to questioning what the unconscious can tell us about those timeless sources from which archetypal patternings of events have, universally and cross-culturally, produced our species' storying mania.

It will be helpful, in this exploration, to articulate distinctions between storied-meanings and storied communications; presentational and *re*presentational modes of storied-reference; between the enacted voice of the body, the subjective voice of discourse, and the objective voice of narrative; between a recounted recollection and the *narrativization* of recollection (Mink, 1980, p.237); between narrative modes, narrative form, and narrative process; and finally, to see what can be learned from psychoanalytic recountings and reconstructions that is implied by the traditional "story" form. It remains a problem for the scientific basis of psychoanalysis if we are more concerned with what the stories are about than with the forms and processes of their narration. Elements of content—storied or otherwise—are infinitely variable, yielding only what is commonly referred to as the "soft" data of an interpretive framework. If, on the other hand, we focus on the speech-forms and interactive features of the dialogue's course in relation to its aims, we are lead to a morphology of conscious and unconscious narratizing *processes* whereby "we find ourselves simultaneously on two planes; that which is and that which was" (Vygotsky, 1978 p. 64).

Let me state at the outset that I perceive a functional continuity, an isomorphism, in processes of symbolization, so that I understand narrative to be the verbal communication of signified and symbolized meanings that are *already* storied, temporal, relational and processual in nature. The classic Piercean triad — object/sign/interpretant — first encountered in language is now equally applicable to the more complex, storying organization of meaning. (Scholes, 1980) "Story" is as intrinsic to mind as meaning: narration, on the other hand, "to give events an aspect of narrativity" (White, 1980, p. 4) is an ordering and sequencing of certain elements in a particularly *linguistic* way. From a psychoanalytic perspective, however, we cannot stop at the idea of narrative as a "sequencing structure" (Kermode, 1980); a "temporal device" attempting to "establish human action at the level of genuine historicality" (Ricoeur, 1980, p. 176); a "place" (Scholes, 1980, p. 200) a text, a retelling (Schafer, 1980) or even, most minimally, as "verbal acts consisting of someone telling someone else that something happened" (Smith, 1980, p. 228), because all of these definitions equate a form of knowledge with its medium of representation. They fail to distinguish between an organization or a structure of meaning, and a mode of discourse, a way of recounting. Yet stories, as has cogently been stressed by Goodman (1980), Chatman (1980) and others do not need to be told: they can be dreamt, painted, mimed, danced, composed, pictured, or otherwise conveyed non-sequentially in the simultaneity and immediacy of presentational form. Sequence, or the illusion of sequence, is less a function of "story" than the result of the temporal and temporalizing activity of verbal narration.

The above definitions confine the idea of narrative to the subjects and sequencing of a linguistic semantic and to the categories and elements of content that language designates best, hence reference to actions, events, happenings, etc. But psychoanalysts are less interested in events and happenings themselves than in how these were experienced and recorded in the sutures and embroiderings of psychic life. We understand much of what is being said by what is being done, how it felt then by its expression now, and what this engenders in us; each of these discrete, informative elements qualifies the other. As Schafer (1980) says "there is no hard-and-fast line between telling and showing, either in literary narrative or in psychoanalysis" we deal with "telling as a form of showing and with showing as a form of telling. Everything in analysis is both communication and demonstration" (p.34). Action and language are so intermingled in analytic discourse that the *way* something is told *is* often the story itself!

The prototypical psychical story, however, is the dream: and the way we go about deciphering its code and interpreting its meanings encapsulates the core paradigm of our theory of mind. Multidetermination has taught us that polyvalence is the norm rather than the exception, that all meanings are "storied" in some way. Every element of content, each wayward word or sigh, is a condensed expression of many contributing, related signifiers converging within it as spokes of a wheel point to its hub. And we recognize that multidetermination also implies "stratification," reference to multilayered contributions from different stages of development, that for unconscious "meanings" the temporal/linguistic distinction between past and present is erased — the past is embedded in the present. We listen along multiple dimensions: and we apply to ordinary anecdote, account, narrative or dream, extraordinary interpretive criteria. Manifest story-lines are significant for their latent meanings, meanings that are implied, displaced, disavowed, signaled, contradicted, metaphorized. For psychoanalysts, the relationship between surface form and deep structure, and the Freudian distinction between "thing"-presentation and *re*presentation, are psychically real, the stuff of our interpretive activities. Psychoanalysis is not interested in either "narrative" or "historical" truth, but in *psychical* truth, the subjectively experienced and unconsciously formulated versions of personal life experiences. Our attentional stance is tailored to be receptive to the dominant patterns and significant repetitive referents that stand out from the verbal fray, as charcoal sketches demarcate figure from ground.

Yet the pull toward structuring content in "polished," "conclusive," "textual," or consciously cohesive ways, seems irrepressible. So we find Spence (1982) writing; "The act of constructive listening is largely in the service of strengthening the narrative voice of the material: we try to give it narrative form in order to better understand" (p. 279). He maintains that "active" listening rather than 'evenly hovering attention' as advocated by Freud is "necessary" because "the patients associations — fragmentary, ambiguous, and allusive — lack the coherence we would find in a fully naturalized text" (p. 279). They must, therefore, be "supplemented with other associations before they can be understood…and these additional meanings are projected onto the material," (p. 279) because, Spence asserts, "they do not speak for themselves" (p. 279). But from my perspective they *do* speak for themselves, such as they are; perhaps not to tell a fully "narrativized" account but certainly to tell *their own* story. Contiguity, pause, gaps, interruptions, abrupt shifts in subject matter or thematic line reveal dynamic relationships; an interplay of discontinuous narrative modes exhibits topographical dimensions, and the linking of form and content to contextual *process* yields a complete experiential picture of what is going on unconsciously. Exploration further tells us what is *on* and *in* the speaker's mind, and how and in what ways it is known. This, in my opinion, is how a psychoanalytic inquiry gradually co-constructs a psychologically complete account.

If one tries to impose the structure of coherent narratives onto modes of communication inherently lacking this kind of order, one is bending the phenomena to fit a verbal semantic rather than allowing their emergent patterns to inform via their own forms. This latter approach, recommended by Freud — *not* to impose structure or meaning but to *find* it — leads to filling in the gaps of conscious accounts by receptivity to, and an understanding of, differentially organized unconscious modes of communication. This in no way entails a projection of extrinsic associations *onto* the material, as Spence (1982) suggests, but rather necessitates an attunement to meanings that are, or have been, transmitted unconsciously. The scientific value of our method as a research venue for studying how discourse transforms knowledge is precisely in understanding these very transmutative processes.

Narration is always a sequencing of something for someone: we cannot therefore logically divorce narrative or story from the discourse and occasion of its telling. As Smith (1980) forcefully emphasized, "no narrative version can be independent of a particular teller and occasion of telling and therefore…we may assume that every narrative version has been constructed in accord with some set of purposes or interests" (p. 215). Choice of subject matter, alignment of elements, selection of categories and meanings that are relevant to or are made relevant in a particular discourse, are all situation-specific and subject to the referential perspectives and interpretive lens of the listener: "World structure is heavily dependant on order of elements and on comparative weight of kinds: and reordering and weight shifting are among the most powerful processes used in making and remaking facts and worlds" Goodman reminds (1980 p.11). The psychoanalytic enterprise has as its supraordinate goal the exploration of psychic-reality, the world of the mind; the facts that it uncovers have to do with unconscious processes and the ways these are made conscious. To understand how psychoanalytic versions are constructed, and how they differ from other stories, we have to identify what kinds of elements, categories and referents are emphasized and realigned within our semantic of the unconscious, and compare these to those of other narrative constructs.

There are those, with whom I agree, who view narrative as "a primary and irreducible form of human comprehension" (Mink, 1978, p. 128); "a metacode, a human universal" (White, 1980, p. 2) for organizing "structures of experience" (Turner, 1980, p. 139); a "mode of making sense of reality" (W. J. T. Mitchell, 1980, VIII).They view narrativity as "the central function or *instance* of the human mind" (Jameson, 1981, p. 13), a solution to the general human problem of "how to translate *knowing* into telling" (White, 1980, p. 1).

Before proceeding it is necessary to make a few definitional distinctions between a 'structure of meaning' and the communicative and linguistic processes by which that structure is recounted. We distinguish between a "narrative," a cognitive construct, the symbolization of a temporal sequence, a form of knowledge; "narration," a speech activity, a mode of communication, a way of giving account, a type of telling; "narrativity" and "narrativ*izing*," those linguistic or cognizing processes by which a sequence of elements is organized in a storied way, or fashioned into a narrative structure.

To refer to something in a "narratized" way is quite different from an ordinary account or telling. However, a sequencing of events is not a narrative until it has been structured into the story mode, that is, until its constituent segments have been endowed with storied-meaning. An historical account, moreover, is required to do more than merely register a series of true events honoring their chronological sequence. These events must be "narrated" as well, so as to reveal them as "possessing a structure, an order of meaning, which they do *not* possess as mere sequence" (White, 1980, p. 5). "Without temporal relation we have only a list. Without continuity of subject matter we have another kind of list," writes Scholes (1980, p. 205). Annals and chronicles, both of which are composed of lists containing temporal relation and continuity of subject matter, however lack "narrativity," according to White (1980), because they do not present these events as "possessing a structure, an order of meaning," and thereby "fail to achieve narrative closure" (White, 1980, p. 5).

Although many things that can be sequentialized can also be narratized, not all things can be *narrated*: "One cannot narrate a picture, or a person, or a building, or a tree, or a philosophy," writes Scholes (1980), "Narration is a word that implicates its object in its meaning. Only one kind of thing can be narrated: a time-thing, or to use our normal word for it an 'event'" (p. 205). Strictly speaking, more than one event is necessary to realize a narrative construction. These events have to provide enough continuity of subject matter to make their chronological sequence meaningful and they must be presented as having already occurred. When the telling gives this sequential ordering a certain kind of shape and elicits a certain level of human interest, "we are in the presence not merely of narrative but of story" (Scholes, 1980 p.206). Scholes' (1980) definition is hard to improve on; "A narrated event is the symbolization of a real event: a temporal icon. A narration is the symbolic presentation of a sequence of events connected by subject matter and related by time" (p.205).

The requisite "coherence" and "closure" of narrative form are created retrospectively resulting from the selection and alignment of elements that in their presentation draw toward an intelligible conclusion. In this sense, the end is the "pole of attraction of the entire development" (Ricoeur, 1980 p.170). Only after the ending is known can one grasp the overall causal implications between each of the parts as these relate to the outcome; a *storied* account then is the narration of something that has already been narrativized. Narrative orients backward from an ending to its early foreshadowings: its propulsion forward is fueled, paradoxically, by this retrospective vision; accordingly, "narrative is past, always past," (Scholes, 1980 p. 206). A story, then, is a unit of meaning taut between two interacting poles; the end prefigured in the beginning, the organization of its segments governed by its end. This, no doubt, is how narrative impels our interest forward, enticing us onward and onward with every compelling "and then" inviting us to follow around another bend to its final outcome and conclusion. Yet precisely because of its non-linear configuration — that it is both a whole *and* a sum of its parts — I suspect that "story" is a unit of symbolization, encoded as such.

Since I am neither narratologist nor connoisseur of literary genres, I have had to borrow heavily in the above from specialists, availing myself of their knowledge to reach solid ground from which to draw comparisons. The yields, so far, reveal that narrative and narrativity are cognized according to certain very specific rhetorical requirements including a grammar of sequence, continuity of subject matter, the selection of certain types of main referents grouped and organized into segments, and a significant-enough order of progression, complexity and coherence. A "story," even more specifically, is a narrative with a distinct syntactic form; it must have a beginning, a developed middle, and an end. It requires a central subject, the unfolding of a plot leading to a conclusion or, as Scholes (1980) puts it, a "situation-transformation-situation" design with a "subject matter which allows for or encourages the projection of human values upon its material" (p. 206), "Virtually all stories are about human beings or humanoid creatures." he continues, and "Those that are not invariably humanize their material through metaphor and metonymy" (Scholes, 1980 p.206).

That narrative might be thought of "less as a *form* of representation than as a *manner of speaking*" (White, 1980, p.3) has been proposed in discussions based, primarily, on a linguistic analysis stressing certain grammatical distinctions between the subjective voice of discourse and the objective voice of narrative. From my perspective, however, rather than a "manner of speaking" narrative is the "speaking of a manner of knowing," a mode of cognition that is at the heart of the human compulsion to pull things together and make sense of them causally. Narrative is that form of knowledge stemming from a deep paradigmatic, patterning of meaning that condenses within its structure a temporal cause-and-outcome-sequence. And this is really the central point; narrative or storied-meaning, a *presentational* temporal schema, is primary; its exposition and exegetic *representation* through a symbolic medium, secondary. This follows logically from principles of symbolization and condensation and explains how stories can yield multiple versions or variants as well as sustain projections onto them of multiple interpretations. We ought not to confuse a *presentational* form with its medium of *re*presentation, and therefore need not ask what language teaches us about narrative but what narrative can teach us about mind.

We learn this in psychoanalytic discourse from our prototypical exemplar of storied-meaning, the dream, and from studying our method of dream interpretation. As Freud (1900) emphatically stressed—and this is still true today—we have failed to grasp the far reaching metatheoretical implications of his account of dream-formation and interpretation in understanding symbolic functioning and the role of discourse in the translation from unconscious to conscious. The dreamer's first account is often fragmentary, disjointed, episodic, a series of vivid iconic elements, intensely felt, tentatively described in segments and loosely strung together. A secondary revision usually sees it grow word by word, clause by clause, into discursive order while slowly gaining narrative strength: it becomes linear, segmental groupings grow more coherent and intelligible, they acquire a distinct shape and often, with new details, quite different meanings. Freud (1900) cautioned against this conscious "filling up the gaps in the dream structure with shreds and patches" (p. 528) saying; "It is in the nature of our waking thought to establish order in material of this kind, to set up relations in it and to make it conform to our expectations of an intelligible whole" (p.537). Yet only after abundant associations to each element, and to the discrete features and feelings that are caught up in these elements, and to the unconscious links between parts to each other and to the whole, will a newly *narratized* version of the dream's multiple latent meanings yield a complete, coherent storied-account. This is why the narrative voice of discourse is, in a sense, the inverse of a dream: the essence of a story is culled and condensed from a sequentialized exposition, while the meaning of a dream has to be unpacked and linearized, its narrative given fullness of exposition via the *narrativization* of each part in relation to the whole. Both are complex patterned equations, "temporal icons" (Scholes, 1980, p.205), created and encoded as such, but originating from opposite directions.

This confirms the fact that storied-meanings, the roots of signification and symbolization, are already evident in the simple act of "naming" which encapsulates the quintessential 'mental' activities of condensation and pattern-recognition that are characteristics of human cognition. Confirmation for this way of thinking is found in the works of A. Marshack (1972). In his explorations of the prehistoric origins of cognition, Marshack (1972) suggests that when names were first used by early humans they would have implied a story, whether this was the name of a person or not, because naming would have embodied reference to a "*relation* or *process* which was understood, teachable, and communicable" he writes, "It was a recognition with a meaning in time and space" (p.119). "Story," Marshack asserts, "refers to the nature of the communication of meaning and, even more, to a certain sort of meaning which is time-factored, relational, and concerns process" (p.119).

In answer to his own question, "What then is 'story'?" Marshack (1972) comes up with the best definition yet:

> ...it is the communication of an event or process — that *is* happening, *has* happened, or *will* happen....It is in the nature of the "story equation" that it must always be told in terms of someone or something. There is, in fact, no other way to tell a story....This holds whether one uses words, mime, dance, ritual, or refers to the symbolism of dream and trance. It holds in the more primitive "storied" communications of lower forms of life, and it holds in the evolved and specialized human "story" categories: magic, religion, ceremony, rite, law, reportage, history, science. In the hominid on the way to becoming man, the time-factored and time-factoring content and complexity contained in story would have evolved as the brain itself and human culture evolved (p.119).

So here we have it: in what, perhaps, began as the simple observation of daily events and life processes; in birth, maturation and death, illness and recovery, the rotation of lunar and calendric cycles, seasonal change; in the series of actions required to make a fire, hunt, kill and prepare an animal, in the urge to indicate, *re*present and transmit this process or lay it down, can be found an essential trait of human cognition. "A good story," writes Marshack (1972), "not only helped the hunter learn, but the human ability to recognize or see a story helped him to recognize and see a pattern *in terms of story*" (p.133). The predisposition to see everything as 'story' and this tendency for storied-thinking, Marshack (1972) suggests, has probably not altered significantly in the last 40,000 years because story form is an "*equation*" that helps organize and "unify the extraordinarily diverse phenomena and processes of...life" (p.133). What has changed are the kinds of stories that are told and their order of complexity. And what is continuously changing, within the course of each life span, are the functional structures of cognition, apperception and symbolization to which these stories are assimilated. Our ability to recognize complex patterns is innate, but our ability to discover new patterns alters according to our apperceptive abilities; "the recognition of a pattern is one thing...its explanation is another" (Marshack 1972, p. 132).

From the above exploration of the origins and features of narrative form, we have learned, among other things that; (a) the principal subject matter of stories are events which can be organized and recounted in terms of a succession of occurrences leading to an outcome; (b) these categories or types of referents can be arranged as elements in a storying format that will orient the narrative toward an ending or conclusion; and (c) that temporality, sequence, coherence, and closure, are key requirements of narrative form.

Consider then the problem with too hasty an application of the conventional idea of narrative or story onto psychoanalytic discourse: 1) we are not immediately interested in "story" elements or events themselves but in their subjective and continued unconscious significance to the subject; 2) derivatives of unconscious or psychical experience—i.e., the unrepresented, the dynamically repressed, early imagoes and identifications, internalized interactions and psychological defenses—are the referential categories and interpretable material from which we derive psychological information. Each of these dimensions tells its own story or history, if you will, but none presents itself directly or sequentialized. Rather, all appear simultaneously, woven deeply through the contextual process and web of words that skims along its surface content; 3) unconscious manifestations are characterized by condensation, displacement and simultaneity, they appear when they will, often concomitantly and in different forms all of which resist linear, linguistic sequencing and closure. Psychoanalytic work depends on a commitment to continued exploration. It proceeds much like a serialized novel with an implicit "to be continued" at the end of each meeting, a conclusion is unforeseeable; 4) the kind of free associative tellings that we invite are unprepared, loosely structured, sometimes storied but for the most part more like monologic ramblings, neither particularly cohesive or logical except in a *psycho*-logical sense yet quite revealing of what is emotionally dominant on the unconscious horizon of the speaker's mind. The organization of a storied narration, which is retrodictive, runs counter to the essence of the free associative and psychoanalytic process both of which are anchored in the subjective present. In fact, the kinds of communication that result from an invitation to say whatever comes to mind turn in the opposite direction from storied structuring, in the formal sense, unveiling unconscious, dynamically motivated contiguity, unusual sequencing, and discontinuous ideation, until this all pieced together. Similarly, supervisory reportings are *most* telling when they are *least* structured, allowing those unconscious transmissions and parallelisms most relevant to our discourse to display themselves; 5) the semantic field for many of our primary referents is not linguistic, so that if narrative is 'a way of telling what is known', we have to find ways of interpreting what is 'shown' but neither told or known. The kind of information we gather to trace our psychological mappings is culled from variously transmitted, projected, enacted, depicted and recounted data which, cumulatively, begins shaping the contours of a complex, intimate psychological portrait of the nature of an "inner world."

In light of all this, I believe it has been misleading and detrimental to the progress of a scientific psychoanalysis to refer to the yields of our dialogues as "stories" while the locus of theoretical advance would have required an inquiry into narrative *form*, not narrative *versions.* Were relevant theoretical data to be found in story lines the exegesis of a clinical text ought to suffice. But the range of communicative phenomena and sources from which information is derived in our semantic go well beyond what any text is likely to contain, requiring, for a full dynamic account, a live reporter and an equally live interpreter of unspoken communications as *essential features* of the discourse. Our method adopts the human observer as *instrument*. We cannot really avoid the implications of this specialized attentional stance.

It seems evident from the above examination of narrative form that one cannot recount in the objective voice of narrative what remains outside of awareness. This means that, in our interpretive framework, we consider the subjects verbalizations as incomplete, unreliable, or partial accounts, requiring completion via the contextual analysis of what is communicated unconsciously. This contextual co-construction grows out of the negotiated input of the analytic dialectic and is constantly being fashioned, refashioned and expanded by the influx of experiential material as it becomes accessible to verbalization. Based as it is on sequence and conclusion, narrative form is contingent on the syntax and grammar of language for the unfolding of a storied line. Psychoanalysis turns this model upside down. Due to the simultaneity of the unconscious, our 'material' has no 'time', no coherence, no sequence, and no closure. We see and reconstruct a hi-story in the experience of the current moment. Many of our elements are not narrated but 'demonstrated' as we go along so that the storying of the psychical tale takes place during the construction of the story of the analysis. None of this achieves completion until after its ending.

Now if we reconsider the analysand's and the supervisee's recountings along narrative lines, we note that they proceed by way of two broad dimensions; a linguistically *re*presented mode and a presentational enacted mode through which are transmitted and projected unconscious, nonlinguistic meanings. What is consciously known or remembered is talked about in the objective voice of narrative, what is preconscious emerges 'represented' in some way, sometimes verbally but in the subjective voice of discourse, its implied or disavowed meanings not fully available to consciousness; and what is completely unconscious or has never been represented, tells itself, but in forms so condensed, displaced, disguised, or projected, as to make its detection and verbal translation very difficult. By interweaving elements from both presentational and representational narrative modes our interpretations look backward from the present and forward from the past, making past and present converge in the experiential moment of a discourse process that mirrors the atemporal simultaneity and repetitiveness of unconscious reality as it honors the time-bound reality and cumulative transformations engendered by the analytic process itself. These dual forms together, and in complementary ways, provide continuous commentary and illustration of the psychical history of the experience of the current moment.

What emerges from our interpretive efforts is a psychoanalytic *narrativization* of the yields of this integration, a tale retold in the objective voice of narrative, unbroken by gaps in consciousness, a life history inclusive of its unknown or disavowed, psychical underbelly. Strictly speaking, then, only after an analysis is over can its *story,* and the psychical biography it generated, be told; and only after a supervisory experience has ended can its full triadic impact be assessed, because the complete transformational pattern required of "story" — its beginning-middle-and-end paradigm — emerges only after a conclusion.

That said, it bears repeating that the content of stories or the fact that people tend to tell tales, is less important than an awareness of the "generalized use of the symbol and of the storied-equation" (Marshack, 1972, p. 280) as being inherent in our cognitive heritage, essentially, in the way we think. And from this basic starting point we can begin again to identify and reexamine the referential and discourse processes which use "symbols and symbolic relations to indicate story and process and which always make the participant, artist, dancer, viewer, or dreamer a part of the story" (Marshack, 1972, p. 280).

I close with the words of another great anthropologist, Victor Turner (1980) who, in tracing the etymological roots of 'narrative' sought a common pathway for the social and cultural instruments that structure human values and meanings as we, who in the formative, structuring roots of the psychical, seek an understanding of mind.

> "Narrate" is from the Latin *narrare* ("to tell") which is akin to the Latin *gnãrus* ("knowing," "acquainted with," "expert in") both derivative from the Indo-European root *gnâ* ("to know") whence the vast family of words deriving from the Latin *cognoscere*, including "cognition" itself, the "noun" and "pronoun," the Greek *gign_skein*, whence *gnosis*, and the Old English past participle *gecnawan*, whence the Modern English "know." Narrative is, it would seem, rather an appropriate term for a reflexive activity which seeks to "know"...antecedent events and the meaning of those events...hence narrative is knowledge...emerging from action, that is, experiential knowledge (p.163).

V
THE PSYCHOANALYTIC SITUATION

> If we survey our psychological data once more in all their variety and over the whole field, from the strongest expression of emotion to the imponderabilia, we become aware that we are treating them as if they served no other purpose but to tell us something about the inner life of another person. I mean to say they aim, among other things, at communicating to us something about the hidden processes in the other mind. We understand this primary endeavor; it does serve the purpose of communication of psychical disburdenment. T. Reik, 1948, p. 142

Freud's (1912) papers on technique candidly reveal that he arrived at his therapeutic method progressively by trial and error until he settled on a set of relatively broad interpretive principles and procedural rules designed to establish and maintain dynamic conditions that would maximize therapeutic leverage while simultaneously bringing into sharp relief the unconscious, experiential world of the analysand. His therapeutic "conversation" was tailored to set in motion and heighten the visibility of certain emergent phenomena which, as Freud (1912) stated, arise because of "the psychological situation in which the treatment places the patient" (p.107). This situation he called the analytic "method" and the phasic progression of events that unfold therein we commonly refer to as the analytic "process."

In this case the "method," to which Vygotsky's (1978) words so readily apply, is "simultaneously prerequisite and product, the tool and the result of the study" (p. 65) It is also true that the method, and its internally generated processes, are *dialogical* phenomena, propelled by the dynamics that originate the encounter and sustained by the semantic and referential perspectives, the nature of the verbal transactions, subject matter and unique interpretive goals of this special discourse situation

This exploration reconsiders the analytic situation as a specialized dialogue defined by its unique semiotic and referential features. The assumption is that its speech patterns, highly personal subject-matter and procedural rules; its specialized interpretive perspectives, activities and purpose, all combine to create an 'interpsychical' semantic field that is especially conducive to intrapsychic restructuring. A detailed examination of its communicative patterns, principal subject matter, and discourse features, ought to yield new understanding of the particular dynamic factors engendering the "therapeutic alliance;" the flowering of transference and persistence of resistances; the development and use of the 'observing ego' and the integrative, therapeutic action of working-through in psychoanalytic insight. If we assume that outer process influences inner structure, we note that this dialogue patterns its communicative conventions to circumvent the very differentiating structures that linguistic form creates thereby providing the conditions for a *de*construction and *re*construction to take place within its aegis and the means for observing the stages in this process.

Discourse situations function in a circular manner: language and speech patterns establish joint referential focus and meanings that are subject to negotiation and reshaping according to evolving interpretive strategies. Communications and referential activities thereby transform discourse situations in order to serve their overriding interpretive and situational goals. The relationship between outer process and inner structuring is an organic one, mutually adaptive and reciprocally transforming. Under certain conditions, the dialogical features, referential activities and overall purpose, can impact lastingly on intrapsychic functional organization. It is these conditions we are about to explore.

Given the marked discrepancy in viewpoints from which the two interlocutors set out, and their disparate expectations and understanding of the situational definition, the entire process might be reconceptualized as an introduction into and continuous negotiation toward a concordance of referential activities in a discourse which must, quite literally, be "lived out" in order to be internalized. This coincides with the generally acknowledged truism that one learns psychoanalysis best by experiencing it. However the psychoanalytic process is extremely overdetermined, its effects impacting on many layers of the personality. To understand specifically how the dialogue exerts its multilayered effects it is helpful to invoke Vygotsy's concept of 'intersubjectivity' in its *semiotic* sense, to define those special points of contact between participants that, in psychoanalytic interpretive frameworks, are subject to linguistic mediation.

The supposition is that there are distinct semiotic and referential mechanisms that must be learned and internalized, in conjunction with the contextual experiences of the dialogue, for the full transformative effects of the analytic experience to produce lasting change. First, then, a description of the unique features of this discourse: This is fundamentally a ***therapeutic*** situation, bound by the ethical responsibilities that structure the basic, real, analyst/analysand relationship. The purpose of the encounter defines the interlocutor's roles in a quintessentially professional situation which determines their respective reasonable expectations and intent. The contractual underpinnings establishing constancy of time, place and fee, confidentiality, the routinization of schedule and the firm boundaries set to this situation, further anchor the special, artificial aspects of the dialogue in its professional purpose. Stone (1961) emphasized the singular dynamic significance and transference valence of the doctor/patient relationship remarking that "to the extent that its latent psychic content becomes available" it is "a uniquely strategic starting point for the development of a profound understanding of basic and general human psychological reactions" (p.17). It has now been amply born out that the same dynamisms, insofar as they are latent and pressing for expression, are engendered by any emotionally tilted encounter where one person seeks help or psychological guidance from another. It is easy for this universal dynamism to recapitulate the primal human condition of helplessness with its corollary wish that conjures an idealized caretaker.

This is therefore an inherently ***tilted*** and ***uneven*** situation from the outset, in which the procedural rules and dialogical conventions impose constraints that further accentuate the extreme emotional imbalance and communicative inequality underlying this dyad. The strict rhetorical specifications and restrictions adhered to are considered to be the best means by which to serve the situational goals. As Stone (1961) put it, "the psychoanalytic attitude (indeed...the whole situational structure) is best understood by *both* parties as a *technical* instrumentality." (p.33) Given their special preparedness in guiding the discourse, and the fact that analysts are required to use their personal sensibilities and responses to understanding their analysands, it makes sense that the recommended stance and speech patterns would have evolved out of the need to reinforce boundaries that, for technical purposes, are otherwise continuously being crossed. This is truer than ever today when both the stance and the technique have been stretched to include interventions designed to repair deficits as well as restore psychic wholeness.

For the most part, the tensions created by the disequilibrium and inequality of the dialogue are balanced by an awareness of their technical expediency, particularly with respect to the analyst's withholding of personal information, "certainly and most stringently, his specifically personal reactions to the patient" (Stone, 1961, pp. 35-36). Stone spoke of the "symbolic anonymity" (p.35) of the analyst and of the high value of the "vacuum" it provides for transference and fantasy development. Unfortunately in today's climate this valuable and important feature is often overridden, resulting in an impoverishment of 'imaginal' material and the degredation of an 'interpsychical' into an 'interpersonal' field grounded in 'reality'. Nevertheless, this is a context in which one person is to remain opaque while the other is to reveal all: where one person is required to initiate and maintain a virtually unmonitored verbal free flow while the other's communications are sparse, select, focused, and dosed. The extreme lopsidedness of disclosure and response, and the persistent frustration of ordinary discourse gratification in the sense of expectable rhythms of reciprocal exchange, spontaneous verbal or emotional reactions, or the offering of guidance, feedback or the like, place the analysand in a position of considerable psychic exposure, vulnerability and strain which, paradoxically, further propels the funneling of mental activity more and more through the verbal communicative channel.

As Stone (1961) depicted it, the formal stringencies and limitations of the communicative conventions of the therapeutic dialogue by which both members of the analytic dyad are burdened, weighted even, are counterbalanced by a recognition that the rigors and rules of the analytic situation are "subtle and cumulative, importantly operative, *whether evident or not*" (p.22). In order for the situation to maintain maximum therapeutic leverage and continue to foster motivational impetus toward continued symbolization and working-through, it must remain optimally frustrating to the patient. The formal parameters of our technical method prohibit extraneous social contacts or any other physical, emotional, or personal exchanges which might be excessively gratifying or significantly stimulating to the patient's transferences.

Yet once the dialogue has gotten underway their settles in a speaker/listener duet,which builds and deepens over time, of remarkable efficacy and plasticity. The unevenness and frustration of normal responsiveness begins to show its yields: an externalized monologic-like version of inner speech, half-reverie, half-communicated, leads inward, to unveil unconscious connections, meanings, beliefs, longings, fears, conflicts and incongruities, as richly and consistently as does the dream. It is this form of speech and the value of its self-selected, self-ordered subject matter and modes of presentation, together with the complementary stance from which it is heard and interpreted, that establishes the *inter*psychical semantic field through which evolve the events of the analytic process.

The social privations imposed by the situation are amply compensated by the development of a connection that is felt, paradoxically, to be deeper, more intimate by far than any ordinary discourse could generate. While retaining its elusive, symbolic character; their springs from within the hub of this fluid, multi-stratal connection, an extraordinarily powerful ***dialectic***. As both the "indispensable driving power" (Stone, 1961, p. 69), as well as the sustained, pivotal resistance of the analytic process, "the transference" is ignited and fueled by tensions facilitated by the situation itself, and therefore is subject to increases or decreases in intensity that can be gauged and titrated according to how the dialogue is conducted. To be sure, for some, establishing and maintaining a genuine connection will be the therapeutic work of an entire pre-analytic experience. But for those who can really use the situation, the reflexive reflectivity of the analytic dyad is an extraordinary vehicle for self-discovery and springboard for self-modification.

The intense dynamisms aroused, over time, by adhering to the dialogical protocol, produce a state of "intimate separation" (Stone, 1961, p. 91) stimulating a series of experiences that are quintessentially ***dialectical*** in nature; we witness the present as reflective of the past, the self discovered through the other; an amplification of desire, and both regressive and progressive strivings; an interplay of de-differentiated enactments and differentiated linguistic self-observation; simultaneous adherence and unwitting resistance to the fundamental rule; basic struggles between union and individuation, understanding and confusion, repeating and working-through, disillusionment and development, all of which underlie the dialogues' progression.

Its inherently dialectical character makes this an ***incomplete*** dialogue insofar as it requires the reflective and reflexive participatory-input of a skilled listener. Yet it is also open-ended, self-propelling, linked from session to session by elusive thematic threads that appear momentarily and are dropped only to reappear later in different form, to be picked up again and again and painstakingly woven into the verbal cloth of the analysis in the knowledge that even after there will always be new and different threads to be identified, processed and spun into words. Due to its multileveled dynamisms, its multiple interpretive perspectives, and the experiential immediacy of its interpretive processes, this is also a ***subversive,*** deviant dialogue, the listener constantly shifting referential focus from content to form, form to process, linking past with present, affect with word, image with emotion, experience with meaning.

The analyst's mandate is to understand everything in terms of its unconscious implications. The speaker's intended meaning is thereby juxtaposed to the listener's interpretive intent, so that what is heard and observed, will always be more and different from what the speaker believes to have communicated. This creates a semantic field that disrupts dialogical expectations by subverting the scope of referents to encompass a widely divergent range of unconscious communications thereby generating an exploratory inquiry that is constantly revising and amplifying itself through negotiations and renegotiations that identify, investigate, deepen, and reword everything unconscious that comes its way. By so modifying the semantic field to include affect-states, paralinguistic signals and signs, projective transmissions, as well as ambiguous or conflictual symbolic communications, psychoanalytic dialogues will always gain from the input of a qualified observer who, like a mirror scanning the rear view, can see more of the unconscious dynamisms than can any of the participants.

This is also a uniquely ***reflective*** and ***reflexive*** dialogue. The establishment of an "observing ego," with its corollary gains in impulse restraint, the capacity for delay, observation, reflection and, most importantly, for its role in enabling emotional "working-through," might well be considered key operative factors of the psychoanalytic method. The "observing ego" and capacities for "working- through" function in tandem; the former by observing unconscious reactive-patterns, the latter joining emotional content and verbalization, literally trans*forming* its expression through communication. Working-through might be conceptualized as a process of "emotional referencing," thereby anchoring *"affective referentiality"* in speech activities that coincide with other referential processes of psychoanalytic dialogues. From a neurobiological perspective, this involves establishing "new neural networks through gradual habituation" which, from the standpoint of cognition, amounts to "learning new skills in communication, the mastering of mounting unpleasure, and the expansion of 'referential activities'" writes Gedo (1991 p. 339). Only these new intrapsychic capacities, he asserts, enable the achievement of the kind of insight that is requisite "for continuous adaptation through self-inquiry" (p.339).

The unique demand to participate while oscillating between observing and reflecting on ones contextual experiences begins in the personal analysis and attains technical status only after lengthy practice in the clinical stance. Once understood as a dissociative splitting of the ego (Sterba, 1934) this unique bi-directional, analytic referentiality that looks both outward and inward simultaneously, sets up the preconditions for deep psychological self-inquiry. For the analyst, this implies a steady self-vigilance, a quickened ability to identify, assimilate and privately refer to a wide range of nonverbal and verbal stimuli, and to store this reservoir of information for use at a select time. For the analysand, the entire analytic process entails becoming more and more adept at maintaining governance over this reflexive capacity in the face of a deepening and increasingly detailed exploration of powerful, often derailing, contextual experiences.

This leads to another unique characteristic of the situation, its ***multileveled, multidimensionality***: in the opening phase, transference manifestations are spread throughout the whole personality, remaining relatively subdued, until their "latent potentialities" (Stone, 1961 p.68) are stirred by the disintegrative effects of free association and the intensification of the analytic relationship. The psychoanalytic situation stimulates the arousal of a multileveled *transference continuum.* Manifestations of transference derivatives emanate from diverse developmental points along this continuum, from the earliest, most archaic, physio-affective discharge patterns, to increasingly differentiated conflictual configurations and symbolically determined ideation, each stratified over the other. Transference expressions come into sharp relief in light of their unsolicited inappropriateness in this context and due to their dramatic persistence. As a unitary psychological phenomenon, however, "the transference" may be identified, observed and analyzed, only insofar as it stands out, and to the degree that its patterns, forms, and impulsions, can be identified, interpreted and worked-through. Hence, the 'observing ego,' ally of the analytic process and secure anchorage for its reflexive tasks, is essential for effective analytic work. It provides moorings in the *real* and *actual* analytic relationship when the eye of transference storms threatens these holdings.

Analysts ought to be able not only to distinguish between, but also appreciate, the variability of semiotic and pre-semiotic organizations expressing different aspects of their analysand's personalities and must strive to articulate communications that are tailored to reach both the phenomenological level of experience to which they directly refer as well as the more ego-centered intellectual capacities to which their analysand may reach. There is, as Stone (1961) commented "throughout the process, the presence of the patient as an integrated adult personality, larger than the sum of his psychic parts or functional systems" (p.55). Stone spoke of the multidimensionality of this dialogue and of its various coexisting patterns of interaction with wisdom and eloquence that is to be savored as it is to be handed down:

> In over simple terms there are three discernable patterns of relationship between analyst and analysand, no one of them

> obliterated (although it may be ignored), coexisting and intimately interrelated in contrapuntal fashion: the real and actual integrated personal relationship, which includes the basic vocational...relationship; the transference-counter-transference relationship; and finally the unique system of routinized activities, deprivations, and prohibitions which find origin in the requirements of analytic technique....Unfortunately, these cannot be separated in fact, as they can be by a few lines in schematic representation; and an error or lapse in one section is reflected in all. (p. 55).

And earlier:

> There is every reason to assume that anything which the analyst does or says impinges in some respect on all topographical levels, on the three psychic structures, gratifies (or otherwise) both rational and nonrational current and infantile strivings, in extremely varied and complex economic distribution. (p.49)

Concluding:

> ...it is an inescapable fact that there is more in the patient, and more in the doctor respectively, than patient and doctor or child and parent, and the extra factors can weigh heavily indeed. (p. 44)

Another important characteristic of this psychoanalytic semantic field is its ***atemporality.*** The dialogue's dissolution of normal social interchange, its special subject matter, purpose, and interpretive focus, together, create a space echoing the transitional space of ritual. Carved out of ordinary daily life, in a suspended time and place governed by its own internally generated operative laws, both the analytic and ritual processes are designed to engender specific contextual conditions that are conducive to psychological transformation. They differ fundamentally, however, in the ways they implement this, specifically in terms of their semiotic functions: ritual depends on formalized, symbolic *actions* to transmit its wisdom and elicit change; whereas psychoanalysis insists on a purely semantic space based on emotionally worked-through and verbally communicated personal insight to exert its impact. Yet both share the well defined, triphasic design, or "*schema,*" in Van Genep's (1909/1960) words, of transformative dynamics: typically, an initial phase demarcating entrance into a transitional realm at variance with daily life and conventional behaviors; a middle, liminal phase of deconstruction or "dismemberment" and ambiguity, with a dismantling and gradual reconstitution of the personality with new attributes; and a terminal phase of reaggregation and completion marked by a return to societally mandated roles, with the functional transformations obtained through the process now fully internalized. [In a sense, this entering-and-exiting from the timeless unconscious is also repeated microgenetically every analytic session, an exercise that seems to have a beneficial, even important, effect on psychic pliance and integration.] Both settings are specialized situations, set apart yet sanctioned by society as mediational devices to facilitate transition, maturation and change.

Time, in the passing of the analytic hour, stands still in an ever current present that accommodates tellings that move in "temporal circles" (Schafer, 1981, p.38) oscillating between enactment, recollection, working-through and narration, spiraling discontinuously around and around, again and again, as the discourse gathers what it can and spins and grinds all into its communicative blend governed by words and verbalization. The breakdown of conventional codes of discourse in conjunction with the disorienting effects of free association apparently engender a kind of fluid, dissolution of the public veneer and concomitant excitation of the inner eye, with a corresponding de-differentiation on the interpsychical plane. Mired as they are in misidentification, transference revisitings resist verbal representation and recollection. The chain of repetition is blunted only by a situation that modulates their impact and automaticity through reflection; the interpolation of thought and language, mediational means that can temper action and reaction, stilling the past with a grammatical turn of tense.

From this timeless nexus of condensations, displacements, contentless moods and imagery, the stuff of psyche, through the persistent analytic focus and sheer semanticity of the dialogue, more and more unmetabolized or banished thematic threads emerge to be named, worked-through and finally understood, in that integrative, transmutative process of personal knowledge that is psychoanalytic insight. Not only are "the conversion of primary-process elements into directed thought, the extension of the integrating scope of the ego" and the preservation of the relational tie in the face of transference distortions, all "mediated...through the indispensable function of speech" (Stone, 1961 pp. 100-101) but, most importantly, it is the degree of referential distance, the essentially abstractive quality of secondary process speech, and the depth and breadth of referential scope reached by means of the dialogue's exchanges, that sets psychoanalytic inquiry apart, rendering it far more comprehensive and superior to other forms of self-knowledge.

With speech as the primary instrument, different types of language functions come sharply into view, particularly, the figurative, descriptive, expressive and conceptual. It is important for analysts to distinguish between these different forms of verbal communication, to be aware of the different responses in state, imagery, or ideation they elicit since each is indicative of different levels and types of semiotic organization, different cognitive styles, and qualities of thought. Genuine insight, that results from having worked-through many archaic and defensive elements, that gives evidence of linking past with present, affect with intellect, comes slowly, only after the complete analytic triad — identifying, naming, and working-through — has been repeated many times. This, I believe, is what it means to replace Id with Ego, to reconfigure intrapsychic organization, and to establish new neuronal connections (Gedo, 1995) by forging referential skills that facilitate selective responses.

As "the sole psychobiological bridge" (Stone, 1961, p. 86), speech becomes heavily overdetermined in this situation, taking on the indicative, denotive, descriptive, conceptual and abstractive functions of language, as well as subsuming the expressive repertoire of an entire spectrum of communicative modalities that ordinarily are spread among various organismic channels. In addition to motor inhibition, eventually, eye contact, facial expression and even hand gestures — as expressive or discharge channels — are curtailed in favor of linguistic articulation. Virtually all of the considerable tensions aroused by this situation are to be funneled exclusively through the vehicle of speech. In this way, the externalization of ideation, the regulation of action and modulation of affect, the negotiation of response and mediation of the entire semantic field, is filtered through the muted and focused vehicle of verbal symbolization. As Stone (1961) commented, with reference to the secondary process language of insight, "we superimpose speech on speech" (p. 86).

Insofar as the psychoanalytic process is generated by a situation created entirely by language, it seems to me that we have focused too little on the diverse forms and functions of linguistic communication to which the dialogue gives rise and upon which it specifically depends for its therapeutic action. It is important to be able to differentiate between talking that is serving pre-semiotic discharge, attachment, exhibitionistic, restitutional or other developmental needs, from communications that reflect the kind of conceptual and abstract articulation resulting from genuine insight, with its ancillary integrative and transformative effects over the whole personality.

This leads to the last three interrelated, predominant characteristics of the clinical situation; namely its ***integrative, transmutative*** and inherently ***maturational*** properties. It is ***integrative,*** by virtue of its knitting together past and present, emotion with language, impulse and reason — the "broad psychobiologic sweep of the analytic situation" (Stone, 1961, p. 105) — and insofar as it sets up the conditions for the mediation, "through the complex psychosomatic activity of speech" (Stone, 1961, p. 105), of a vastly expanded range of emergent experiences. It is in this sense, I believe, that Gedo (1995) refers to working-through as a treatment "modality," emphasizing that the "crux of analytic work is changing those biological functions we call thought processes" (p.339) The discourse is integrative, also, in so far as it harnesses and supports whatever innate developmental drive toward autonomous, functional wholeness is present. Personal insight, moreover, is integrative — a "correlate of biological maturation, a phenomenon of integration" (Stone, 1961, p.106) — because it spurs the whole personality toward favoring higher levels of conscious, symbolic organization.

That the discourse is inherently ***transformative***, by its very purpose and functions, is self-evident: it radically transforms archaic, infantile impulsions, beliefs, and repressed emotions and ideas. But the clinical situation is transmutative in a deeper and more fundamental way; we do not merely point to unconscious phenomena and enacted behaviors, we are expected to facilitate a complete transmutation of their form; not only to signify but to *symbolize* their unconscious sources and meanings. By our inquiry and communications we strive to catalyze a more general movement toward a functional transposition of the very modes through which unconscious experiences are expressed. It is to this trans-morphological action of the semiotic processes of this dialogue, and their correlate intrapsychic restructuring, that I would especially draw attention.

The analyst in the analytic situation represents a symbolic order. One of the main responsibilities of this role is to serve as a model or guide fostering the high value that is placed, in this process, on verbalization. As the bearer of this symbolic order the analyst insistently renders the therapeutic dialogue reflective and reflexive for both participants, engendering, from within the experiential center of the situation, an inducement to stand back, inquire, reflect, conceptualize and understand. In addition to vigorously exercising the indicative, representational and communicative functions of language, the combination of subject matter and this emphasis on speech, fosters continuous efforts at symbolization, so that in both a functional and formal sense, the semiotic activities of this dialogue are inherently *maturational.* Language forces differentiation and delay in its articulation of ideas, promoting degrees of conceptualization that strengthen self-regulation, autonomous thinking and self-expression, through communication.

This group of qualities transmitted by the analytic attitude, in conjunction with the unconscious dynamisms the situation rekindles, potentially provide a therapeutic spread that spans from the most basic attachment and containment needs to the highest inducement toward self-knowledge and cognitive-abstraction. It is as though the multiple functions of the situation parallel the multiple dimensions of material that flows from pre-symbolic and symbolic spheres, reemerging as though in order to be revisited. The fact that the analyst strives only to "understand" and, by inquiry and interpretation alone, to translate and "give back" in words the analysand's unconscious presentations, evokes a transference dynamism harking back to the earliest fundaments of basic trust, the capacities to attune and interact, and to that array of multifunctional transactions that simultaneously converge in the ministrations of good-enough early care. I have in mind the crucial impact of the maternal gaze in the development of the self—the visual mirroring of the mother of infancy – and the visual vigilance, protective, admiring and affirming, of the mother of toddlerhood.

One has the impression that in this semantic space, where most para-linguistic interactive gratifications have been barred, that the acts of listening and understanding — even the still presence of the analyst — may become substitutes for a variety of intensely cathected and developmentally crucial, nonverbal, communicative functions. In semiotic terms, however, there is an enormous functional gap between *equating* with and representing. At the least differentiated non-verbal end of the transference continuum, the space itself can become a reliable, holding, pacifying, organizing environment, in which talking, and the analyst's interpretive activities, become *equivalents* of the "seeing" and being "seen" dialectic of early mirroring. In fact, at the deepest levels, the setting may quite regularly call up and provide gratification for a universal transference configuration actualized in many archetypal care-giving situations. Here the analyst is cast in the role of healer, Promethean guide, shaman, priest confessor, rabbi or any other earthly stand-in for an all-knowing, parental protective deity, the analyst's activities taken in and appropriated as substitutes for an array of care giving ministrations with eroticized undertones; words may be serving as stand-ins for milk, sustenance, kisses, pills, drops, sap, semen, omens, directives, blessings, or any other derivatives of love to which the individual human mind may turn.

Where language is the only currency of communicative interchange, its use may become endowed with substitutive value, its very functions cleverly exploited to serve the purposes of resistance. As the most efficient and effective bridge connecting one mind with another, talking "lends itself all too readily to hidden trends of the transference resistance, to a sort of paradoxical 'acting out' of primordial transference tendencies within the framework of the actual analytic work" (Stone, 1961, p.103). Thus desymbolized, 'talking,' has been diminished to a restitutional means rather than an instrumental medium, the situation itself reduced to a form of self-indulgence rather than a dialogue of self-examination.

Yet from this same primordial pre-semiotic plane, along the transference continuum, there also spring buoyant urges, equally compelling, pointing in the obverse direction, toward separation, differentiation, autonomous thought and mastery. The counterpart to those de-symbolizing regressive tendencies pushes progressively for the relinquishment of restitutional substitutes, toward the redirection and transformation of primitive aims through sublimatory fulfillment on a semantic stage where a cluster of individuating activities induce differentiation, self-knowledge and, consequently, the use of the analytic dyad for *symbolic* exchange. Stone (1961) considered this trend as representative of the "mature" (I would say progressive) wish of childhood, a legitimate source of gratification paralleling the "whole great complex of instruction" and benevolent parental lessons of early years, in which the "teaching of language in its representational and communicative functions is of basic importance" (p.50). Stone (1961) poignantly captures what has to be the common essence of the deepest of these human developmental longings, in this passage:

> A wish for help in mastering the baffling and challenging outer world of living and inanimate objects and forces, the pressures of somatically experienced discomforts and urges, and most of all the mastering and directing of a dark and mysterious inner psychic world. (p. 50)

One is impressed by the extraordinary pliancy and plasticity of the whole context and by the breadth of reference and multifunctional potential of the dyad's communications. It is astonishing to note how the fortuitous fit between the recommended stance for the analyst and the required speech form for the analysand gradually create a semantic matrix of exquisite verbal intimacy fostering ideal conditions from which to safely plummet the subjective depths of human experience, as has never been done before. One marvels at the modernity of Freud's vision, who, more than half a century before relativism had definitively pointed our gaze toward the sovereignty of language, devised a dialogue that would simultaneously subvert the limitations of linguistic signification while pushing to outer referential limits the potential reflexivity of verbal exchange. Freud invented a discourse, I would add, that by its self-generating, ever expanding scope, would, of necessity, eventually lay bare the very semiotic building blocks that produce the phenomenological underpinnings of all human experience.

The basic analytic attitude — an attentional stance of sustained benevolent interest, "excluding the slightest nuance of exploitation," (Stone, 1961, p. 42) — is able to communicate the analyst's primary function, namely, to understand. Whether in silence or through words this multidimensional attentional stance reflects the biopsychical amplitude of reference from which the analyst 'attends' to the analysand, a disposition which, given the now widened scope of psychoanalytic therapy, can transcend even the most deeply barred recesses of private isolation and desolation. This emphasizes all the more that the analytic attitude embodies a *symbolic* stance which must stand at full referential distance from a multitude of unconscious manifestation.

Given its breadth of reference, the analytic situation brings into play a spectrum of therapeutic potentialities all operating simultaneously: constancy of time and place and the creation of a safe semantic space; the analysts nonjudgmental stance, careful inquiry and willingness to use him/herself receptively; and the insistent orientation toward bringing everything that appears on the analysand's preconscious horizon into the interpretive domain — all factors pertaining to the basic situational rhetoric and formal conventions — are inherently therapeutic factors, regardless of the particulars of every communication or each analyst/analysand pair. In this way, the clinical situation is able to function therapeutically according to the functional level through which it is currently experienced by the analysand. An accurate assessment of what that organization or dynamic need is, however, whether it is resistive, restitutional or collaborative, or (more likely) a combination of all three, and of how best to formulate a focused yet encompassing intervention, is contingent on the analyst's personal sensibilities and communicative skills. Recognizing which of the current threads of content is most dynamically pressing, and the choice of how to understand this or intervene, at any given moment, rests entirely on the analyst's theoretical frame of reference, timing, and verbal discretion. And this, given that the analyst is both instrument and medium, has as much to do with *who* the analyst is as how much he/she knows. It is a given, in this profession, that everything about the analysts age, sex, tone, knowledge, and subtle nuances of expression, all contribute to the shaping of the process.

Contrary to current popular trends that encourage a more or less spontaneous communication to the analysand of the analyst's private contextual responses, in my view, this habit, which takes a good thing too far, is not only undesirable but potentially even harmful. Claiming this to be an appropriate use of the "countertransference" (in its generic sense) those advocating this practice, in my opinion, fail to recognize the value of the dynamisms created by the unequal tilt of self-disclosure. Due to the analysand's fluid and fluctuating functional organizations within the dialogue, moreover, there is no telling in what way or how such personal pronouncements will be heard. There is a big difference between being cognizant privately of ones responses—personal or evoked—and using this information to increase ones understanding, and blurting this out precipitously in a communicative field where the analyst's every word ought to be measured. The analytic stance and interpretive commitment is poised toward understanding the analysand: excessive self-referencing tends to undermine the entire dialogical structure, obfuscating its primary intent. Whether conscious or unconscious, intent, is of prime importance in this context: the analyst's special preparedness and expertise are used in the service of understanding the patient. Precisely because personal responsiveness and communicative skills function as *technical instrumentalities,* in this situation, the stance advocated by Freud proves again and again, to safeguard the requisite, referential distance from which to do analytic work.

We seem to have lost sight today, in ways the earlier analysts had not, of the extraordinary power of this situation. Paradoxically, the more we have come to understand the subtle complexities emanating from this discourse-matrix, the less we seem to remember the necessary precautions; as Loewald (1970/1980) cautioned, "Psychoanalysis is...as dangerous and as promising an understanding as atomic physics, depending on how we use this emerging power of understanding the formation, composition, decomposition, and reorganization of the human psyche" (p. 282).

The therapeutic encounter begins as analyst and analysand agree to work together: this basic treatment contract serves as the foundation from which to observe and assess all that will subsequently emerge within it. The clinical process thereby set in motion is contingent on the interpretive activities of the analyst who initially orients and continuously steers the dialogue toward fulfilling its superordinate treatment task "to make conscious everything that is pathogenically unconscious" (Freud, 1917, p. 282) and to strengthen the ego. In our exploration of the unique features of this communicative field we noted that by its formal conventions it subverts and violates ordinary codes of dialogical exchange; it is uneven, emotionally tilted from the beginning and, by its odd speech patterns and purpose creates a dynamism whereby the expectations of the analysand, to be helped, are dynamically opposed to the analyst's, to understand. The "fundamental" rule only exacerbates this central dynamism initially accentuating the sharp discrepancy between the analyst's special preparedness and the analysand's vulnerability and unclear view of the situational tasks.

This creates a situation in which the two participants start out with apparently antagonistic aims: the analysand wants to *feel* better rather than *get* better, strives to elicit response rather than free associate, to act out rather than reflect, and is compelled to reproduce rather than verbally represent. The entire dialogue becomes devoted to a reconciliation of these discrepant goals. Analysands are further disadvantaged by their scant understanding of the discourse's main referent "the unconscious." For most educated people this word is merely an abstraction, a fascinating "idea," distanced from anything real, that is, until they come face to face with experiencing their own! Then it becomes a threatening internal presence, slippery, potentially overwhelming, very difficult to articulate verbally, to be both guarded against and avoided, simultaneously. For analysts, this is familiar turf, "the unconscious" an umbrella term for a group of multidimensional manifestations expressing powerfully active facets of their analysand's psychical makeup and experience. The analyst is in his/her interpretive domain, and its referential dominion is ample. For the bewildered analysand the "unconscious" has suddenly become what is being pointed to and interpreted of his/her own unbidden behaviors, attitudes, feelings, dreams and words.

But this is a no fault situation for the analysand; the fundamental rule was made to be broken. Indeed, it is a verbal task contrived in such a way that neither can it be accomplished nor can it fail because, in one sense, it functions much like a decoy: it was set in place in order to become the "target of the attacks of the resistance" (Freud, 1917, p. 288), designed to elicit and make accessible to observation and analysis everything the analysand cannot, and could not, possibly say. It makes sense that a dialogue designed to uncover "the unconscious" would have to be devised in such a way as to itself become the means by which to bring all that is unconscious sharply into view. And it is here that Freud's genius inspired him to take every apparent obstacle to the process as it arose and turn it, instead, into a vehicle of cure. As his understanding of the regularities and dynamisms of the dialogue grew he harnessed the "resistances" and made them the objects of interpretation; "the greatest threat to the treatment, becomes its best tool, by whose help the most secret compartments of mental life can be opened" (Freud, 1917, p 444).Understanding and overcoming the 'resistance', as it arises, becomes the central function of the treatment.

Resistances are of many different kinds, often "extremely subtle" and "hard to detect"; they exhibit "protean changes in the forms they take so that the analyst must be distrustful and remain on his guard" (Freud, 1917, p. 287). Moreover, resistances, are fluid, constantly fluctuating in intensity, typically increasing "when we are approaching a new topic…most intense when we are at the climax of dealing with this topic" and dying away "when this topic has been disposed of" (Freud, 1917, p.293); and, resistances are of inestimable value in bringing to life and exposing dynamisms that are still actively contributing to current psychological problems; they "include so much of the most important material from the patient's past and bring it back in so convincing a fashion that they become some of the best supports of the analysis if a skillful technique knows how to give them the right turn" (Freud, 1917, p. 291).

It ought to be said that the concept of "resistance" springs from a dynamically oriented etiology, maintaining that were it not for such dynamically motivated impediments analysands could remember, acquire insight, and be rid of their problems. Given what we now know of the broad range of psychological phenomena, all unconscious, to which we refer in our discourse this, would, of course, be an impossibility. No one can recall their unrepresented past, verbalize their identifications or tell us about their defenses. Most people have considerable difficulty fathoming the meanings of their own dreams so alien to conscious awareness is the vast vocabulary of the unconscious. But not everything that cannot be communicated verbally is necessarily repressed, in a dynamic sense; early identifications, compromise-formations, and the unrepresented past are pre-semiotic organizations, bio-psychically encoded, to which we have access only through their contextual derivatives reemerging in the transference. In effect, not all resistances are actively "resistive" in the same way.

All the various dimensions of the unconscious to which we refer in clinical discourse are, by definition, inaccessible until one has some familiarity with psychoanalytic referential perspectives and the special reflexive, semiotic steps required of psychoanalytic work. The preliminary two are the same universal means by which all verbal denotation singles things out, separating figure from ground, and those familiar with the microgenetic progression of symbolization will recognize the sign function in *identifying* and *naming*. But psychical phenomena are not "things" or objects. Dreams, transference expressions, unconscious affects, ideation and introjections, are experiential phenomena, emerging unbidden, their qualities and attributes notoriously difficult to name. These experiential referents—the material of our analysis—are derivatives of intricately and deeply interwoven dynamic networks of archaic patterns, defensive attitudes, early identifications and primitive affects, which, in order to "catch the eye of consciousness" (Freud, 1917, p. 296), require the catalytic interventions of a skilled analyst accompanied by the additional inner eye of an "observing ego."

We can appreciate the extraordinary efficacy of this goal-directed dialogue which, paradoxically, must both generate *and* analyze away the 'obstructive' material upon which it depends for its task. It accomplishes this by so arranging it that the interlocutors perform the requisite steps jointly in a dialogical dance that advances the communicative stages through the interpretive process. In order to both circumvent yet utilize the bi-directional tendencies running through the entire process, the analytic dyad functions toward a single aim by assigning complementary roles, participants sharing the burden of a persistent dynamism that pulls in opposite directions: forward toward knowing and understanding; backward to enacting and repeating.

The analyst's task is to keep the discourse moving towards its primary goal and he/she provides the momentum through an untiring, nonjudgmental spirit of inquiry. The dynamic complementarities operating within the dyad, through their joint tasks and discourse goals, produce the characteristic oscillations and cyclicity of clinical process, as phases of heightened resistance swell, rise to prominence, are worked through, and subside again temporarily. This pattern repeats itself over and over again until the discourse matrix has gathered unto itself myriad threads tied to unconscious issues that continue to emerge, pressing for integration. What the analysand gradually learns is the full scope and nature of the 'situational definition' — or, how the discourse actually works. And, given adequate reflective capacities, what are ever so gradually internalized, are the reflexive referential means and semiotic steps to be able to continue the analytic procedures independently, after the transference has been resolved.

In this sense, the analytic meetings could end when the analysand has grasped the situational definition and fully internalized the prerequisites of analytic inquiry and introspection, and can perform them autonomously. This, however, does not occur until the full force of the personality dynamisms have emerged, as it were, to tell the whole genetic tale and see it through. Perhaps, psychoanalytic contexts serve the very purpose of providing a consciousness-raising "stage" where the personality can be seen and reworked; *both* the internalization of the semiotic functions *and* the working-through of emergent material, *together,* are operative in bringing about the radical psychological restructuring that results from the analytic process.

It is here that Vygotsky's concepts and approach to the study of learning can be immensely helpful in understanding the particular stages and forms of semiotic mediation that operate in the transition from interpersonal dialogue to its intrapsychic structuring. We approach our examination through two interrelated semiotic concepts; the 'situation definition' and 'intersubjectivity', loosely defined as "what the context is all about and how we establish a linguistic basis to get where we're going." Our overriding goal in clinical discourse, is to put everything into words; yet, as I have been stressing, the experiential nature of the principal referents of the 'unconscious' are notoriously resistant to verbalization, as are the defensive reasons for not 'saying all'.

In early development, when there is yet minimal mediated accord regarding situational definitions, 'intersubjectivity' cannot be established through abstract, linguistic formulations but has to be grounded in context-bound signs (Wertsch, 1985, p.161). A very similar situation is recapitulated in clinical discourse where points of intersubjectivity are transiently established at the level of contextually-bound (and often subliminally transmitted) signals and signs before they are negotiated linguistically, their meanings investigated and articulated in verbal terms. The analyst's stance and attunement to unconscious communications promotes points of intersubjectivity at presemiotic levels before they are brought into the dialogue and negotiated upward, as it were, where their meanings can be explored through linguistic exchange. The dialogue begins with a minimal level of shared 'situation definition' demanding of the analyst continuous acuity in identifying enacted/resistances which, if not identified and worked-through, may threaten to derail the process.

In order to be theoretically useful, the concept of 'intersubjectivity' has to be understood and used in its *semiotic* sense, not to signify a permanent or fixed condition (as in its current, misconstrued use) but as a fluid, constantly fluctuating range of provisionally-established mediated states that are, to greater or lesser degrees, created, lost, renegotiated and reestablished, lost again and recemented continuously, through continued verbal transactions. The issue of how and in what ways different forms or levels of intersubjectivity between interlocutors in the clinical dyad are established, lost, renegotiated and maintained, lies at the heart of a semiotic analysis of clinical process which examines the actual operative steps of the dialogue's functioning in the transition from communicative exchange to intrapsychic restructuring. Observed developmentally, it is clear that internalizations are intimately related to degrees of psychic-differentiation and to the nature of the discourse reference.

These several semiotic/referential steps to which I have been referring as the 'analytic triad' — identifying, naming and working-through — reflect three points in this transition from dialogical exchange to intrapsychic internalization. The final phase of this referential process, which consolidates in the personal formulation of psychoanalytic insight, fulfills the primary goals of this discourse. Initially, the requisite referential steps leading to insight have to be dynamically apportioned between the analytic pair. But ultimately, the ability to do this independently indicates that the dialogue's very functional processes have been fully internalized.

If we return now to the beginning: it's as if, upon listening to the analysand's presenting issues, the analyst were to ask: "Why do you suppose you are currently experiencing these problems? Any idea what has led up to them?" and the analysand, throughout the course of the process, proceeds to revive and show instead of tell. We can now fully appreciate the extraordinarily effective instrumentality of a dialogue founded on a paradoxical necessity: that it must itself engender the contextual arousal and demonstration of everything that it must analyze away. In this sense we would expect to find, along its course, as many kinds of resistances to verbalization as there are referential perspectives in our semantic, since each perspective points to a facet of the unconscious that resists linguistic formulation in a different way and for different reasons. A typology of resistances, aligned with logical principles of symbolization, would greatly enrich a theory of technique.

Three broad phases are discernable in the course of the analytic process. Each is characterized by its own predominant forms of resistance and breakthroughs, deepening and shifting the nature of the material that rises to prominence. Passage through each phase takes place by navigating through specific emergent issues and transference constellations. This occurs in minute to minute transactions (microcosmically) as well as more slowly over time (macrocosmically), the analyst gaining familiarity with the analysand, the analysand with the dialogue's procedures. Roughly speaking, the situation engenders three major phase-specific resistances: i) to its speech patterns; ii) to the feelings it arouses; iii) to its ending.

At the outset difficulties around free association and the analyst's sparse responsiveness often take center stage. Informed of the fundamental rule, Freud (1917) describes:

> The patient endeavors in every sort of way to extricate himself from its provisions. At one moment he declares that nothing occurs to him, at the next that so many things are crowding in on him that he cannot get hold of anything. Presently we observe with pained astonishment that he has given way first to one and then another critical objection: he betrays this to us by the long pauses that he introduces into

> his remarks. He does admit that there is something he really cannot say — he would be ashamed to; and he allows this reason to prevail against his promise. Or he says that something has occurred to him, but it concerns another person and not himself and is therefore exempt from being reported. Or, what has now occurred to him is really too unimportant, too silly and senseless....So it goes on in innumerable variations... (p288).

Working through of the typical initial-phase issues concerning basic trust, anxieties around disclosure, intrusion, commitment, the validity of the method, and fears of the unconscious, resolve in the establishment of the "working alliance," an indication that a rudimentary 'observing ego' has sprouted along with a good-enough attachment to the analyst, both signals that the analysand has entered into a process that will now gather momentum.

The central, or middle, phase of the process is dominated by the appearance and rise of profound feelings and emotional attitudes toward the analyst who, now the fulcrum of the maelstrom, is able to meet the ebb and flow of its dynamism with technical expertise:

> Thereafter...we are no longer concerned with the patient's earlier illness but with a newly created and transformed neurosis which has taken the formers place. We have followed this new edition of the old disorder from its start, we have observed its origin and growth, and we are especially well able to find our way about it since, as its object, we are situated at its very center. All the patient's symptoms have abandoned their original meaning and have taken on a new sense which lies in a relation to the transference; or only such symptoms have persisted as are capable of undergoing such a transformation. (Freud, 1917, p. 444)

Transference is a ubiquitous human tendency. But only psychoanalytic treatment invites the full resurgence of its latent potentialities (Stone, 1961), identifies its infantile origins, and cultivates a situation wherein to analyze its constellations, taking something that is "still growing and developing like a living organism" (Freud, 1917, p. 444) and opening it up to interpretive intervention. The analysis of transference and resistance are shibboleths of the 'psychoanalytic process,' a situation constructed to highlight and examine a vital phenomenon that, by affording a unique panorama of the vicissitudes of a developmental story, also provides the analyst with the necessary leverage and means to modify its course.

By the beginning of entrance into the third phase, most major transferential issues have been worked through and, in the classical model, the transference neurosis is reaching resolution. Listening to the free associative flow during this last phase one can hear that the analysand has internalized the dialogue's reflective attitude and spirit of inquiry and is able, in large measure, to carry on the analytic functions independently.

Relinquishment and internalization are two faces of a termination process weighted by transient recapitulations of principal issues and transferential themes, and the working-through of feelings of loss, separation and mourning. Just as the process was instigated by the dialogue's procedures, now its closure is contingent on the dissolution of the analytic contract and the internalization of the analyst's presence and functions. A full resolution of the transference—and any residual forms of infantile attachment—concludes with an awareness that the analytic meetings and the analytic relationship too must irrevocably end, both having fulfilled their purpose. Closure, in this psychodynamic setting, parallels the inevitable departure of offspring from the parental home toward the fulfillment of a personally chosen and independent life beckoning from beyond home and the analytic couch, as well as the irrevocability of endings.

Both the relinquishment of emotional ties to the analyst and the internalization of the discourse's referential activities, in my opinion, are necessary for the complete consolidation of intrapsychic reorganization. But it is only after the meetings have ended that the full benefits of the psychoanalytic situation, and all that transpired within it, are fully felt, and the narrativized memory of the whole experience, fully constructed.

The clinical narrative began with the analysands presenting problems: everything that followed was taken as an exhaustive illustration and exposition of the genetic origins, contributing dynamics and current meanings, of the analysand's symptomatic picture. From the outset we have listened and observed in a special way and, from our particular viewpoints, have taken two interweaving narrative threads — the presentational-enacted and the represented-told — and woven them together to form one psychoanalytically coherent, life-historical tale. The merit of this version is not in its newness but in its amplification and completeness, having integrated much that would otherwise have continued to divide, defeat, fragment and weaken the integrity of the self.

What we have pieced together of the analysand's principal themes, sub-themes, recurrent refrains, archaic anxieties, mini- and meta-myths, that strike keys guiding beliefs that fuel the life-motif, have not appeared in temporal or chronological sequence. In order to complete a psychoanalytic narrative we have had to ferret out and make use of the contextually arising signals and signifying behaviors that provide us with a psychical, shadow subtext. The value of the presentational narrative for those aspects of our understanding that involve reconstruction is that it informs us of everything the analysand cannot re-member or 'say'; it fills the gaps of the *re*-presented story line by including hidden elements of the plot that had to be rekindled before they could be told — a narrative relived in order to be narrativized.

We have yet to systematically explore or fully understand just how many different therapeutic factors are operating simultaneously, at multiple levels and in diverse ways, in the clinical situation. From the yields of this exploration, it is safe to say that, when in good hands, the situation is pliable enough to be used in whatever way will further the analysands growth.

Referring to this multiplicity of functions, Frank (1998) writes, the reason the "search for common ground regarding the conceptualization of the analytic process has failed, is that there is no single "universal (common) process"" (p.301). Grouping analytic goals into three loose categories, the narrow, the broad and the existential, Frank states, these have "different appeal for different analysts and apply differently for each patient"(1998, p.301). These dimensions, furthermore, "vary from analytic experience to experience" (1998, p.301) depending on such factors as the formal arrangement of the setting, the nature and degree of the analysand's ego disturbances and the quality of fit between analyst and analysand. In emphasizing the broad scope of the analytic process, Frank stresses an important point. In my opinion, the common ground is to be found less in the details of each singular process than in the specific and highly specialized features of the semiotic and referential activities that generate and propel the events of any given psychoanalytic situation. In other words, in the *operative* features and unique communicative factors of each dialogue.

Freud discovered and developed a situation that by words alone enables adult individuals to alter the course of their lives by becoming aware of the psychical patterns that have carried them to their current predicaments. Never in the history of human evolution have the transmutative potential of dialogue and the transformative power of language been put to more momentous use than in the talking cure. We have, in the psychoanalytic situation, "an instrumentality of unique scientific productiveness," a dialogue of "tremendous psychodynamic range and power" (Stone, 1961, p. 111).

VI
THE SUPERVISORY SITUATION

> The supervisor is a representative of the institute, and beyond that, the institute and its committees help form the frame of reference in which the interaction between the therapist and the supervisor takes place. Against this background, what is essentially unique in the supervisory situation is the opportunity to observe, all at the same time, a group of simultaneous interactions; the interaction between patient and therapist, between therapist and supervisor, and finally the subtle effect of the organizational relationship to the institute.
> Supervision is a special type of learning process based upon the joint examination of the record of a therapeutic interaction between a patient and his therapist. Like any learning process, its possibilities and limitations are to a very large measure determined by the nature of the situation itself.
> Arlow, 1963, p.577

The supervisory situation offers an unparalleled view of the kinds of replicative phenomena and inter-transmissive dynamisms that characteristically arise in psychoanalytic semantic fields. It is also a teaching and learning situation embedded in a training setting in which the goals are to further a candidate's capacities to think analytically, understand analytically and communicate analytically. As a *research* venue, supervision is a veritable laboratory for the observation of the unconscious phenomena that arise in its semantic orbit.

In addition to sharpening complex diagnostic, clinical and interpretive skills—the "analytic working ego"—this is a dialogue that must foster personal and professional growth, quickening those sensibilities and interpretive competencies that till the soil for the use of language as a therapeutic medium. And it must do this seamlessly via exchanges that model analytic inquiry and observation as they point inward and outward to current interactions that are to be investigated and understood in an analytic way. This is, therefore, more an *educative* than a *didactic* setting, in which everything a supervisor says or does is geared toward advancing the candidates understanding of the analytic process and how to use him/herself in it: "The skills which lead to successful teaching are essentially the same which the student needs to develop in himself for therapeutic work," write Fleming and Benedeck (1966), "The supervisor, like the analyst in the therapeutic process, is the instrument of the teaching-learning process and simultaneously the observer of it." (p.2) In the truest sense, the supervisory situation is a dialogical process that must impart analytic competencies *in* process and through process.

I am not the first to stress the potential value of a thorough analysis of the supervisory situation. Early on Searles (1955) advocated an exhaustive study of the interplay between the patient/therapist and therapist/supervisor inter-dynamics, the former reflected in the latter, stating "the results of such research might well be applicable…to human relationships in general" (p.176). Subsequently, Doehrman (1976), Gediman & Wolkenfeld (1980) and Caligor (1984), all stressed the importance of studying the multidirectionality of reciprocal unconscious dynamisms in a network where there is no apparent set point of origination; Person (1989) drew attention to the uniqueness of the supervisory vantage point for observing the transmissibility of affects, the general porosity of mind, and the reemergence of internalized dyadic interactions; Luber (1991) and Baudry (1993) pointed to the tendency of the supervisory constellation to elicit displaceable and split transferences, and Dewald (1981) and Schlessinger (1981) focused on the investigation of the specific goals and phases of the supervisory process: Arlow's (1963) analysis of the features of supervisory interactions was an attempt to uncover a theory of supervision, while Ekstein & Wallerstein (1958), Fleming & Benedeck (1966) and Ornstein's (1967) works testify to the belief that an analysis of the supervisory experience, from both sides of the teaching/learning engagement, could become the point of departure for a psychoanalytic theory of learning.

Papers focusing on the problems and vicissitudes of the supervisory situation have mushroomed in the last thirty or more years. But these tend to chop up the issues addressing only one facet of a complex, dynamic situation that in order to be thoroughly understood has to be analyzed in its entirety with an eye toward examining each of its interdependent aspects in relation to the whole. Typically, rather, these papers focus narrowly either on the goals of the learning process itself, on the parallel process phenomenon, or on problems of supervisory technique and methodology. No one (with the exception of Arlow, (1963)) has attempted a methodical analysis of the unique phenomena engendered by the singular nature and purpose of this dialogue. Consequently, there is no clearly defined supervisory model anchored in principles of supervisory technique; no clear understanding of the similarities and differences between phenomena that emerge and orient the clinical process versus those that arise in the supervisory dialogue. More seriously, few strides have been made to break down into operative terms precisely what has to be taught in supervision or how, exactly, it is learned. It is still true today as Ornstein (1967), and Rapaport (1960) before him, noted that progress in this area is hampered by the absence of a psychoanalytic theory of learning. In my view, this persistent lack is a reflection of the absence of a viable theory of *psychoanalytic knowledge*, an acceptable, integrative theory of mind.

Despite a general recognition of the immense value and importance of scrutinizing the supervisory exchange in all its dimensions the supervisory situation remains largely uncharted territory. The field lacks a vocabulary through which to articulate a comprehensive analysis of dialogue: and one cannot investigate or understand what has no name. Not until we are in the supervisory position, faced with the multiple tasks and responsibilities of the supervisory role and the different kinds of experiences and processes engendered by this setting, are we confronted head on with the necessity of being able to identify and refer to discrete phenomena for which there is no name and no clear methodological guidance. Certainly, different kinds of unconscious manifestation, once differentiated, each require different interventions. This would imply having made clear distinctions between three broad classes of unconscious supervisory phenomena; 1) obstructions to understanding originating in endogenous, characteriological or neurotic problems, namely, blind spots, collusions, distortions, defenses, etc. (and countertransference proper); 2) various kinds and degrees of responsiveness, resonance and/or attunement, to exogenously originating projections and/or inductions; and 3) those non-referential forms of information transmission or parallel processes, through which unconscious interactive dynamisms from the clinical situation are reproduced in the supervisory setting. Given today's broadened scope of analytic treatment and the fact that virtually any analyst working with patients of less than neurotic organization will be exposed to the powerful tug of multiple counter-reactive forces, clear distinctions between desirable and undesirable responses in the analytic field, well overdue, are now essential.

The analysis of transference and resistance, two shibboleths of analytic technique, provide interpretive principles for clinical psychoanalysis. Basic principles underlying a supervisory method can and ought to be found by drawing from parallels and differences between the speech patterns, referential activities and goals of these two situations. Just as multiple therapeutic factors operate simultaneously at different levels in clinical discourse so, in my opinion, does the supervisory dialogue function educatively in various modes and along multiple dimensions. The old dichotomy "therapeutic or didactic" breaks down when we conceptualize our dialogues as regularly serving multiple functions simultaneously, addressing different phenomena and levels of organization through different communicative strategies. Increased understanding of the operative functioning of discourse situations and of the discrete phenomena in each, will lead to finer conceptualizations and to the use of principles of communication that reflect precise situational goals at different stages of the supervisory process. The premise is that all learning takes place in dialogical settings with unique semantic and referential foci, and that through a gradual internalization of their subject matter and formal interactions, learning that has been deeply assimilated can take place. In order for the supervisory situation to fulfill its multiple functions seamlessly it must be guided by a mounting awareness of the diversity of the unconscious phenomena it gives rise to.

At this point we might revisit the question of our philosophy of supervision, since a detailed analysis of the features of the supervisory dialogue will have to orient toward understanding the relationship between its primary referential focus and joint aims, and the phenomena that arise to facilitate or obstruct, these primary aims. My view of this is that supervisory discourse must operate dialectically moving between a contextual, experiential exploration of what emerges unconsciously in the supervisory account and hour; the specific details of the clinical case and process; and the articulation of principles of clinical analysis referring to, but also above, levels of content. In my opinion, only a referential perspective that insistently oscillates between viewing current interactions as informative of dynamisms from the clinical process and understanding the supervisee's experience of these, exercises the requisite reflexive referentiality that is the *sine qua non* of analytic work. Realizing that supervisory discourse — and particularly teaching/learning exchanges — must operate at a different, higher level of abstraction than does clinical discourse, safeguards against the following, classic supervisory pitfalls: 1) the supervisee becoming a conduit for the supervisor's analysis of the patient; 2) derailment into an analysis of the supervisee's character; 3) becoming mired in content; 4) being swept away by parallelisms instead of using them informatively; 5) becoming bogged down in theoretical discussions at the expense of process.

To some degree and in various ways, the above supervisory derailments are brought about by an inappropriate supervisory stance with insufficient referential distance from the process. But, more seriously, unclear referential focus and fuggy understanding of the supervisory contract and parameters of supervisory responsibility are, once again, primarily caused by our scant understanding of what exactly is to be taught in supervision and how it is learned. We are not helped in this by a profession that has now proliferated so many incongruous approaches as to engender an atmosphere in which virtually "anything goes," without having established shared principles for achieving precise aims. It goes without say that differences in method, beyond personal style and penchant, result from differences in theoretical orientation and where there is no generally accepted unifying theory there are, consequently, no unified methodological principles of teaching or of practice.

I agree wholeheartedly with Levenson (1984), that "in any process that is both performed and talked about, what is said and what is done are not in direct relationship to each other" (p.155). We cannot learn how to do anything well or independently by instruction alone, and "no one who knows how to do something well can transfer that knowledge by telling the other person how to do it" (Levenson, 1984, p.155). We learn by experiencing, understanding and practicing the necessary skills under the watchful eye of someone who knows more about it than we do and by familiarizing ourselves with the principles of the method. The art of learning, then, is also dependent on the ability to construct an internal model of the requisite knowledge and skills involved in the activity and being able to refer to this model as an ideal standard from which to measure different degrees and dimensions of proficiency that can be assessed along technical and aesthetic, or artistic, lines.

This applies equally to the teaching and learning of a craft as to the refining or perfecting of any interpretive art that relies on the technical, specialized use of an instrument or medium: the art of teaching, as Levenson (1984) points out, *"operates at the interstice between the word and the act"* (p.155). But what of an interpretive, therapeutic art that has no foothold in a systematic approach to the "instrument" or medium of its method? That has through years of "instrumental" metaphors confounded the difference between instrument and instrumentation, with, as Ornstein (1967) stressed, an additional difficulty "stemming from the fact that interpretation is still often referred to as the *major tool* of analysis, rather than as a *major operation* of the instrument — the analyst" (p.454). Interpretation, today, is actually only one of many different communicative forms used therapeutically. How then are we to disentangle the conceptual confusion that stems from having clung too long to preliminary metaphors connoting but not pointing to the specific attributes of psychoanalytic knowledge and the personal sources from which this specialized understanding is wrought?

What Levenson (1984) and most, however, have failed to emphasize, is that in psychoanalytic situations words *are* deeds. Our dialogues are made of speech acts: we are the instrument, language and communication our instrumentation. Given our tasks, we are required to use language focusedly, precisely, expressively, therapeutically, and to teach this purposeful, measured use of speech through supervisory exchanges that are the experiential building blocks for modeling analytic skills. Since how one speaks reflects how one thinks, supervisors have to explicitly verbalize how they are exercising their analytic skills, steering the dialogue in such a way that the supervisee will learn to do the same. These skills include focused inquiry and reflection on current interactions, an ability to discern non-indexical, enacted transmissions (i.e., parallel processes, projections, etc.) as well as identifying whatever resistive obstructions to understanding and/or learning that may originate in the supervisee's characteriological difficulties. Although this entire discourse takes place and orients toward higher levels of abstraction, the supervisory situation elicits unconscious dynamisms and phenomena in phasic progressions that in many ways are formally parallel to those of clinical process, though not *identical* either in focus, content or purpose.

Again, we will turn to Vygotsky's (1934) "zone of proximal development" to denote the distance between what the supervisee is able to understand of the clinical process independently and what cannot yet be reached without supervisory assistance. The anchoring of this concept in dialogical factors contingent on the establishment of an "interpsychical" connection, referring to that mysterious "dynamic region of sensitivity in which the transition from interpsychological to intrapsychological functioning" (Wertsch, 1985, p.67) takes place, makes it an exceptional tool for studying the elusive, "experiential learning" that takes place in supervision. Applying the concept of a "zone of proximal development" to the study of the supervisory process makes it possible to pinpoint the specific referential factors and failings that generate hurdles, hitches or obstructions to the joint purpose of the context. Otherwise stated, a detailed examination of the interactive phenomenology of this "region" exhibits those points of supervisory "intersubjectivity" that are jointly established and maintained, how they break down, derail, are renegotiated and reestablished, and their functions eventually internalized. It enables us, also, to define the unique referential activities exercised in supervisory exchanges that have to be internalized in order for their 'cognitive' operations to function autonomously. The establishment of an "alliance" and other dialogical phenomena that are tied to gradual progressions along this triphasic process, might also be rethought along semiotic and discourse lines.

Before embarking on this analysis, a brief descriptive foray: the supervisory situation is both more complex and less well understood than the clinical situation. Embedded in an institutional setting, supervision represents an important, integral, formative part of every candidates analytic training. Because it takes place when inexperience, anxiety and the general psychical strains of analytic training converge, it is subject to the infiltration of systemic dynamics. This makes it particularly vulnerable to becoming a matrix for the expression of displaced or split transferences and projections issuing from tensions originating in a number of other settings. For these several reasons, the supervisory exchange engenders a multidirectional, polypsychical field in which direct communications and unconscious transmission are occurring simultaneously at multiple levels, and different forms of information are constantly being exchanged. This is, therefore, a dialogue in which different channels of communication and different modalities of interaction are all brought into play.

In addition to becoming a veritable laboratory for observing an array of evocative, replicative and inductive forms of recounting, supervision, for the supervisee, provides a sheltered context in which to first witness and weather the disruptive battering and infectious potency of less differentiated dynamisms, from the very epicenter of the storms, and from the obverse side of the analytic dyad. Supervision, moreover, is an encounter into which both participants enter with already shared semantic and referential perspectives, a pool of shared knowledge (albeit unevenly understood), where the reflective competencies requisite for doing analytic work are familiar, if not equally, to both parties, and the capacity to sift out, disentangle from, and identify what is coming from where, are tested to ever greater degrees. It is a situation where the power and reciprocal impact of one mind on another becomes a palpable reality and where one can witness the fluid, transferability of unconscious interactive patterns as the dynamics from one dyadic encounter pervade another, and the dynamics of this triadic field can permeate an entire group.

The opportunity to observe live supervisory sessions from a one-way viewing room, on a regular basis, greatly reinforced, for me, a necessary observational di-stance from the experience. I am not the first to be impressed by the ripple-effect or inductive power of reciprocal and parallel processes (see Searles, 1955; Gediman and Wolkenfeld, 1980; Luber, 1991; and particularly Caligor, 1984, all of whom shared this interest). However, in noting parallelisms arising during group discussions immediately following the observed sessions, I was repeatedly struck by the extreme mobility and displaceability of unconscious interactive patterns, by the fluid alternation of roles in subgroups they elicited, and by their persistent impetus toward replication, until their charge was interfered with by verbal analysis and attempts at bringing their dynamisms to conscious awareness.

Suffice it to say that the supervisory situation offers a wealth of potential investigative avenues: it is a complex multidimensional context in which intersystemic and interpsychical crosscurrents intersect, and most communications are condensed, polyvalent and highly charged, making for the frequent turbulence that surrounds supervisory experiences. It is a situation that engenders uniquely varied reportorial phenomena, maximizing their emergence and visibility; and it is an educative context in which the exchange and assimilation of different kinds of information employs multiple modes of learning, a setting that lends itself to studying the vicissitudes of its triphasic teaching/learning processes.

The following comparison of the dialogical features of the clinical and supervisory situations ought to help isolate what is unique to supervision: Both situations are governed by the same overall semantic and referential scope and methodological approach; both employ the contextual exploration of emergent unconscious transmissions as a way of investigating the unconscious; and both situations are premised on the understanding of current interactions as recapitulative of unconscious dynamisms transferred from other contexts. Insofar as they attempt to make conscious what is unconscious both dialogues meet with formal and dynamically motivated resistances that obstruct these primary goals, however, both dialogues also use these apparent obstructions as a means for negotiating their aims and hence require initial, preparatory phases during which, among other things, shared referential perspectives and their particular foci of interpretive interest are established. Understanding the unique features of this referential focus in relation to different situational goals is important in establishing an appropriate stance and is quite central to understanding how the discourse functions.

Similar principles underlie two situations with very different purposes and goals: and different purposes imply different roles, different frames and contracts, different formal speech patterns, and referential activities that engender different types of dynamisms, problems and resistances. In keeping with the supervisory agenda and in order to clearly differentiate the two settings in the context of proposing a process-centered supervisory model, Eckstein and Wallerstein (1958) defined these as the supervisee's "learning problems" and "problems with learning." Accordingly, in 1966 Fleming and Benedeck proposed a model of "pedagogical diagnosis," whereby maintaining a "diagnostic" attitude toward the supervisee's learning process was advocated as part of the supervisory task. (Schlessinger, 1981). While such a stance effectively safeguards against any temptation to analyze the supervisee's character rather than catalyze learning, it elicits a cumbersome disposition and fosters a top down approach in a communicative network where multidirectional parallelisms with reciprocal impact render the supervisor subject to the very same dynamisms as the supervisee. This factor offers a wonderful opportunity for the supervisor to bring his/her own self-observing inquiry and expertise into the dialogue or to "think out loud," as Dewald (1981, p. 79) put it. Ideally, wrote DeBell (1963) supervision ought to provide the supervisee with "the opportunity to observe in reflection his own conduct of an analysis and thereby readjust and refine his observing instrument," adding, "He should in this process be constantly occupied with the translation of the clinical material into theoretical forms, and with the reverse," this exercise being "vital if the student is to become more than a rule of thumb technician" (p.548).

This statement draws attention to a number of key points: it stresses the importance of that aspect of analytic skill and knowledge that is contingent on self-monitoring and the characteristic rapid oscillations of self and other observation; it clearly identifies the importance of relating practical experience to theoretical formulations; and, it points to the dialectical nature of supervisory discourse. Nowhere is the recursive embeddedness of unconscious dynamisms between interacting systems more evident than in the semantic field created by supervisory discourse. Actually multiple dialectics are at play in this triadic field with reverberations echoing from and into its institutional setting: one dyadic encounter is echoed in another; the supervisee understands more of the clinical process through what is reflected back with supervisory assistance; the patient experiences more of him/herself through the supervised therapeutic interchange; the supervisor learns how and what to teach the supervisee through what transpires in the supervisory exchange, and this increased understanding, in turn, filters down affecting the quality and progress of the therapeutic process. The supervisory situation, moreover, is replete with uncanny triadic interpenetrative phenomena that come to light through reflective observation: "The most effective supervision, then" Doerhman (1976) concludes "depends on active insight into the interplay of forces in the parallel processes of therapy and supervision" (p.17) since the resolution of difficulties in the supervisory exchange will frequently encourage supervisee's to have more confidence in their own clinical intuition and offer more spontaneous interventions. And this, of course, highlights the profoundly dialectical nature of all psychoanalytic insight: the more one can consciously observe and understand of oneself, the more one is able to observe and understand of another.

Different kinds of insight and different dimensions of understanding, however, are sought by the two situations. And it is the *purpose* of the dialogue that determines its primary referential spread and focus as well as the kinds of unconscious dynamisms that are engendered between its participants. Clinical discourse is a therapeutic, transmutative situation, designed to bring to the fore, examine and work-through the analysand's unconscious: personal insight is its principle vehicle. Supervision is an enabling, educative dialogue: its task is to advance understanding of the clinical process and elevate self-awareness and interpretive acuity to levels of technical proficiency. Both use insight — employing those key referential steps that lead to it — but in different ways, with different foci, and for different purposes.

The goal of supervision is not to unveil or interpret the supervisee's personal unconscious but to refine those personal and communicative skills employed for analytic work while dispelling emergent impediments to learning and understanding how to analyze the case. Neither the supervisee's personal history nor personal affairs belong in this context and if the dialogue should regularly digress and degenerate to this type of content something is amiss with the frame or the supervisee is insufficiently prepared and requires further analysis. However, the widening scope of inquiry in supervision of recent years, as Teitelbaum (1990) has pointed out, has led to two major developments; "it has encouraged supervisors to take a greater interest in and be more attuned to the emotional needs and state of the therapist" in supervision, and it has "led to a greater interest in exploring and acknowledging the anxieties and interferences which emanate from the side of the supervisor" (p.249). This more interactive, process-approach to the supervisory dialogue invites supervisors to pay equal attention to their own possible contributions to a supervisory stalemate or misalliance.

One of the fringe benefits of this growing trend from the late fifties that has shifted our attention away from a patient- and technique-centered, *textual* approach toward a *contextual*, process-centered model, is that it has promoted closer scrutiny of emergent resistances and difficulties within the supervisory exchange, from within the hub of the exchange itself, and from both sides. This has resulted in a growing interest in and appreciation of the reciprocal impact of less differentiated transmissive dynamics created by psychoanalytic semantic fields and has pointedly heightened the need to make new phenomenological distinctions between the different kinds of phenomena that supervision brings to the fore. It is now essential to differentiate between defensively motivated problems in learning, collusive selective inattention (Epstein, 1986), blind spots and *genuine* countertransference reactions, from the subliminal registration of unconscious dyadic interactions reproduced in supervisory parallel processes.

One of the principal functions of the teaching/learning exchange is to sharpen and hasten the ability to make these very distinctions. This suggests that a supervisory participant-observer stance requires an active technique whereby supervisors explicitly carry out the processes of their own thinking, namely, efforts to identify the sources and understand the significance of various facets of the current presentation *in* interaction. The observation, inquiry and referential activities involved in this — the "essentials of our professional role"— as Tyler (1974) writes, are "usually at least two-thirds within the professional's mind and only a small fraction...overt where a novice could follow...effectively" (p.91). Exteriorizing some of what is going in an analyst's mind is, in fact, an effective way of modeling important steps in our professional skills, namely, the continual integration of various forms and sources of information. Yet supervision entails more than distinguishing between different types of unconscious phenomena; among its many objectives are the capacity to perceive micro- and macro-processes; to move from emotional experience to verbal formulation; to relate contextual events to theoretical concepts; translate theoretical knowledge into practical application(and vice versa) and, most importantly, to formulate and articulate timely, effective, spontaneous communications.

In order to be able to do all this effectively there has to be a vocabulary of terms in use that clearly defines and differentiates these phenomena, within a viable conceptual framework (a cognitive map) providing an idiom that recognizes formal differences. Continuing to apply the umbrella term "countertransference" to *both* the analyst's undesirable reactions to the patient's transference *as well as* to those forms of attunement and unconscious resonance that provide essential, even crucial, information, only perpetuates conceptual confusion, notwithstanding the exceptional contributions to this topic by Herman (1950), Racker (1968), Spotnitz (1979), Kernberg (1984), Springman (1986), and others.

In fact, we are encountering two different classes and levels of semiological response, the one unanalytic, the other eminently so: to 'react" to a stimulus (whether internal or external), or "reactivity" of any kind, in our discourse situations, implies a signal to signal interactive equation. This is a nonanalytic attitude indicative of insufficient symbolic distance, or a faulty attentional stance. On the other hand, resonating with or pointing to and interpreting unconscious meanings from a fully differentiated position, implies signal to sign, and sign to symbol equations. To be aware of these distinctions implies some familiarity with principles of semiotic transformation. And steps in the indexical referencing of non-referential processes (enactments, inductions or projections) can, in fact, be identified, along the lines of progressive symbolization.

The methodological confusion created by dichotomizing "teaching *or* treating" in supervision, arises, also, out of a lack of understanding of how discourse works: a dialogue does not have to be exclusively "didactic" in order to teach, or solely "interpretive" in order to impart insight (consider how much is learned in the clinical setting). Different referential forms and tactics with different communicative agendas produce different kinds of intervention that elicit very different responses. Intent and referentiality impact quite formidably on how something is known: to indicate by pointing out or to identify by inquiring, are quite different from alluding to or interpreting meaning; the former establishes joint attention, the latter invites thought.

In his incisive critical review of the supervisory literature DeBell (1963) concluded that "extensive interpretation is not the task of the supervisor" (p.555) citing various authors who proposed "confrontation" as the most appropriate supervisory form. But confrontation, today, has other connotations and, to me, appears as a last resort communication. Ideally, the supervisor does not even point out but points *toward*, the goal being to catalyze attention and enable the supervisee to do the rest. Without the personal genetic dimension or the analysis of transference and resistance, as such, neither psychoanalytic "interpretations" nor the travail of working-through, in the clinical sense of the word, are present. Yet supervisory discourse presupposes that those reflective/reflexive referential activities acquired in the personal analysis will have already considerably expanded the accessible dominion of personal awareness, and be, at least partially, in place and ready in this context to be harnessed for technical purposes.

Supervision further expands and stretches these referential demands by adding several new dimensions to them, and, more generally, sharpening and quickening the supervisee's ability to integrate multiple levels of information and translate these into focused communications. Fleming and Benedeck (1966) put this very well: "To know what one knows and how one knows it becomes part of the process of learning, and to be able to express this level of insight in words becomes a significant (albeit often ideal) part of the interaction between teacher and student" (p.27). This gap between the supervisee's current independent awareness and understanding, and what requires supervisory feedback, constitutes Vygotsky's (1934) "zone" of proximal development. It is this gap, giving rise to dynamic fluctuations and special interventions designed to bridge emergent lapses in "intersubjectivity" that creates the terrain for teaching and learning exchanges.

As in all creative ventures where background, pause, silence and stillness, relationships between intent and expression, and protocol and spontaneity, produce aesthetic moments, supervision teaches not just how to know but also how *not* to know. The competent analyst knows how to doubt, hover, wait, inquire, suspend closure, be silent, and also when not knowing is the wisest form of knowledge. All of these communicative skills have to be learned and practiced in the heat of the experiential moment, at the heart of dialogical exchange. A dialogue that actively and repeatedly exercises these skills ensures that they will become internalized in such a way as to promote the accessibility to unconscious stimuli and fluidity of response required of analytic listening.

Both clinical and supervisory situations are dynamically tilted and uneven, but in different ways and for different reasons, and, in both, analysts and supervisors have greater expertise. But whereas analytic abstinence and sparse responsiveness are technical tactics that foster a therapeutic regression and tend to increase anxiety, in supervision neither apply or are desirable. Maximum learning occurs where there is minimal fear and optimal arousal: the supervisee's level of anxiety — and identifying its sources — ought to be a supervisory priority for a number of reasons. Inevitably new and old transferential issues will be rekindled and the situation will inherently draw unto itself split and displaced transferences from other contexts. However, signs of personal growth are evident in their decreased intensity and duration, their rapid resolution (Dewald, 1981) and uninterrupted, progression of the supervisee's learning. Active feedback and engaged responsiveness are counter-regressive exchanges fostering the alliance and a type of dialogue where the panoply of supervisory processes and phenomena can be safely experienced and explored in mutually satisfying ways. Dewald's (1981) recommendation is even more incisive: "The feedback system should provide quick information about the adequacy of the performance, both positive and negative, and a constructive analysis of the ways in which behavior was inadequate" (p.80).

While the personal rigors and abandon of the analytic situation are counterbalanced by an absence of judgment and extreme confidentiality, supervision — neither as circumscribed or clearly structured — is certainly neither confidential nor judgment free. Evaluation and assessment underlie the whole situation, a factor that complicates the supervisee's communications which may be compromised by a dynamic of *suppression* rather than repression. The supervisee in a training setting is often anxiously torn between multiple educative requirements including learning how to carry an analytic case while *being* an analytic case; how to report process and conceptualize clinical events in relation to theoretical understanding; how to appear knowledgeable enough while stretching, deepening, expanding and negotiating, a host of conflicting new, personal and professional demands. A great deal hinges on the outcome of the supervisory encounter, and while the supervisor's evaluative edge can be moderated by a system of mutual evaluation, given institutional politics, most supervisees work hard to remain in their supervisors' favor.

Inexperienced, anxious to both show and hide, eager to learn, and especially to be helped in processing and organizing an onslaught of impinging stimuli, understandably, this entire complicated admixture of unmediated and dynamically tinged information emerges in the supervisory report.

Based on the "joint examination of the record of a therapeutic interaction" (Arlow, 1963, p. 577) the supervisory process begins and pivots around the supervisory report. Like any narrated account in the oral tradition, this is a unique telling minted from a particular perspective, for a particular person and situation. It is, in other words, a version of something embedded in a genre. In this case it is the supervisee's version of a clinical encounter recounted in the psychoanalytic case-report tradition. Of course it is edited, filtered and formulated through the supervisee's subjective experience and further dynamically slanted to both reveal and conceal what really went on, to put the supervisee in a favorable light. All recounting is retrodictive, the raw materials of the experience having already undergone some selection, classification, sequencing and packaging. But the overall form of this verbal account cannot really be considered apart from the kind of information that is to be derived from it, namely, its specific semantic and referential orientation, its conventions, constraints, and the interpretive sensibilities and focus of the listener. Any criticism of this type of reporting that does not take into account the *whole* interactive interplay of verbal and paralinguistic means, in this situation, is invalid because it will necessarily have failed to recognize the full yields of this reportorial form. In fact, the supervisory account is replete with information so highly condensed that it is hard to unpack it linearly. In terms of "relevant" data for psychoanalytic inquiry, the tapestry of the supervisory report is a densely embroidered cloth with damask lining!

It is true, as Kubie (1958) has written, that a candidate is required to "record and recall both the patient's free associations and his own, and simultaneously to record and recall the 'how' of their expression, and also to evaluate these, while at the same time he must be responding to the patient's free associations with his own...asking him to be free and bound in the same moment of human interchange..." so that, as Kubie continues, the supervisee has "simultaneously to be a free reactor, a participant in a complex emotional interchange, an observer, a recorder, and an objective recounter of this whole intricate chain of events" (p.229). However impossibly complex this task may seem, the supervisee's mandate is exactly the same, writes Bromberg (1984) as is that of supervisors, who are obliged to articulate out loud their mental activities: "Say what occurred; present what you do, but also share your conceptual perspective of what you are presenting; reveal all, including the experience of your own participation" (p.36).This is how analysts have to think; it is therefore also how they have to speak about what they are doing.

The fit between evenly hovering attention and free association was established to bring the unconscious of analyst and analysand closer together, engendering a sort of implicit communicative matching. Were Freud to have been searching exclusively for repressed memories he would surely have missed the transference, now the operative fulcrum of the analytic experience. Clearly, his attention was spread evenly enough over the whole interactive field for him to realize that relevant information was issuing from different sources. In fact it emerges in the expressive confluence of words, feelings and actions, so that if "analyzing the relationship between what is talked about and the behavior that goes with what is talked about" (Levenson, 1984, p.103) constitutes the analysts activity, it is also the supervisor's activity in the supervisory process. The dynamic tension between what is recounted verbally and what is reproduced and induced contextually, generates a continuous account narrated by discontinuous means: this interplay of transmissive, enactive and linguistic means tell us how something was experienced and how it is currently known

Psychoanalytic situations generate a type of discourse that reveals the phenomenology of how different kinds of experiences, differentially processed, are registered, unevenly mediated, assimilated and internalized. They call attention to the emotive ignition that sparks recall, the way memories sprout from and cluster around a single trigger, and to the highly subjective, selective nature of memory, the tenacity of affect, and how experiences are reconstituted, revived and relived as they are recounted. Just as the transferential dimensions of the clinical encounter bring into the present the developmental drama of the analysand's past, the play of voices and parallel enactments shadowing the supervisory report carry the clinical encounter into the new context.

Psychoanalytic accounts cannot be treated as decontextualized scripts that can be transmitted via flattened verbatim transcripts or analyzed like texts. The contrapuntal tessitura of their dynamisms necessitates a live teller and a skilled listener trained to recognize the polyphony of voices and medley of meanings that characterize versions of psychical tales. The receptive supervisor has before him/her a display that in many respects is a replay of what went on in the clinical process, and of communications that mirror the dynamic organizations that progress toward conscious awareness.

If the report has retained any creative spontaneity at all it will make use of a broad range of semiotic options and devices to embroider the vital texture of the account. Typically it will harness a spectrum of inductive, indexical and lexical narrative instruments that shed light on a number of interrelated processes such as attention, perception, thought, verbal symbolization, and narrative form. If a slice of supervisory process of approximately 3 to 5 consecutive utterances were selected for micro-analysis, we would be able to observe microgenetic advances in symbolization progressing through verbal exchanges that lead increasingly to the awareness of being aware. It ought not be overlooked that this is possibly the first dialogue in which the dynamic organization of consciousness has itself become a subject—we are interested in knowing *how* the supervisee knows what he/she is reporting.

Yet this type of reporting has been severely criticized for being imprecise, non veridical, even "unanalytic" (Kubie, 1958, p. 229) in its requirements, the supervisory system itself inherently flawed. No one can validate the "accuracy" either of the report or of the supervisor's assessment of the candidates "performance," writes Kubie (p.228), adding that "on these imprecise impressions, whose validity is wholly speculative, has depended the success or failure of every student who has gone through the mill since analytic training was formalized"(p.228). The supervisee's anticipation of emotional stresses upcoming in the supervisory exchange, Kubie notes, are "superimposed" on the emotional interplay of the clinical encounter creating a "continuous background of distant and faintly ominous music" (p.228) during sessions, so that what "actually" transpires in the charged supervisory situation is that the candidate "recalls and reproduces screened, biased, and altered versions" (p.229) of what occurred in the therapy. That there is any "true" resemblance between what actually took place and the candidate's report of it, for Kubie, is "almost a miraculous accident"(p.230) and it remains a "constant source of wonder" that anything at all can come of "such a procedure" (p 230) although, he concedes, it does.

Were these condemnatory remarks not prefacing his presentation of a supervisory system based on group discussions of live clinical and supervisory tape-recorded sessions — a method clearly favored by Kubie — one would have to marvel at the uncharacteristic, unanalytic emphasis on the value of "precise" impressions, "true" resemblance, "accuracy," "performance" and the importance of knowing what "actually" happened. While I would agree that the supplementation of supervisory accounts with occasional joint examinations of taped sessions is a useful, often highly informative additional tool in an ongoing supervision, this is also a procedure wrought with its own problems and pitfalls. For one, the merit of introducing an inert recording instrument to be replayed "later on" into a highly confidential context and a highly dynamic, delicate process of human interchange is open to debate.

But what is more troubling about Kubie's criticism is that it indicates a failure to recognize the informative value of the very characteristics and features of supervisory reporting that he most condemns — their spontaneous composition, dynamically infiltrated partly enacted constitution, the fact that though psychoanalytically incomplete they contain a play of voices that renders a very personal version of what transpired in the clinical encounter. Supervisors ought to be as interested in the form and style of the report as in its content, in how it is retold as much as what is selected for retelling, since both, in a supervisory sense, are "diagnostically" informative. Are we listening to an engaging, lively, interesting delivery or one that is dull, disjointed or detached? Is its compositional structure coherent, narratively filled and interspersed with relevant comments, or is it clipped, staccato, incongruous, reticent and uninformed? Does the account yield a rough sketch, can we picture the client and the interchange, or is it wordy, factual, intellectualized? Is the supervisee absorbed in it or self-absorbed? Does he/she respond to inquiry with thoughtful or flighty responses? Is he/she stimulated or made anxious by supervisory comments? Does he/she become more involved in the inquiry or become aloof, withdrawn, hesitant, etc.? It is precisely the supervisee's capacity to compose, recount, comment upon, and continue to investigate the clinical exchange that is of interest to the supervisor, to observe how open and receptive or how submissive or defensive the supervisee becomes during the joint exploration of the reported material.

The supervisory report is not a "fixed" immutable text (like a transcript) but an organic source-point for a vita dialogue wherein the speaker, who and what is spoken about and the person it is spoken for, soon form a tight, interconnected triadic network. The supervisory report as-narrative-version is an open, fluid account subject to embellishments, rejoinders, reminders, inquiry, commentary, clarification, associative expansions, modification and alteration according to the listener's listening style, referential orientation and the particular interests and conventions he/she adheres to. The supervisor's multidimensional stance and the supervisory dialogue will inevitably contribute added values and perspectives, it will uncover new meanings, make new inferences, offer technical suggestions, invite reflection and, in general, enrich and transmute the earlier version as the new voice is added to the mix.

We need to appreciate the formidable impact of the listener's stance and responsive comments on the speaker. In supervision the nuanced exchanges of the joint inquiry will themselves draw out what went on, how it was experienced and is now understood, what was "actually" said, how, when and why. If it is skillfully conducted the supervisory dialogue reveals the supervisee's current technical and theoretical sophistication or lack of it, his/her capacity for reflection, ability to move from micro- to macro-process elements, shift nimbly between various referential perspectives and positions, generating well conceptualized and articulate communications. These are the set of interests that enable a supervisor to assess how full and insightful, how psychoanalytically coherent and complete a clinical account the supervisee has been able to compose according to the reconstructive conventions of the psychoanalytic case report genre. We produce versions of versions: and a version need only be "true" to itself.

This takes us to the heart of the question of what is the primary or relevant data of supervision, a question directly related to what we consider to be the primary objectives and tasks of supervision. If we believe that our objectives entail knowing what "actually" happened, in order to compare this to the report, then we may have slipped into the detective story genre. Veridicality, or "truth" correspondence, is not a psychoanalytic concern. All that we need to know is already there, in the dialogue. A truly skilled supervisor, whose attention is keenly folded in the process — and I have seen but a few at work — will pick up almost imperceptible patterns of information from the parallel process alone. Not only interactive dynamics and affective states are reproduced and transmitted unconsciously, but also tone, volume, vocal style and physical expression, the use of particular words, a turn of phrase and even specific content. It is possible to pass "cognitive material from one mind to another," Person (1989) comments, because "the same potential for cognitive processing exists in different minds" (p.60). In fact, the parallel process is far more informative and far less disguised than is a blanched out, drearily recited verbatim transcript — of the "courtroom" (Arlow, 1963, p.588) variety — a supervisory practice I find particularly pointless so far does it take us from the vital, dynamic, interpenetrative dialogicality of spontaneous oral narration. It succeeds, in effect, in removing from the report precisely it's most important and essential aspects.

Perhaps this current vogue results from a misguided pursuit of "manifest" precision. Unfortunately, the more standardized and stylistically or defensively removed from spontaneity is an account, the more camouflaged will it be, and the more will it bar access to those very spheres of human interchange that psychoanalytic dialogues peruse. The only form of information the verbatim transcript can report is verbal content — word for word. Yet the phenomenological wealth of the supervisory account and the semantic scope of psychoanalytic referentiality reach well beyond the verbal stratum, teaching us that we have to look, listen and sense transmitted and communicated meanings that are spread among many referential and non-referential transmissive modes. An utterance in psychoanalytic discourse is like a chord or an arpeggio in a musical phrase, with resonating overtones and undertones of which one strain, the verbal line, is but a single tonal strand.

The idea then in supervision is to keep as many channels of communication (in Rapaport's (1951b) sense) open as possible, and to unblock those that are closed. The more we understand the nature of narration—the "gnosis" of narrative forms—the more will we understand that the "data" of supervision is not encased in a polished, linear "linguistic" chronicle, but is interspersed, continually called up and scattered throughout the dialogue, and will appear unevenly organized, partially digested and only partially lexicalized. It is a mistake to think that without *actually* hearing the two voices one may miss the "subtle changes in pitch and placement of voice, in enunciation, volume and pace," the "running counterpoint to the words themselves" (Kubie, 1958, p.232). The qualities of aggression, spite, anxiety or deceit, that this counterpoint reveal are relevant to us only insofar and in the ways that they have impacted on the narrator/supervisee. And it is precisely these expressive qualities in vocal interplay, with their dynamic and inductive effects, that will reintroduce themselves through subtle evocations in contextual patterns of interchange. The more we remain receptive to the subtleties of these inductive forms, considering everything as, in some way a replay, the more will we have access to the inherent wealth of information in supervisory discourse. In order to carry into the fray of supervision as much of the clinical process as possible, then, the freer, the more spontaneous the report, the better.

Typically the supervisee will begin with a thematic overture connecting recent sessions with past process, perhaps revisiting the case as a refresher for the supervisor or returning to some previously raised issue, and then, from brief notes to aid recall, will select a sequence of loose utterances including exchanges and interventions, for "starters." This sampling may be chosen from the opening and closing sequences of a session or from the middle, at random. And all of this will already be accompanied by a running commentary—explicative, descriptive, diagnostic, contemplative—replete with impressions, evocative phrases, reflections, modulations in tonal inflection, technical and theoretical queries, assessments, doubts, etc. If the report has maintained any creative license it will generally *not* proceed in chronological order, but will already give evidence of some "analytic" thinking; it will jump around exhibiting associative linkages, observations of process, assessments of meaning, it will relate present to past, the particular to the general (and vice versa) connect anecdote with dream image, focusing now on content now on form now on interaction, citing what the patient said, how it was heard, what then transpired, what the supervisee said, thought, felt, etc.,….Some things will be augmented some diminished, some embellished, some omitted…but the principle point is that the report will build on itself, recomposing and transforming its contents as it unfolds and includes supervisory input. And as the spontaneous supervisory account gathers narrative momentum it will become enlivened by a play of narrative modes and devices that alternately recount, cite, recite, describe, enact, project, impersonate, dramatize, parody, evoke, induce, and reproduce both sides and multiple levels of the dynamic patterns that characterized the clinical interactions, quite literally, *carrying in* the unconscious undercurrents of the clinical process into the new situation.

We are in the presence of a "hybrid" (Bakhtin, 1981, p.304), polyformal and polypsychical composition, whereby the speaker's voice is infiltrated by the voice of who is spoken about and the unspoken frequencies of their interactions interpenetrate the unmediated dynamisms of the current exchange, suffusing this new encounter with the subliminal texture of the other. At times the report includes formal markers between the voices but at others, where assimilated experiences are less differentiated or as yet unmediated, no formal markers separate the speakers so that the voice of the supervisee also contains and expresses the patients transmissions and the supervisor is put in the supervisee's place, thereby bringing the supervisor in close contact with the supervisee's unconscious experiences. Projective inductions[8] take hold where psychical boundaries and semiotic demarcation lines are temporarily weakened or delayed, or when the quality of attention renders the listener particularly vulnerable to their reception. In fact parallel processes manage to accomplish a number of transmissive feats including replicating an interactive pattern in its entirety, from all experiential vantage points, inducing in the supervisor feelings and reactions originating in both the supervisee and the patient *and* their interactions.

At these profoundly undifferentiated strata of interchange unconscious dynamisms pass fluidly between participants; roles are constantly alternating, a dyadic encounter transforms into a multidirectional inter-psychical field. Until identified and understood, the parallel process may draw into its sphere of influence as many people as enter its semantic orbit, engendering the ricocheting of a cast of characters and their central dynamics among all participants.

In addition to its "interanimation of voices" (Bakhtin, 1981, p.304) and inductive-presentational potency, the supervisory report enlists a hierarchy of referential forms to deliver its unevenly organized information. This play of referential modes produces a multistratal composition: according to how something is known, the report will alternately and simultaneously tell, show, transmit and comment: At the verbal level the report retells several thematic threads corresponding to the patient's "intended narratives" as Makari and Shapiro (1993, p.1004) refer to them, perhaps including a few remarks on the content. On another plain, the report reproduces some of the feel and tone, the rhythms and style of the patient's utterances and the clinical interchanges, perhaps pointing to the implicit and metaphorical sense of what was said while indirectly indicating the felt qualities of the interactions by replicating them. At still another level, the relevance of the spoken content will be superseded entirely by the emotionally charged, completely unconscious, parallel process interactive patterns that may temporarily envelope the supervisory situation. And finally, at still another level, if the supervisee is endowed with a sufficiently functional "observing ego," the working-through of these contextual experiences will trigger reflective comments indicating increasing cognizance and insight into the corresponding transferential impasses and dynamisms of the clinical process. One might say that the contextual experience and symbolic mediation of the parallel process is as essential to the supervisee's learning as is the working-through of transference for the analysand in the therapeutic situation.

From the supervisory perspective: not only do we observe an interplay of material communicated at different stages of semiotic mediation, but we also come to understand that for certain types of experience — particularly subtle emotional *qualities* — the message is most convincingly conveyed when it retains its original form. Alter the means and you alter the nature of the message altogether — alter the form and you alter the effects of the message on the listener: different functional organizations and formal compositions reflect different ways of knowing. And this factor is of great consequence in human communication.

In order to disentangle from this hybrid, multiform account and the various voices speaking from within it, it is helpful if the supervisor is familiar with the interplay of transmissive and communicative forms. In addition, the supervisor has to be skilled in selecting from the current account and interactions the most relevant thread or salient problem and respond to it in such a way as to further the *supervisee's* learning. At the height of a highly charged parallel process, only if the supervisor can hold his/her bearings and remain committed to understanding what arises as reflecting the nature of an impasse or undetected problem in the clinical process, can the supervisee follow suit and begin to observe and understand the force of these triadic phenomena. Recall (p.124) how my supervisee had become embroiled in a powerful parallel process from which we emerged only very slowly through weeks of continued reflection and discussions that served to process the multiple strands of her experience when caught at the epicenter of this stormy dynamic. The gradual working-through of this experience brought her much closer to understanding her patient's psychology and his communications to her. It seems self-evident that none of this can be done without considerable preparation and understanding of the informative significance and inductive power of the multidirectional dynamisms of this psychical field. In my opinion, just as it would be unthinkable to undergo an analysis with someone unfamiliar with the analytic process, so is it undesirable for supervision to be conducted by individuals who are unfamiliar with the referential forms and dynamic phenomena *of dialogue* that rise to prominence in this situation.

The contextual significance of reciprocally inter-penetrating dynamisms is surely one of the things that render psychoanalytic dialogues so charged and complex, making it imperative that the technical fine-tuning of analytic and supervisory skills emphasize resonance and sensitivity to the function and form of communications in terms of the nature of responses they call up in oneself. Nowhere, as in supervision, is it more evident that in psychoanalytic semantic fields process simultaneously contains and reflects content, and vice versa: this interplay of modes spins a narrative web telling and replicating a clinical tale in which non-referential evocative, exemplative and inductive replays are *taken* to refer to unmediated aspects of the encounter. Of course the supervisee is trying to put as much as possible into words: but a psychoanalytically complete and fully narrativized account of a clinical process is a slow accomplishment, requiring the articulate inclusion of many dimensions of awareness, insight and formulative skills that are developed only slowly with experience and over time. Until it has been psychoanalytically "filled out" and collaboratively, fully narrativized the supervisee's report appears through a medley of disorganized forms that mirror forms of unconscious, preconscious and conscious awareness, a report replete with thematic lines, dialogical threads, enactive spouts and the whole family of blind spots, collusions and dynamic obstructions to awareness and learning.

As previously mentioned, the already complex interrelationships between content, form and process reach a peak of complexity in supervision, where the principal subjects of reference and analysis keep shifting. The characteristic oscillations between participating, observing and formulating that take place continuously in the psychoanalyzing mind yield a verbal account that mirrors a type of thinking that must rapidly pull together many stimuli and a lot of information from different source points. A polished and complete psychoanalytic report will weave multiple dimensions of contextual experience, inference, interpretive understanding and rationales for interventions, into a seamless narrative. Students betray their novice status by presenting reports that reflect large gaps in awareness, flaws in technique, and an incomplete mastery of the integrative, formulative skills required of the narrative specifications and conventions of this compositional structure. But even a seasoned analyst, presenting a well documented clinical process, providing a psychoanalytically full and compelling commentary, with multiple dimensions woven skillfully together, will still give evidence of blind spots and lacunae in awareness that others are often only too happy to point out. Bromberg (1984) refers to this ubiquitous phenomenon as "case-conference cleverness — the uncanny ability of the members of a case conference to discover what the presenting analyst 'missed' and to hear what he did not hear" (p.37). It is common knowledge that in this impossible profession, it is as impossible to grasp *everything* as it is to observe the back of ones head, unaided. Depending on the particular function of the discourse, the purpose of its communicative interventions will vary, but the semantic sweep and referential requirements of psychoanalytic dialogues will always be contingent on a reflective dialectic that always benefits from the insightful impact of another skilled participant/observer.

If one of the primary objectives of supervision is to fine tune and reinforce the integrative functioning of sensory-apperceptual faculties and communicative competencies, a second is the initiation of the supervisee into the art and refinement of psychoanalytic case reporting. By speaking about and pointing to certain things consistently in a psychoanalytic way, supervisory discourse simultaneously models and teaches how to maintain an analytic attitude toward ones own analyzing activities. The more ably the dialogue is conducted the more smoothly will its referential patterns be assimilated.

To engender an effective learning experience with lasting educative results, the entire dialogue must fuse function with form, embodying and practicing the principles it teaches. Bromberg (1984) advocates a method designed as much to improve the supervisee's hearing as to teach principles of clinical psychoanalysis (p.34). Supervision must take place in a climate that fosters collaborative inquiry, providing the optimal conditions for self-disclosure, self-observation and discussion: "In supervision the student must be able to scrutinize what he *already* does" and "What he hears must be more than that which fits comfortably into his current perspective" (Bromberg, 1984, p.35). The accommodation and integration of supervisory input will benefit by a setting that encourages the student's active "questioning and disagreeing, comparing the supervisor's opinion and perspective with his own, freedom to comment in an ongoing way on the supervisory process itself and the supervisor's impact, and in general, an atmosphere that encourages self-regulation rather than passive ingestion" (Bromberg, 1984, pp. 35-36). It is important to realize that supervisory learning is not a given, thanks to its built in reciprocal tasks, but a dialogue created, negotiated and continuously steered by the focus, theoretical slant, and the dynamic and stylistic sensibilities of the supervisor.

It seems self evident that a dialogue contingent on the establishment of mutual trust, concordant expectations, shared referents and joint objectives; that can make use of obstructions, move through impasses and weather a crisis through sustained, educative exchanges, can only develop and take place over time. In fact, like its analytic counterpart, the supervisory process exhibits the same triphasic design characterized by 1) a preliminary or entrance phase when working goals and familiarity with personal style and professional orientation are negotiated and established; 2) a middle or central, working phase, during which teaching and learning exchanges take place in a "zone of proximal development," generating a dialogue that mediates the gaps between the supervisee's current understanding of clinical process and more complex, advanced levels of understanding; and 3) a closing phase, moving toward the termination of the meetings with increased awareness of what has been learned, concluding with a mutual assessment of what learning has taken place.

The set of conditions created by psychoanalytic dialogues are such that their successful unfolding and outcome is contingent on the formation of a solid "working" alliance. The "learning" alliance of supervision proves crucial not only because it safeguards ongoing negotiations and resolutions of potentially disruptive problems but also because it anchors the dialogue in its purpose during the demanding middle phase, when "teaching and learning" take place primarily by engaging in an often turbulent, complex triadic field. The supervisory "learning" alliance—which can alternately be viewed as the establishment of shared referential perspectives—is both the catalyst and *sine qua non* for the joint examination of those interpenetrative influences that begin to pervade this multi-psychical field. It is really only after this ubiquitous, initial phase in supervision, as Bromberg (1982, p.99) has also noted, when participants have familiarized themselves with the nature of the communicative exchanges and with each other, and when *both* have fully entered into the ways and business of the dialogue, that mutually satisfying "teaching and learning" interchange yields growth, mastery and advancement in the difficult art of clinical insight and therapeutic communication. In the language of discourse, this means that only when verbally mediated exchanges have succeeded in integrating the dialogues' subject matter, referential perspectives and purpose, consistently and long enough to generate various levels and forms of "intersubjectivity" in this field of reciprocal influence, can the full "teaching" function of the dialogue, in a psychoanalytic sense, bring lasting results.

Gradually, the expanded referential activities of supervision together with the supervisor's theoretical position and personal style will come to bear on the supervisee's thinking and, as the supervisory work deepens, we will observe different kinds of information being assimilated and internalized at different rates and in different ways. We also observe imitative and identificatory modes of learning taking place. During the course of this multidimensional experience, many different facets of clinical work will be addressed with particular aspects and issues rising to ascendance at different stages. Throughout the dialogue, however, information is negotiated regarding 1) real management, scheduling or bureaucratic issues; 2) clinical, historical data, diagnostic skills; 3) emergent process-dynamisms and phenomena, including transference/countertransference, issues; 4) technique, wording of interventions and phases of treatment; 5) technique in relation to theory, or a body of knowledge that informs how to understand process and clinical interventions. These areas of learning and knowledge constitute the referential foundations informing clinical work.

Progress in supervision is mirrored in the clinical setting and will be apparent in the supervisee's increased tendency to conceptualize, question and discuss clinical material along various dimensions using his/her responsiveness as an index of unconscious meaning. Progress will also be reflected in the fluidity and fullness of the psychoanalytically narrativized report, now predominantly *re*presented, with comments interspersed throughout indicating a broader grasp and ease in clinical formulations with more tellings than showings. In other words, progress in supervision is gauged by observing how the supervisee is speaking about the case material and by the degree to which a number of personal faculties have been integrated, shaped and honed to function in a specialized way, as professional skills. In this way the situation truly fosters personal and professional growth while teaching without being 'didactic' and treating without being 'clinical,' the old confusions regarding these two overlapping functions having collapsed into a stance that recognizes that "a great deal of information and experience must be combined with a considerable degree of psychic freedom in order to insure that the intellectually and emotionally demanding task of working successfully at the creative act of psychoanalysis can be accomplished" (DeBell, 1963, p.554).

Fleming and Benedeck (1966) and those before and since, approached their investigations of psychoanalytic supervision by studying a teaching and learning "process" the goal of which was defined as "clarification of the analytic instrument" (Isokower, 1957, in Fleming and Benedeck, 1966, p.19). Cumulatively these works have enhanced our understanding of the supervisory role, supervisory goals and the emergent problems and phenomena of supervision, which in many respects parallel and call up the very processes supervision is designed to oversee and teach. Yet the conceptual framework and language governing the formulations of these investigations both delimits and constrains the scope of their yields to what that vocabulary can, or has already, defined: we end up enriched but inevitably led back to the "instrument" metaphor.

My approach here has been to view supervision as a particular psychoanalytic situation and to study its operative dialogical phenomena and referential features in relation to its purpose and goals. This avenue led to an exploration of the many dimensions of a situation which proves of unparalleled richness and complexity. During this course, we have examined; 1) its expanded referential perspective and activities in relation to its particular focus and primary goals; 2) the triadic (and systemic) inter-psychical field of reciprocal influence that this generates and the ricocheting of parallel processes thereby engendered at unconscious levels; 3) the inductive, replicative and verbally mediated narrative modes through which the supervisory report first appears, and the development of a jointly negotiated, more complete narrativization of clinical material achieved through supervisory exchanges; 4) the subdivision between supervisor and supervisee of microgenetic steps in verbal referencing (symbolization) of emergent unconscious problems or communications leading toward advancements in clinical awareness and understanding; 5) different kinds of information being assimilated at different rates and via different mediational activities; and 6) the triphasic design of a "learning process" that concludes with the internalized structuring of the referential practices and orientation of the dialogue which can now be carried out autonomously.

It seems to me that the study of psychoanalytic supervision approached in this way provides a window into those discourse events and mediational stages that first translate and then transform the raw tissue of human interactive experiences into meaningful, intelligible, communicable exchanges. I would also emphasize — and I believe it is safe to surmise this — that referential activities of verbal symbolization that are used to mediate unconscious experiences to conscious awareness, and that come to light in psychoanalytic dialogues, reveal universal modes of human assimilation, semiotic processing, dialogicality, and narrative construction — that is, ways of knowing, — the building blocks of which rise to prominence due to a semantic with referential perspectives that is poised to identify them.

INSTRUMENTATION OF THE PSYCHOANALYTIC SEMANTIC

> I imagine I am listening to an orchestra. I hear the instruments of the orchestra one after another play the same pitch, with the same degree of loudness, and for the same duration. Although I do not hear a music of melody, of changes in pitch, yet I do not hear a sameness. I hear a music of colors, of qualities, a music that moves not from one pitch to another, but from one timbre to another. No matter what note is played, nor how loudly or long it is played, I recognize the instrument — the flute, the piano, the oboe — that plays it. No matter what melody is played, I hear beneath it the music that is the result of the passage of the melody or any part of it from one instrument to another.
>
> M. Edelson, 1975, p.169

Musical analogies are called on when words are wanting. Edelson's (1975) passage describes an innominate experience; the analyst's listening and hearing of multiple, different qualities of meaning, as he puts it, to a music of "timbres" (p.170) that lies too deep for words, in which, nevertheless, he recognizes every instrument. In his attempt to find a verbal way to capture this subterranean music he searches for "patterns of language sounds in any linguistic object" (p.171), likening the different frequencies and combinatorial qualities of linguistic communication to the subtle, tonal shades and harmonic sound waves that create music.

Yet earnest explorations of meaning cannot evade the force of form. In recognizing the power of pattern we have to realize that 'signifying' attributes differ from medium to medium, imposing their own limitations on what can be expressed, so that key constitutive elements tied to one medium cannot easily be transposed onto another. Sound and rhythm, as such, for instance, are not as centrally signifying in linguistic meanings as they are in music. A translation from one medium into another necessitates a transposition that subsumes comparable but not identical qualities and structural principles that make such a translation possible. In order to do this, a measure of fluency in the vocabulary and grammar of both is needed: where such principles are lacking, they must be found.

Although long sought, no fruitful parallels between music and language could be drawn until the common origins of their subverbal, resonant frequencies registering deeply within the human organism had begun to be traced and understood. It is here, in searching for these parallels, not only in language, or even a linguistic semantic, but in an expanded communicative framework including expressive frequencies and meaning-forms well beneath the verbal line, that a real avenue toward meeting this challenge appears. Parallels between these two vast vehicular systems can be found in the shared characteristics of those primary, most basic expressive/inductive processes that nourish linguistic and musical meanings alike, once these have been deciphered, systematized and, in some way, laid out.

The hierarchical model of human communication presented readily calls to mind an orchestral score, with its multitiered instrumental lines all played simultaneously. It provides a visual and conceptual analogue for density and continuity, the vertical and horizontal dimensions that music and human communication share. Its schematic overview (p.129) displays a visual representation of conceptual parallels that are rooted in formal and structural similarities between two systems that combine multiformal condensation with progressive transformation. Both systems possess similar structural constitutions combining depth, complexity and sequence, in compositional phrases and passages that build upon each other. They also share performative similarities: both proceed linearly in time achieving their overall effect additively; are subject to an array of interpretive possibilities including the listener's response; and both are endowed with an astonishing array of potential qualifiers, so that sense, impact, and especially emotional induction is significantly determined by timing, tone, pitch, volume, phrasing, and intent, or the particular *manner* in which elements are strung together and delivered.

Hierarchic designs are particularly effective in depicting this multistratal, crossmodal quality of communication whereby the functional dominance of language as primary communicative channel does not preclude the enduring participation of earlier modes, all of which continue to contribute, albeit in abbreviated or vestigial ways, to the full meaning of any utterance. In this sense, every utterance is a densely packed, multifaceted composite (like a dream or a musical phrase) of multiple possible meanings, to which sense and significance are given by the interpretive orientation or goals of those participating in the speech context in which it is spoken.

We have before us two vast combinatorial systems of immense complexity, dexterity and seemingly unlimited variability.

But whereas music is handed down and taught via a rich vocabulary of terms and a notational system reflecting a superbly articulated body of theory, we, who are encharged with the understanding and interpretation of human meanings, possess no comparable theoretical framework or vocabulary. This comprehensive study of human communication begins to fill this void. The conceptual analogy I am proposing makes visible a conceptual framework exposing the key formulative, combinatorial and interactive principles, along functional and formal lines, that constitute unconscious and conscious dimensions of human communication.

To apply this directly to communication: through its vertical and linear vectors the model accommodates enormous combinatorial complexity while accounting for three closely interrelated characteristics; 1) the *simultaneity* of multiple forms, multiple voices and dynamic multidetermination of meaning that typify psyche; 2) formal transformations encumbent on functional development in ontogenesis, as well as enduring *formal heterogeneity*; and 3) the idea of *correlate interactive modes*, or morphic-matching, an attunement to the overall functional organization underlying communications. This points to a listening stance that is resonant to, and aware of, form in relation to content and functional organization, an attentional disposition that is attuned to different frequencies transmitted by different formal combinations of pre-semiotic and semiotically mediated meanings, often all communicated simultaneously. The *nature* of response engendered by an utterance in our semantic field becomes an informative indicator of the phenomenological experience from which its unconscious meanings issue.

This tells us how we are to understand it in order to respond in a therapeutic manner.

A technical stance that is attentive to interrelationships between actions and words, that adopts correlative matching as a technical means to apprehend different types of unconscious information, leads to greater understanding of communicative forms themselves and of how to use communication as a versatile therapeutic tool.

The model offers a schematic viewing of the course of verbal symbolization and the impact of psychoanalytic semantic and discourse referentiality on the expansion of conscious awareness. It provides the means for conceptualizing the interdigitation of expressive, projective, enactive and ideational strands that participate in mnemonic and narrative processes, while drawing attention to the informative value of the nature of induced responses based on principles of semiotic differentiation: the signal induces reaction; signs indicate or point to; symbols invite ideation and conceptualization. Only *symbolic* denotive reference leads to conscious awareness. In naming and systematizing correlate modes of interaction within a developmental framework, and identifying the logical semiotic basis for the nature of induced responses, analysts are provided with integrative underpinnings for an internal working model that anchors clinical and supervisory experiences in viable metatheoretical principles.

Having redefined the functional activities of the "analytic instrument" in operative terms puts us in a position to assess a spectrum of personal and professional competencies that are essential for playing this "instrument" masterfully. With the help of this knowledge analysts can become aware of the specific functions and sensibilities involved in the "instrumentation" of their instrument. They acquire a referential system based on formal laws of relationship and interaction, a vocabulary that identifies the notes, their timbres and tones, range of keys, chords, tempi, and principles of composition, providing guidelines for how this instrument is to be played. As with any other instrumental training, teaching can occur only while the instrument is being played.

For this reason the model is particularly useful in supervision where it provides experience-near referents and differentiated terms pointing to contextual phenomena and speech interactions that also help structure the learning process itself. By laying down conceptual foundations that identify referential activities and dialogical processes the study generates a vocabulary to speak about multidimensional interactive events *in* process and through dialogue. It offers the means to observe, name and use current exchanges for teaching while assessing a candidate's capabilities. This helps construct a more objective frame of reference with discernible criteria through which to establish and evaluate basic standards of analytic competence while eliminating the artificial cleavage between "experiential" and "formal' learning. Rooted in still deeper false dichotomies polarizing feeling and thinking (emotion and reason) these misconceptions, if perpetuated, are particularly thwarting to an interpretive semantic that requires resonance to psycho-dynamic patterns and the ability to use felt-thoughts or emotional-cognition for analytic understanding

The instrumentation of our instrument engages sensibilities and formulative skills engaging the entire human nervous system. Playing it well, as with any art, is an organismic activity culminating in the verbal symbolization of complex, polyvalent meanings from the communicative span of our semantic field. Unconscious communications seep through psychic pores, showing themselves to us with immense persistence and intensity, relentlessly repeating their thematic messages until we are able to grasp their intangible forms and transpose them into linguistic terms. Proficiency as a psychoanalyst, in conducting clinical or supervisory dialogues or any other kind of psychoanalytic investigation, signifies — as basic minimal requirement — the ability to bring together, within oneself, all modes and forms of human apprehension in order to resonate with, observe, hear, and understand, what is communicated unconsciously.

How do psychoanalysts come to hear, understand and interpret complex meanings issuing from this vast, multiformed, multivocal composition that is human communication? By becoming aware of the contributing information transmitted by each of its informative levels and lines; by becoming deeply familiar with the special attributes and inductive qualities of each of its informative modalities and identifying their relative weight, in any given passage, in relation to the whole.

To be a competent musician entails, among other things, having become familiar with a body of theory and achieving sufficient technical ability to play the repertoire. It entails having learned to sight read; being able to translate instantaneously what is on paper into playing notes that make music, measure by measure, phrase by phrase, movement by movement. Countless details of musicianship enter into this, from the rudimentary principles of fingering to the subtleties of touch, timing and style, from dexterous precision and sensitive phrasing to inspired spurts of interpretive brilliance. As in the course of any instrumentalist's training, eventually theoretical knowledge, technical abilities and artistry will all come together. And we distinguish between the incompetent, the mediocre, the accomplished, and the great, by general standards that can be measured along various dimensions, some of which appear self-evident, others that are intangible.

A conductor, however, has to do more: what the instrumentalist must accomplish with one instrument, the conductor must achieve with a whole orchestra. He/she must not only be able to look at the long page of an orchestral score and mentally hear the combined sounds of all the instrumental lines, he/she must also be able to shape that orchestral sound in such a way as to draw out and express the composer's musical intentions. It is the conductor's job to select, sustain and titrate tempi, tone and volume; to accentuate or attenuate and balance the relative weight of one instrument group against another, and to maximize the dynamic tensions and suspensions of the music; to interpret the whole while being aware of all of its parts. And a great conductor is great not only by virtue of skills and musicality but because he/she strives to enter into the composer's mentality in order to interpret what is already there, inherent in the music itself.

The parallels to the supervisory position are obvious and the analogy need not be belabored. Suffice it to say that when theoretical foundations and practical application are epistemologically concordant, they work in synergy cross-fertilizing and enhancing each other. The model breathes theoretical life into psychoanalytic phenomena by the reciprocal nourishment of metatheoretical principles that can inform dialogical events and processes of both clinical and supervisory situations and vice versa, by contextual observations that can feed back into ever expanding theoretical frontiers.

Finally, a last word regarding the hierarchic design of the model which, despite the analogy, is not to be taken literally but merely as a visual representation for the simultaneity of multiple forms: Like all schematic images, it can convey and impress in one instantaneous, figurative moment what has taken me lengthy labor to develop in sequence.

FOURTH MOVEMENT

PRINCIPLES OF APPLICATION

The psychoanalyst has to learn how one mind speaks to another beyond words and in silence. He must listen "with a third ear."

One of the peculiarities of this third ear is that it works in two ways. It can catch what other people do not say, but only feel and think, and it can also be turned inward.

Reik,1948,p.144,146

INTRODUCTION

> In psychoanalysis we act upon the transference itself, resolve what opposes it, adjust the instrument with which we wish to make our impact.
>
> S. Freud, 1917, p. 451

The most obvious benefit of a comprehensive model of communication is that it provides a framework, unifying principles of theory and practice, and a prism through which to further study the yields of the method. Its more subtle value is in pointing toward a clearer view of psychoanalytic knowledge—how it is arrived at and by what personal means. This can lead to an analytic breakdown of the "instrument" metaphor in terms of its functions and interactions, which, in turn, makes possible a genuine psychoanalytic theory of learning. The following sections will test the applicability and usefulness of the conceptual reorientation embodied in the model.

Clinical psychoanalysis pivots around the centrality of transference/resistance, and understanding the developmental organization, the particular qualities and constellations of even the most subtle or primitive transferences, is now a technical necessity. In addition to being a tool of treatment, however, transference/resistance can also be used as a methodological vehicle of research. Attending to the 'transference', in fact, teaches us that we must stretch our instrument considerably in order to attune to the various patterns and forms that transference can take. A developmental understanding of transferences that includes different modes of attunement and interpretative-understanding that are tied to each form—the "adjustment of our instrument" to which Freud referred—can become the cornerstone of a tailored technical approach. Freud recommended an attentional/listening stance for a method that was destined to build upon itself, to expand and evolve. And so it has. He also repeatedly pointed to the fact that "What characterizes psychoanalysis as a science is not the material which it handles but the technique with which it works" (Freud, 1917, p. 389). With the help of a developmental model of communication, informed by principles of semiotic mediation, we are equipped to examine the interactive phenomena illumined by our technique along a continuum from nonverbal transmissions to dialogical speech activities; the model provides a template for correlate modes of attunement (interactive-matching) and the logical basis for how to listen, understand, and intervene.

The principal interpretive referents of Freud's unconscious were; the unrepresented infantile past (infantile amnesia of the first five years); the presentational or "creative unconscious" of dreams and fantasies; the secondarily repressed, dynamic unconscious; and the persistent "resistances" that appear to counter analytic work. These were all subsumed and came into sharp relief through the activation of a clearly circumscribed new version of an old story, "the transference neurosis" of the classical model, of which the resolution of the "Oedipus complex" was the principal treatment objective. One cannot, in my opinion, overestimate the methodological sophistication and coherence of this core dialogue out of which so many variant, psychoanalytic genres have sprung. And we have yet to establish a modernized treatment model of such methodological precision.

Today our referential base has greatly expanded to include innominate, pre-semiotic spheres of affect-and state-transmission, projective/introjective processes, the subtle push and pull of broad attachment and withdrawal patterns and of intense merging and disconnection. From Kohut we acquired the idea that only empathy and introspection were optimal ways of engaging transferences of damaged or fledgling selves, the restoration of which flourished not through 'interpretation' but through interventions that serve mirroring, affirming functions. The etiological roots of many disorders in treatment today originate in the cumulative impact of non-specific empathic failures and repetitive pathogenic interactions with primary caretakers the toxic effects of which were woven daily through communicative patterns that are re-experienced in the fine tessitura of clinical exchanges. Similarly, the catastrophic reactions and psychotic-like transferences that characterize the borderline classification, point to etiological origins in disintegrative traumata of primary attachment in the first two years of life. In none of these groups does the treatment process clearly resolve in the dissolution of the Oedipus complex, and we have come to appreciate the etiological significance of wholesale introjections of very early, real, pathogenic experiences and interactions that require careful contextual inquiry and reconstruction founded on developmental sophistication. Introspection and empathy, in this technical sense, are indispensable aids in broadening a listening stance that must now capture experiential-transmissions of deep non-verbal dynamic patterns from the earliest sensory-affective anlage.

As the operative fulcrum of the therapeutic encounter, in all their diversity and complexity, transferences have taught us that different modes of attunement are required to hear and engage with different developmental constellations underlying more archaic states. An incremental move away from a focal interest in conflict, content and the reified "transference" of the classical neurotic has led to encompassing various kinds of transferential manifestations arising in minute to minute clinical transactions, spread throughout the process. This has gradually shifted and expanded investigative focus to the minutiae of interactive exchanges occurring in the organic latticework of the current process. The scope and modes of attuning to these "unverbal" (Kern, 1995, p.307) process-elements have now extended our interpretive purview to experiential referents at bio-psychical spheres of mutual influence that go well beyond the range of unconscious derivatives accessible to the pioneers of our field, the domain that had heretofore defined the legitimate province of psychoanalytic investigation. Schisms have arisen precisely over these issues. Yet thread throughout our literature can be found the truly common ground of analysts from all eras and persuasions, in a general consensus regarding our approach to how we listen to the unconscious. Growing cross-fertilization within the field and the gradual broadening of the parameters of analytic therapy over the last fifty years have led to increasing modifications in technique, with a corresponding amplification of an "instrument" now required to register referential categories and deep transmissive frequencies in keeping with new therapeutic challenges.

Functional impairments originating in the pre-semiotic anlage tend to produce unstable, archaic psychoneurotic transferences whereby the analytic situation and the analyst in it are enlisted to serve the most basic quasi-maternal integrative and holding functions. In phases or areas of heightened dysfunction, when the capacity for self reflection and the symbolic use and function of language appear lost, therapeutic interventions may range from state- and affect-regulation through inquiry and joint verbal referencing; the educative co-management of time and daily activities; joint examination of cognitive processes and linguistic communication, to the juxtaposition of past and present with intermittent reconstructions in which "calmness, firm realism and quiet competence" are the principal "effective agents in the analysts attitude" to use Stone's (1954, p.586) pithy phrase.

While it is true that neither in form nor function do these kinds of communication correspond with the complex, symbolically organized conflict-interpretations of the classical repertoire, the analytic intent to co-identify, name and understand qualities of distress, the systematic invitation to give verbal expression and ideational or mnemonic representation to these experiences, or indeed even to share them, in my view, provide rudimentary exercise for mediational activities that are requisite for later forms of working-through. The polarization of interpretive vs. reparative interventions is further complicated by the impact of the philosophical *zeitgeist* of our age ineluctably showing us that *everything* is interpretation, and hence, that nothing that comes within our formulative grasp is, strictly speaking, "beyond interpretation" (Gedo, 1979).

Insight is the singular psychoanalytic form of knowledge obtained through a clinical analysis, and working-through the crucial intermediary stage in an otherwise unremarkable semiotic progression — identifying-naming-working-through-insight — that is initially divided between two dialogical lines in a continuous contrapuntal duet. The defining feature of psychoanalytic insight is that it cannot be given, it must be earned; hence, while this painful, slow, laborious integrative effort cannot be bypassed, it leaves deep and lasting gains.

Analysts provide critical catalytic communications moving this dynamically resisted mediational process forward as it spirals, ever more consciously, along in micro- and macro-genetic sequences, again and again grinding each thematic thread that emerges and reemerges into the dialogical fodder. But analysts could not so steer or conduct the dialogue were they not themselves intimately proficient in processing and verbally referencing a broad range of stimuli issuing from a spectrum of different informative sources. Hence the truism that analysts can take their analysand only as far as they themselves have gone. Now that transference-analysis has reached these deepest regions of human intercourse, our attentional stance similarly has had to expand commensurately to register forms of communication that are not mediated linguistically. Considerable evidence from neurobiological studies (Schore, 1996, 1997a, 1998b) suggests that it is precisely these profound chambers of unrecorded, yet deeply registered, experiences, imprinted at the dawn of life, that are to be revisited and given verbal account in the analytic treatment of certain conditions. Characteriological defenses producing empathic inhibitions constitute serious professional deficiencies in analysts of all eras but particularly today, insofar as they interfere with some of the most central interpretive tasks in the analysis of archaic transferences —the capacity to enter into, contain and understand their manifestations and sequelae.

A clinical process is defined as "psychoanalytic" insofar as it adheres to the two shibboleths of the psychoanalytic method, the analysis of transference and resistance—all types of transference and all forms of resistance. Theories of technique are derived from theories of pathogenesis and if our strategies of intervention have now expanded to accommodate new etiologies, these modifications need not, in my view, subvert the essential functional properties of the method. In the same sense, while advocating a "careful study of the 'modifications' and their effects" Stone (1954, p.571), felt that "any number and degree of parameters can be introduced where they are genuinely necessary…so long as they are all directed to bringing about the ultimate purpose and processes of the analytic end requirements" (p. 575).

Yet if all understanding is "interpretive," a term so broadened has lost its psychoanalytic specificity. We may be obliged to reexamine the repertoire of communications employed during an entire pre- and post-interpretive sequence, giving particular attention to the analyst's therapeutic *intent* and the analysand's immediate responses to the communication (see Schlesinger 1995). Psychoanalytic interpretations are no longer isolated, momentous, fulminating pronouncements (although occasionally an utterance may appear thus pithily crafted!) but creative, dynamic, formulative, semiotically differentiated communicative steps in dialogical sequences, that develop partly out of disciplined principles of analytic procedure and partly out of the profound understanding of another person that is the potential of psychoanalytic encounters. Exchanges within the analytic dyad, as Arlow (1993) and others have pointed out, are exceedingly complex, diverse processes "involving much more than resonance and countertransference" (p.1149). The dialogues' therapeutic infiltrations occur in macro- and micro-analytic passages and segments spread out over long phases, as well as in the unpredictable moments of resolution in an isolated exchange. "Analysis," writes Arlow (1995) "partakes of the nature of the creative process"; it is, in this sense, also, a "highly aesthetic experience" (p.1149).

Conversely, it may be important to specify the referential attributes and constitution of an interpretation that is a genuine *psychoanalytic* "interpretation." Some therapeutic processes may be characterized by prolonged periods of working-through via interventions that correspond semiotically to earlier stages in an interpretive progression designed to lead eventually to interpretations, and to the elucidation of that preparatory phase itself. One could say, on this account, that psychoanalytic modes of therapeutic action are interlaced throughout the whole dialogical weave and include, as important collateral operants, the burden of initiative, the capacity for delay, close observation and self-reflection, emotional integration and autonomous thought, as well as a general expansion of experiential referents and personal responsibility to adhere to the formal protocols of the process even through tough moments of working-through. On the analyst's part, sustained restraint and the disciplined application of analytic formulation to therapeutic intent, together with psychological and clinical sophistication, yield what used to be referred to simply as wisdom.

The governing methodological premise on which psychoanalytic situations operate is that current dynamics are recapitulations or reproductive enactments of unconscious internalizations from the infantile past. The rationale for creating an atemporal semantic field is to establish a psychical space, like the stage of ritual, for dramatic replays that provide interpretive material for the analyst's underlying point of view—that what *is* once was, and that what *was* still is. The idea of transfer from one time and context into another is central to the entire enterprise. Without this paradoxical juxtaposition of past and present—the past as *in* the present—and its instructive play of narrative modes, in my opinion, there is no *psychoanalytic* process. And this methodological principle is borne out in supervision by the appearance and use of parallel process as a primary source of unconscious information, the exploration and elucidation of which might well be considered the defining feature of a truly *psychoanalytic* supervisory process.

Analytic opaqueness, neutrality and personal restraint are technical necessities for such an interpretive methodology ensuring the stability of a dialectical, reflective referentiality that is tailored to the tasks of the discourse. They were originally invoked to avert the temptation to inject personal judgments and to temper a general human tendency to bend all input to fit into patterns with which one is already familiar. These procedural recommendations are not, as some would have it, whimsical rules inspired by a misguided nineteenth century illusion of "objectivity," but sensibly grounded semiotic and referential activities serving the operative fundaments and goals of this method. The communicative strategies that generate psychoanalytic dialogues originate in and are steered by the analyst's intent and attitude, both of which are embedded in the analytic stance. These specialized dialogues produce not inter*personal* but inter*psychica*l fields of mutual influence: those compelled to react, counteract, interact, actualize, act-in or act-out verbally in these contexts, rather than analyze, may be using the same medium but they are *not*, by definition, practicing the same method.

Extreme relativism and a passion for self-disclosure, two trendy trademarks of the past provocative 50 years and their wanton offspring, pervasive uncertainty and a disregard for form, have trickled into even our discreet profession. Brandishing what may initially appear to be valid rationales for transforming the Freudian method into a dialogue of personal "intersubjectivities," these new voices have wielded yet another internally divisive blow to the Freudian legacy. But semiotic principles of semantic and discourse referentiality cast a critical light on terms and concepts so hastily pulled together. Without the necessary scrutiny of the operative features and speech activities that create the dialogue, these superficial concepts and borrowed terms end up signifying nothing at all.

Tracing the course of expansion and fragmentation that has characterized the growth patterns of our field, we can see that shifts, rifts and radical ruptures have frequently come by way of departures in the recommended stance, both on epistemological and technical grounds. Yet different ways of listening yield different ways of understanding the method's therapeutic action: to *engage* interactively is not the same as to *examine* interactions analytically; to disclose an inner reaction is not the same as to process it privately, as a source of information; to adopt corrective measures is not the same as to apply interpretive means. These are all formally and functionally distinct ways of using a dialogue as a vehicle of psychological change — the first alters behaviors, the second recomposes functional organization; the former talk through, the latter work-through; the former are corrective, the latter transformative.

I may be exaggerating contrasts that are not in practice as pronounced as they are important in principle. Certainly many unspecific therapeutic events must transpire at the matrix of a multidimensional, crossmodal dialogue that is always impacting at multiple levels. But major fault lines dividing the field ultimately wrest on such personal, ethical, aesthetic, technical and theoretical, positions — whether one wants to be an agent of corrective impact or of transmutative insight. For these reasons I was interested in considering the nature of the modifications in broader terms, from a perspective that preserves key methodological principles while necessitating new forms of intervention for what Stone (1954) referred to as "modified psychoanalysis" (p.575). At the moment we are an unruly community, resistant to the rigorous thinking required of radical revisions; to date the technical modifications inherent in the widened scope of analytic therapy are neither anchored in, nor buttressed by, the unifying principles of a comprehensive theory of mind. This enables our splintered field to advance willy nilly, particularly with respect to the enduring confusion between resonance and countertransference, a term now senselessly serving double duty in its "desirable" and "undesirable" forms.

By providing metatheoretical underpinnings that correlate with methodological activities, and using operative terms that point to referential and semiotically-mediated communications, this model offers experience-near referents backed by conceptual guidelines that can deepen and sharpen our grasp of dialogical processes. The field of observation, from this perspective, is the *entire semantic arena* viewed from *all* sides, and from all presemiotic and semiotic organizations and points of reciprocal impact. The presentation of a continuum of communicative channels through which multiple types of information and meaning are simultaneously expressed opens the door to a systematic reevaluation of how we listen and how we communicate psychoanalytically. The unique tasks and interventions of psychoanalytic dialogues are designed to uncover meanings in semantic fields in which there is no such thing as a "simple" communication: the past is in the present as surely as the ancient etymological sense of a word is subsumed in its current usage; the historical anlage and the sensory-motor response embedded in the current moment *both* suffuse the verbal line with multiple, condensed polyvalent meanings; sources of unconscious communication spread throughout the organism emerge dynamically cross-referenced via different expressive channels; what is explicit will also always contain what is implicit and verbal qualifiers muddle the senses as they contradict what the body is conveying. And we who "attend to the world of the referent" (p. 1004) make our way through labyrinths of words "as if they were not words at all, but invisible, undistorting avenues into another's mind" (Makari and Shapiro, 1993, p. 1003).

That we are able to steer a course through these linguistic mazes may be because we are not unfamiliar with their pathways. The fact is that "mental" phenomena and meanings start in the body, at the outset and throughout the life span, from the same organically rooted matrix. For this reason, psychoanalytic or "depth" listening is, more than ever, an *organismic affair*, employing a full spectrum of mediating sensibilities and referential faculties for interpretive pathways that begin in multisensory registrations and end in complex, symbolically-formulated psychoanalytic understanding. Different types of information conveyed via different modes of communication are apperceived and processed at different rates. Neuroscientists inform that the cerebral processing of sights and sounds occurs in milliseconds while even the simplest of thoughts takes full seconds to develop, a fact that helps explain the frequent time lag between recalling what went on in a session and formulating some understanding of it. Listening in psychoanalytic contexts *necessitates* the capacity to dip, at will, into presemiotic modes of attunement establishing correspondences between verbal content and nonverbal transmissions while giving this underlay discursive form.

The model proposes that each formal organization of communication calls forth its own reciprocal mode of responsiveness; different semiotic organizations, tied to dynamic patterns, are also fitted with correlative interactive modalities. Analytic understanding entails attuning to these and transposing their form as well as interpreting their meanings, so that these naturally paired resonating registrations and responses are to be keenly monitored and carefully mediated by our extensive referentiality and interpretive intent. The problem of remaining attuned to an inflowing array of semiotically uneven currents of information while simultaneously distinguishing between them makes assuming a fully differentiated stance all the more imperative.

One way to begin demystifying the aura of "intuitive," "experiential," "enacted," "projective-introjective," "transmitted," and other less differentiated or nonverbal phenomena, is to begin classifying them and giving them names: "coenesthetic expression" and "ideo-motor replication" are but two such broad categories of non-indexical forms that distinguish between distinct classes of unconscious communications. We will find that "empathy," also, is not a unitary phenomenon, but a mode of attunement with a developmental line that, for technical purposes, must be studied in relation to its specific referential functions and use. There is no contradiction between listening for the dynamic unconscious and "feeling into" expressions of what is unspeakable.

These unconscious interactive phenomena can be understood and logically exhibited through a semiotically informed theoretical lens: my task, in the following, is to discern the broad principles of their correspondences and transmuting organizations. Through the exploration of an attentional/listening stance that simultaneously encompasses and integrates the entire scope of our referential perspectives and mediational activities it is possible to effectively break down the range of operative functions that the "instrument" metaphor so effectively subsumed. Analytic listening exercises prodigious integrative and synthesizing competencies and all skillful analytic communications reflect the power of intentional symbolic condensations to subsume and express multiple levels of meaning. To listen with all of oneself entails utilizing the full stretch and compass of our feeling/thinking/

apperceptual faculties, moving fluidly between different modes of reception while quickening the translation from sense-registration to conscious, verbal formulation through the disciplined use of a vigilant referential device, the "observing ego."

I believe it is possible, once we have understood the highly mediated, specialized nature of clinical empathy, of intuitive inference, resonance and morphic-matching, to satisfy the rationalists among us, by reconciling these modes of attunement and understanding with a rational formulation of human sentience tied to the analytic enterprise. In this last chapter I will continue fusing science and art with the help of musical metaphors wherever conceptually necessary in highlighting the integration of theory, technique and dialogical process.

PSYCHOANALYTIC LISTENING AND EMPATHIC COMPETENCIES

A BIOPSYCHOLOGICAL APPROACH

> ...we react to the unconscious with all our organs, with our various instruments of perception and comprehension.
>
> T. Reik, 1948, p. 143

> The analyzing instrument has two constituents: a voluntary and controlled, situation-specific and goal-specific regressed state of mind in the analysand and a near-identical one of the same nature in the analyst. These parts function together through mutually evocative communication, leading to the elucidation of the analysand's unconscious, fantasy-memory constellations.
>
> Balter, Lothane, Spence, Jr., 1980, p. 474

> The capacity to be unconsciously at one with the patient's unconscious at an emotional as well as an intellectual level, is to my mind an essential feature of what we call psychoanalysis.
>
> J. Sandler, 1993, pp. 1106-1107

In the context of the framework of this study, it is important to reconsider the role and place of empathy in psychoanalytic listening. The following proposes a developmental understanding of empathy and its highly specialized, technical application in clinical listening.

Psychoanalytic discourse-situations stimulate the emergence of multi-modal, hybrid dramatizations in which the principal characters, the plot, and other psychodynamic elements are vividly rendered via the externalization and enactment of a polyphony of unconscious currents that, like the contrapuntal lines of a fugue, are all played simultaneously. The central insight of this discourse remains Freud's (1914) observation that what is not remembered is repeated in action, a tenet that orients our observations and referential perspectives toward viewing everything that transpires within these semantic fields as in some way reflective of the hi-story of the subjective experience of the current moment- as a repetition of some kind.

Accordingly, from the moment I enter an analytic space I am guided by two orienting principles: i) I view psychoanalytic situations as recapitulative *sui generis*, whereby the kind of information that I am to be attuned to will be transmitted and communicated via projective, enactive or verbal channels; consequently, ii) I take *everything* that transpires within them—anything that is said, done, felt, experienced, or exchanged—as meaningful, informing me, in some way, of some aspect or facet of the others' unconscious knowledge and experience. I find that this central vantage point situates me at an optimal equidistance from a hierarchy of modes of attunement all registering different kinds of information simultaneously. At the hub of this "semiotic sphere" there forms a temporal circle that sets the stage for an emergent replay that will yield the transferential material upon which the psychoanalytic process depends. In order to attend and respond analytically to the unconscious meanings communicated through this emotionally-laden re-play, I find that I must remain deeply attuned yet very aware of my own multiple levels and forms of response.

After working with someone for a certain period of time, once I have created a mental map of the key events, relationships and patterns of their history, and am familiar with their thematic and meta-thematic life-motifs, core issues and personal style, I find that gradually, as I listen, most of what I experience mentally or physically, even the particular way I experience my weight in the chair or the quality of air in the room, or the silences between us, in fact, *everything* that transpires in and outside the session, represents a subtle communication of some aspect of the analysand's current material, perhaps its surrounding mood, memories, or ideation. That a similar, reciprocal form of attunement occurs on the part of some analysands is attested to by the uncanny appearance in dreams and/or fantasies, of facts and details of my private life and circumstances, of which they could not possibly know anything about. These regions of interpsychical resonance go well beyond the "unobjectionable positive transference" and are related, rather, to powerful transmissive processes aroused by the semantic field. It is the analyst's job to be able to move fluidly and freely between them, mediating swiftly between more- and less-differentiated modes of assimilation in order to resonate with the full range of meanings that are referred to and interpreted in psychoanalytic situations.

I take Freud's (1912, 1913a, 1914, 1915) technical prescriptions very seriously not only because I believe he knew what he was talking about but because I consider this set of tightly interrelated procedural principles, that work in synergy, to be indispensable for the establishment and functioning of a viable analytic (and supervisory) process. More importantly, everything we now know about the ubiquity and trenchant hold of transference distortions and tenacity of defenses: the porousness and interpenetrative fluidity of projective mechanisms at less differentiated strata of interaction, and inflammability of interpsychical fields; and all that has been discovered regarding deixis, semantic and discourse referentiality, the compelling mediational role of Vygotsky's "zone of proximal development" in learning, and about the intrapsychic structuring of semiotic processes of discourse, point to the prescient modernism of Freud's vision and the wisdom behind his select technical recommendations.

Freud formalized a dialogue to serve the specific goals of investigating and interpreting the unconscious. To these ends he devised a specialized speech form and matching way of listening that, together, generate a semantic field of mutual psychical influence. Freud (1915) recognized the requirements and dangers of a method that instigated, isolated, and made use of a potentially explosive human situation, and all his technical rules and directives were designed to optimize its instrumentality and minimize its pitfalls. The dialogue and the analyst's functioning in it are both vehicles of psychoanalytic methodology: implicit in this instrumentation is the idea of attunement. In order to register, hear and interpret the meaning of another's *unconscious* communications — that is to use oneself "as an instrument in the analysis" (Freud, 1912, p. 116) — one has to be able to use one's own unconscious without unbidden personal intromissions. Freud (1912) put this in a formula; the analyst "must turn his own unconscious like a receptive organ toward the transmitting unconscious of the patient" (p. 115).

Hardly a recipe for the detached, unresponsive, objectifying stance Freud is alleged to have advocated, this personal instrumentation calls to mind words that are in vogue today to describe analytic listening such as resonance, attunement, receptivity, responsiveness. In fact, the degree to which his recommendations have been misconstrued remains a constant source of dismay to me: of his three (1912) now overly used and thoroughly distorted famous analogies—the telephone (p. 115), the mirror (p. 118), and the surgeon (p. 115)—it is, of course, the surgical one (and to a lesser degree the "opaque" aspect of the mirror one) that is most cited, but in such a way as to obfuscate the particular meaning the analogy was designed to convey, namely, the necessity to put aside personal feelings, even sympathy, in order to "concentrate" all of ones "mental forces on the single aim of performing the operation as skillfully as possible" (Freud, 1912, p.115).

Freud used a medical analogy because he was a medical man but its significance ought to be acknowledged for its broader implications inasmuch as a requisite emotional distance from ones material is a technical necessity in any art form or specialized skill. In fact, an appropriate "psychical distance" (Bulough, 1912) combined with immersion in ones medium—to the point of becoming its "instrument'—is the hallmark of great mastery and artistry in *any* field. As any artist will tell you it is impossible to execute a technically or interpretively demanding task while wallowing in personal emotions; only when these emotions have been symbolically represented or verbally referenced and rendered *through* the medium and the material, can one speak of technical acumen and interpretation.

The psychoanalytic listening stance is non-selective but deeply attuned to those prosodic features of tone, pitch and tempo, and to the sudden prosopopeaiec shifts announcing the animation of a wholesale identification; it is a stance from which multiple types of hidden meanings can be recorded, identified, recrafted or newly minted, as it were, from which can be detected even the subtlest, sneakiest sorts of resistances and the mercurial, or as Freud (1917, p. 287) saw them, "protean" changes in form through which they become manifest; a stance that dictates keen surveillance over all of ones own sensory-formulative faculties, inviting judicious personal restraint, opaqueness, sparse interference, a reverence for the individuality and autonomy of the others' psychical stirrings and inner world. It is a stance that predisposes toward inquiry, exploration, the suspension of certainty and closure, caution of thought and word — and self-monitoring of both — verification of inference, confirmation of hunches, the selection of deliberate, purposeful, well-timed communications, and the ability to engender tolerance for ambiguity, ambivalence, unpleasurable tensions and affects, multiple versions, the child, the body, the bad, the ugly, the intolerable, the disavowed in all of us. . . .

What does this stance communicate? It communicates interest, constancy, acceptance, tolerance, respect, forbearance, continuity, understanding, closeness, separateness, and, where there is belief in the effectiveness of the method, it communicates process — the unfolding of outcome over time. By its disciplined, unswerving analytic attitude, and the high value this places on language and the spoken, shared utterance, it is a stance *intrinsic* to a process that plants firm, functional and communicative roots in the integration resulting from struggling to put everything into words, sharpening that transformation into mind that comes of repeated cycles of working- through and insight. If it is anchored in benevolent motives, the quality of analytic attention gradually induces trust, a sense of significance and purposefulness in a collaborative process, increasing tolerance of imperfection and delay, faith in linguistic negotiation, hope in the possibility of being seen and understood and of gaining self-mastery through self-inquiry and communication. I have no doubt that for many, if not all analysands at the most archaic levels, analytic listening functions as a substitute, or equivalent, for the ideal maternal gaze of early mirroring conveying unconditional presence, attention, and acceptance. Gratifications, within the confines of analytic procedure, are plentiful, but they are of an uncommon kind.

We are speaking of situations in which language is the interpretive medium, the analyst its "instrument." In order for this interpretive instrumentation to be effective and incisive, it is essential that it be carried out at the necessary symbolic distance from its material. This fully differentiated quality or requisite referential distance can be logically explained; it is simply "the experience of apprehending through a symbol what was not articulated before" (Langer, 1942, p. 223). We recognize this referential di-stance immediately as an essential feature of the "analytic attitude" and of all psychoanalytic interpretive activities, engendering, by way of their semantic focus and spread, a special kind of echo, so that when something has been "*symbolized*" for us, what this invites "is not emotional response, but insight"(Langer, 1942, p.223).

Once again we find that semiotic distinctions are helpful in understanding specific responses in the listener; the difference between a *signal* inducing reactivity, a *sign* that indicates, and a *symbol* that elicits conceptualization. We do not formulate or articulate our sobs and outbursts as we conceptualize and lexicalize our interpretations: "The laws of emotional catharsis are natural laws, not artistic" writes Langer (1942, p.216). "Psychical Distance" (Bullough,1912) thus contextualized, becomes an *aesthetic* principle of interpretation insofar as it ensures a requisite symbolic distance from the material. But in the clinical setting it becomes an *ethical* principle as well, fortifying the formal character and specialized speech codes of a situation that cannot be degraded or allowed to fall into unmediated expressions of human sympathy. This distance creates the correct referential space to formalize the procedures of a dialogue that has specific integrative, therapeutic and educative purposes. Freud not only used language articulately with the imaginative flare of a literary giant (winner of the Goethe prize) but in its clinical purpose he *medicalized* it, having discerned the healing potential of dialogue that fuses therapeutic artistry with the science of mind.

We have, in psychoanalytic situations, dialogues in which ethical and aesthetic principles converge in an attentional stance that, precisely because it operates in semantic fields where psychical boundaries are thinned, must function at a fully differentiated equidistant position from all forms of communicative stimuli. In fact it must contend with registrations originating from both internal and external sources. For Freud this listening technique was relatively "simple," consisting in "not directing ones notice" but "maintaining the same 'evenly suspended attention'…in the face of all that one hears" (1912, pp. 111-112). This was designed to avert undue strain on ones attention and memory but also to "avoid a danger…inseparable from the exercise of deliberate attention" (p.112), the imposition of meaning rather than the finding of it.

All of Freud's technical recommendations converge in the intent to create for the analyst a counterpart to "the fundamental rule of psycho-analysis" (1912, p.115) and his principle methodological concern was to make sure that neither member of the dyad introduce any obstruction to the establishment of the free flow of communications passing between them. On the other hand, given his reasoned position regarding analytic neutrality and abstinence, he also recommended that analysts be "opaque" to their analysands, reflecting back only what is shown to them (1912, p.118).

True to his style Freud provided loose guidelines for *how* but not really *what* to do: Aside from cataloguing the elements of a fitting attentional stance, offering advice on practical and procedural rules, Freud's technical papers address the relationship between enacting, representing and working-through (the semiotic and referential processes to which I have been pointing throughout), and the development and use, in treatment, of the transference. The closest he came to giving any actual technical instructions is on the subject of when and how to begin interpretive interventions, assigning prime importance to the establishment of a "proper rapport" (1913a, p.139). Much has been written about this "rapport," or the unobjectionable positive transference, an attachment viewed by some (particularly Meissner, 1996, 1998; Adler and Bachant, 1996, recently; and Greenson, 1965, 1967; and Zetzel, 1956, earlier) as that aspect of the "real" relationship through which the 'observing ego' and all important 'therapeutic alliance' are cemented.

One can approach this 'rapport' from a number of perspectives — functional, procedural, formal — not necessarily by finding a formal cleavage in the "relationship" but, like Freud (1913a), by turning to the question of when to begin introducing interpretive interventions. The answer to this is, not until an effective transference has developed; "It remains the first aim of the treatment" wrote Freud (1913a), to attach the analysand to the analyst and the process, a task for which nothing in particular need be done except allow time, carefully clear away initial resistances, show genuine interest, and avoid making certain mistakes (pp 139-140). The next sentence has become a source of controversy due to an apparent mistranslation of a key word in it; "It is certainly possible to forfeit this first success if from the start one takes up any standpoint other than one of sympathetic understanding…"(p.140). *Sympathetic*, is the word in question, apparently mistranslated from the German *Einfühlung*, meaning *empathy*, a word used sparingly by Freud elsewhere (1905, 1906, 1913c, 1918, 1921) yet carefully selected here for its particular significance (Shaughnessy, 1995). If Shaughnessy is correct then in this sentence Freud was emphasizing the importance of adopting an *empathic* stance as an essential component of the attentional disposition in analytic listening. Empathy is to be thought of as a way-of-understanding, a *quality* of attention.

This ought to be enough to dispel the fictional idea that Freud was anything other than humane and interactive in conducting his analytic "conversations," a fact that is corroborated throughout his writings. Freud was undoubtedly familiar with the Lippsian theory of empathy, as his selective use of differentiated terms when referring to understanding, sympathy, or "feeling into" another's experience, clearly indicates. When he used *Einfühlung*, he was using it deliberately for its specific psychological and etymological implications, describing the attempt to come to understand another's experience by *resonating* with it, or putting oneself in their shoes. Since he believed that one could forfeit developing the necessary 'working alliance' by adopting anything other than an empathic stance toward the analysand, then empathic attunement had to have been a central component of Freud's analytic attitude. In fact, in his 1921 study of group psychology discussing the nature of mutual interactions between ego and objects, in a footnote, he offered this definition: "A path leads from identification by way of imitation to empathy, that is, to the comprehension of the mechanism by means of which we are enabled to take up any attitude at all towards another's mental life" (p.110, fn. 2). On several other occasions, Freud used the concept of empathy to convey a particular way of bringing oneself closer to another's experience, "…only somebody who can *feel his way into* the minds of children is capable of educating them, and we grown-up people cannot understand children because we no longer understand our own childhood" (1913c, p.189).

Here, and elsewhere, he points, albeit indirectly, to the ontogenetic origins of this mode of apprehension in the phenomenology of childhood experience when perceiving and feeling are little differentiated and contagional inductions strike swiftly on senses that are impressionable, reactive, unmediated. Throughout life, empathy entails a momentary and "involuntary breech of individual separateness" (Langer, 1972, p.129), in our terms, a transient de-differentiation. I would stress, however, that the specialized, technical application of this mode of apprehension, in the analytic situation, is a highly mediated, controlled, richly referenced and *purposeful* type of empathy, equidistant between participation and self-awareness, issuing from a fully differentiated baseline position through which all emotional responses are filtered and used to better understand another's unconscious transmissions. The distinction between an empathic and a *sympathetic* stance, for psychoanalytic listening, is an important one, clarified by Arlow (1993) in the following:

> When the analyst becomes aware that the mood or thoughts he has been experiencing represent commentaries on the patients' material, he has made the transition from simple identification to empathic comprehension. If the analyst fails to take that step and remains in the state of identification, he is sympathetic but not empathic. This is one of the most common factors in many instances of disruptive countertransference. (p.1149)

Arlow is quite correct: the problem of "countertransference" in its intended meaning, as an obstruction to analyzing can, however, be exhibited on logical grounds; it represents a degradation in the stance, a loss of the appropriate referential, and hence *symbolic,* distance from the material of interpretation.

The same principle applies to the clinical use of empathy: psychoanalytic empathy is that aspect of an interpretive disposition that maintains referential awareness with less differentiated modes of engagement, employing listening, observing and, particularly, feeling to provide direct access to qualities of emotion and ideation. It is a mode of understanding, conveying benevolent interest. Empathic attunement in psychoanalytic discourse is a way of reaching to the heart of the *emotional* sense of another's experience, beyond and beneath surface signifiers, by resonating with its unreferenced, nondiscursive, expressive, and emotionally evocative elements. By its breaking down of linguistic (semiotic) blocks of interactive structuring it is also a way of establishing a mutually interpenetrative dialectical nexus at the core of this "psychical field" (Freud, 1914, p.153). But *never*, in this discourse, is it an unmediated or undisciplined response. While operating in this communicative field, the analyst's function and responsibility is to maintain sufficient psychical distance from all emergent experiences; to be able to *refer* rather than react to them.

The model of communication here presented, can assist us in better understanding the bi-directional quality of less differentiated modes of interaction at the matrix of our semantic fields, and the origins, development and constitution of empathy. The term empathy is a verbal noun making a 'thing' out of an inter-activity: empathy is actually *empathizing*. Like listening or observing, which must be qualified, empathy is a particular *way* of entering into the unspoken dimensions of another person's experience, a two-way interaction that can best be understood by studying its particular attributes as they function in a specific situation. Given its sensory-emotive core, the concept of empathy, in psychoanalysis, has been hampered, thus far, by the absence of a comprehensive developmental theory of affect that would clarify its primary communicative and interactive functions.

In its earliest, most primitive form, the empathic response is an automatically triggered, affect-matching reflex, inducing the contagion of a similar feeling state. Very quickly, however, its reflexive quality is modulated by proprioception and mediated by more controlled mimicry. Early forms of imitation are the first in a series of unconscious introjective and identificatory processes initiating capacities that culminate in the ability to internalize experiences by representational means. Mimicry in childhood involves the whole body, in sensorimotor modes, however, the manifest expressive signs of this pattern-matching become increasingly interiorized and subdued as they are mediated by increasingly differentiated and ever more expedient referential processes. Their intensity diminishes to a mere signal of a signal. Eventually even these go under until only the faintest, merely suggested, neurophysiological trace remains. Yet it is on this minuscule, barely perceptible neurophysiological trace-signal that the activation of *affect-resonance* (affect-matching) or an emotionally like response continues to depend.

I know of no better description of this than Langer's (1967), "…the perception of emotional expression leads the observer to an unconscious, merely incipient imitation of the fleeting act, and…the resulting faint tensions involve an equally faint feeling by which he understands what is passing in the other person" (p.176). The mature empathizer responds to this faint, mirrored arousal as to a subtle signal concomitantly mediating its activation with an array of ideational referents associated with all that is known of this state and that person, and all that is inferred from the other's entire communication. This is an engaged response, implying focus and attention.

The empathic response, therefore, is fed by two vectors; one that responds to perceptual, auditory and emotional cues, the other, by associative inference, that is tied to referential and ideational, interpretive constructs. Degrees of sensitivity and empathic acuity vary from person to person and what to do with it depends, specifically, on what the situation warrants and on ones role and goals within it. Rapid oscillations between emotional-participation and internal verbal-referencing characterize more mature, increasingly differentiated forms of empathizing. As that aspect of a specialized attentional disposition that is deeply in touch with feelings, psychoanalytic empathy has to be integrated with other, more differentiated levels of attunement in order to resonate with communicative frequencies transmitting experiential patterns that are received directly before they are articulated or negotiated linguistically. This implies that transient dedifferentiation is common to all forms of attunement to non-verbal information. But while the attuned attitude responds to stimuli through a sensory-emotive disposition by *feeling into,* it is not limited or exclusively tied to emotional-patterns; it includes resonance to any kind of directly-presented patterns as in ideo-figurative matching or the concordance of images, movements, ideas, sounds and other non verbal evocations. Semantic resonance or attunement may also play an important part in grasping the deeper meanings woven through linguistic forms like tropes, synecdoche, metonymy, metaphor, analogy, anecdote and that great gnösis of temporal and causal belief, narrative form.

Originating in unmediated, automatic, affect-contagion, the empathic response achieves *informational* value in its more mature forms when it combines fully differentiated, internal referencing that formulates linguistic or *conceptual* correspondence with another's experience, without necessarily *participating* in their *feelings*. This is a very important point when considering the disciplined, psychoanalytic use of empathy as part of an interpretive technique. For if its primitive roots originate in automatic affect-matching, its uppermost branches reach sophisticated ideational forms of *conceptual* correspondence that, thanks to language and speech, are able to transcend separateness. Mature and psychoanalytic empathy depend on being able to formulate an *idea* of what the others' experience feels like and of having come to this understanding by way of a synthesis of perceptual, sensory-emotive and ideational referents generated in oneself by the other. The bi-directionality of this process is contingent on the unimpeded flow of emotional information passing through less differentiated channels of communication and, where blockages or defensive obstructions arise, in making these impediments the very targets of interpretive understanding.

Freud was well aware of the power and bi-directional nature of this "new force field" (Loewald, 1970, p. 62). In order to counterbalance the almost magnetic pull toward collusive-reactivity at unconscious levels he advocated analytic neutrality and abstinence as technical necessities. The wisdom in providing a stance in which restraint is built in comes from having recognized the strength of unconscious agendas in their ability to override analytic reflectiveness. My point is merely that "psychical distance" and referential differentiation through linguistic mediation work in tandem producing analytic thinking and focused communications that generate symbolizing activities that are central to the functional effectiveness of the discourse.

But analytic neutrality and abstinence were never intended to imply emotional indifference, detachment or cold unresponsiveness, the cadaverous analyst of caricatured extremes. Originally designed to protect the analyst's emotional life, and to protect the analysand from the analyst's emotional life, neutrality safeguards against unwarranted personal intromissions into the material and the process, just as abstinence guarantees the exclusion of vicarious or substitutive gratifications that might interfere with the specific conditions and aims of the situation. One crucial difference between analyst and analysand at the outset is that the analyst is already capable of monitoring a spectrum of internal and contextual experiences along multiple dimensions, while the analysand, initially, is not. Having generated a mutually impacting "psychical field" it becomes essential to respect and protect the psychical boundaries of both participants in their interlocking yet distinct roles within it.

Freud's (1912) three famous (maligned) analogies, when scrutinized, quite masterfully subsume the specific formal and functional features of a stance that must paradoxically integrate empathic attunement with psychical distance, fluidly adjusting between different modes and levels of reception. Precisely because it must adopt and sustain a linguistic attitude toward many nonverbal meanings, it must be fully differentiated from its principal referential categories. Receptiveness and retransmission (the telephone, p.115); reflectiveness and personal opaqueness (the mirror, p.118); and dispassionate incisive intervention (the surgeon, p.115) convey the special fusion and synergistic functioning of personal sensibilities filtered through technical communicative skills that constitute the professional use of the self as analyzing instrument.

Freud used the term "instrument" (1912, 1923) to describe the analyst's listening and interpretive functions. By 1948 this had become an auxiliary "sense organ" (T.Reik) and by 1963, Isakower had fine-tuned a now fully reified "analyzing instrument" conceptualized as a specialized "team structure" in which both halves work together in one mutually evocative continuous communication (Malcove,1975, pp.7,9). What Freud (1912) had described as *a way* for the doctor to use his/her unconscious "*as* an instrument in the analysis" (p.16) was, as late as the 1960's, characterized as "a very concrete entity" (Isakower, 1963 p. 4). And still in 1980, despite their efforts to operationalize this entity, Balter, Lothane and Spence, Jr., refer to it as a "subsystem" in the ego.

To his credit, Isakower emphasized the intensely dialectical nature of this dyad, singling out the ability to maintain a controlled reciprocally matched "regressed state of mind" (Balter, Lothane, Spence, Jr., 1980) as an essential aspect of creative listening. He stressed the importance for analysts of increasing their capacities of self-observation and the value of using any transiently evoked mood, image or phrase arising in complementary responsiveness when listening. And, Isakower discussed "*fluctuations* in states of consciousness" (Malcove, 1975, p. 9) oscillations between "the intuitive and the cerebral" (Malcove, 1975, p. 9) occurring in both members of the dyad, viewing the analytic "state of consciousness that activates the affect or mood which is associated with the content of experience" (Malcove, 1975, p. 9) as the most essential element of analytic work.

Isakower's musical background, exceptional gifts of self-observation and the special interest he had in "states of consciousness" made him particularly well suited to "systematically and elegantly" formulating "the nature, structure and function of the dyadic analytic activity in the analytic situation" (Malcove, p. 4). By so articulating the de-differentiated quality of analytic attunement and the importance of using all forms of evoked response — in contrast to "countertransference" proper — Isakower did much to legitimize the kind of "interpenetrative" modes of interaction that enable analysts to become deeply in touch with unconsciously transmitted meanings.

But the now tired "instrument" metaphor has been amply exploited by generations of analysts, and understandably so. It was apt and appealing and one is tempted to go on using it since longstanding metaphors accommodate processes that are otherwise laborious to unpack. The problem is that in their reification they end up congealing and concealing the very functional activities they were designed to subsume.

This brings us to where we are today, now highly self-conscious of a listening/attentional stance that through its methodological effectiveness has led to the visibility of more and more differentiated unconscious referents enabling analysts to become increasingly aware of the subtle registrations and complex, synthetic thought activities of the listening process itself. Through the years major shifts in theoretical and technical trends have been reflective of the changing nature and expanding scope of what we hear according to what we know and how we listen. More than ever, we have become interested in investigating the sources, forms and nature of the analyst's knowledge and the means by which it is derived, an interest that parallels a de-emphasis of content and a new focus on process that includes virtually all aspects of the dyad's contextual experience. This work, which reflects this shift in orientation, is part of a greater paradigm change that studies the formal interface of communicative interactions themselves.

Recent years have seen the emergence of important papers detailing the experiences and contributions to the process of the analyst's mind (Jacobs, 1993); the persistent, subliminally enacted or actualized dimensions of the clinical encounter (Katz, 1997); fluctuations between listening modes

(Freedman and Lavender, 1997) and characteristic oscillations between "experiential and cognitive," or "empathic and intellectual," have also been amply documented. Important distinctions between responsiveness and countertransference proper have now begun to be made with respect to originating source and dynamic intent (Sandler, 1976, 1993; Arlow 1979, 1993; Grinberg, 1970; Springman, 1986), and a new technical focus on close-process monitoring requires analysts to be keenly attuned and optimally responsive to minute-to-minute interchanges.

For such a task the whole organism is employed. And while responsibility for carrying the process forward rests on the analyst's knowledge and skills, the working-through of unconscious material and more primitive mentation, representing the analysand's 'analytic labor,' eventuates in that expanded accessibility to experiential referents, bringing personal awareness and integration, that are the yields of analytic work for both. Freedman (1971, 1978) and his co-workers (Freedman and Steingart, 1975; Freedman, Grand and Van Meel, 1978; Freedman and Grand, 1984; Barroso and Freedman, 1992; Freedman and Lavender, 1997) have now produced a considerable body of empirical research on relationships between kinetic manifestations of listening and symbolizing processes, making it plain that the body is involved in gauging degrees of receptivity to input as well as in processing (assimilating) and formulating responses: "The listener not only receives, but retrieves, orders, sorts, and shifts to verbalization, and the body participates at every step" (Freed, Barroso, Bucci and Grand, 1978, pp. 171-172).

More recently, Freedman and Lavender (1997) observed nonverbal behaviors during psychoanalytic listening along the dimensions of the "symbolizing and desymbolizing countertransference." Identifying three relatively distinguishable modes through which the analyst experiences "difficult" and "not-so-difficult" sessions, they document empathic attunement "marked by rhythmicity; a symbolizing countertransference marked by a transitory arhythmicity, and a desymbolizing countertransference marked by continuous arhythmicity" (p. 79). Bodily activities reflecting attunement, misattunement and efforts at symbolic processing during psychoanalytic listening, they suggest, may be viewed as a "bridge," functioning to both express and regulate (Freedman and Lavender, 1997, p.

83). Freedman's work and findings accord well with an organismic view of analytic listening and referentiality offering empirical corroboration for a multimodal, biopsychological model of psychoanalytic listening, combining principles of semiotic progression with those of correlative attunement, such as the one here proposed. We listen, think and communicate at the behest of a nervous system integrating multiple sensory and cerebral *signifying* activities

Freud's loosely focused, receptive stance may well be central in predisposing organismic attention toward receiving and hearing new patterns of meaning and identifying unconsciously enacted and transmitted forms of communication. Part of the difficulty in becoming proficient in this multidimensional listening and synthetic thinking has been the increasingly expanding, poliperspectival referentiality of psychoanalytic clinical discourse, a factor that, as Loewald (1970) pointed out over 30 years ago, places greater demands on the analyst's agility in moving between 'psychical levels' (p. 61) that now descend to quasi organic levels. In a lesser known and infrequently cited passage from his 1912 recommendations, Freud actually spells this requirement out: "The correct behavior for an analyst lies in swinging over according to need from the one mental attitude to the other…" (p. 114). Resonance is the word that comes to mind, both more generic (and less charged) yet synonymous with the more in vogue "empathic attunement," connoting a disposition or, as I am using it, a *mode of understanding.*

The listening analyst is poised dynamically equidistant from a continuum of transmissive, projective and symbolic communications while experiencing, identifying, naming and interpreting unconscious meaning, that is, exercising those semiotic progressions by which experiences are transformed into ideas. Technical dexterity in this attentional stance implies moving fluidly between different levels of interaction and modes of attunement while remaining receptive to an incoming stream of multinuanced, differentially organized material, and relating this to a pool of accrued information and technical knowledge, while assessing how and when to formulate an appropriately phrased, well targeted and timely intervention. Of course, this is an ideal; as Ornstein (1967) commented, and I think most analysts would agree, "It is actually impossible to be 'tuned in' on all systems, on all levels and on all processes simultaneously; to register all that transpires and intervene where intervention is most fruitful, timely or even necessary to enhance the analytic process" (p. 457).

A technical approach that is guided by principles of formal attunement and informed by familiarity with semiotic principles of progressive symbolic mediation leads to increased understanding not only of differently organized meanings but also of the analytic process itself. The model is helpful in making a distinction, in functional terms, between empathy as a reaction and empathy as a *stance*. Formal resonance and synthetic thinking enable analysts to experience the *meaning* of feelings and thoughts arising in the immediate process in relation to all that has gone before and to use this integrative understanding in the broader context of the whole process with its characteristic, yet idiosyncratically orchestrated, progressive and resistive cycles. Given the multiperspectival and multidimensional nature of our interpretive field, it stands to reason that our attentional stance will have to move fluidly between the spectrum of unconscious transmissions and communications of which we are currently aware. Sources of analytic knowledge are derived from a synthesis of sense- and semiotic data issuing from different sources, each registering different kinds of information, all of which are drawn together interpretively through interventions that are simultaneously transmuting form as they are translating meanings. Listening, thinking and communicating analytically, then, are subsumed in an attentional stance that includes multiple referential perspectives. Ornstein (1967) expresses similar ideas:

> ... "How to *Think*" refers to that process that underlies the "How to *Feel, Behave* and *Talk*" and gives these the unifying rationale, the integrating ingredient which makes for a well-functioning analytic instrument. (p. 457)
>
> There is a reciprocal relationship between "How to Think" and "How to Feel, Behave and Talk"... in the sense that not only are the latter three integrated by analytic listening, but analytic thinking itself is enhanced by having acquired the capacity to feel, behave and talk analytically. (p. 457)

One cannot but be impressed by the dialectical power of these inter-transmissive modes of interchange which can be a source of profound understanding and knowledge of another's experience. Empathizers may learn of experiences they have never had by 'entering into' the others communications. This receptivity enlarges the scope of ones range of understanding enriching the pool of referents from which to further understand others, so that while it may be true, in a physicalist paradigm that "...the material out of which I create the other person in me cannot but be my own" (Fleiss, 1942, p. 213) it is *not* true in a paradigm of form, where input and experience — that is *information* — can be 'taken in' and assimilated as part of ones personal knowledge. The role and function of an interpreter, like that of an instrument, is not to so much to partake of another's emotions but to *convey* them, to formulate them and express their translation through a symbolic medium. It is a way of knowing that moves *through* experiencing as a means of witnessing, interpreting and understanding.

I believe it is clear from all the above that the technical, psychoanalytic use of empathy must be founded on the most differentiated of positions, balanced by controlled, evaluative self-monitoring and mediated through verbal inquiry and negotiated exchange. Empathy has its own developmental line, frame of reference, and modes of application. Throughout, I have been suggesting that it is inherent in different organizations of transmission and communication to elicit correlate modes of responsiveness and that it is to these naturally-fitted types of interaction that we have been referring when misusing the term "concordant countertransference" in its totalistic sense considering it a tool rather than a contaminant of the treatment. Awareness of different kinds of elicited response and an ability to detect their differences must figure prominently in our interpretive understanding of the psychical significance and contextual sense of any given communication. These distinctions are not just terminologically discriminating — identifying different originating source-points and modes of interchange — they are logically founded. Perhaps the most important aspect of the analyst's role and responsibility is to create and maintain a semiotic field that is symbolically grounded: the analyst does not respond to signals with signals, but with *signs* and *symbols*. For this very reason analysts must be versed and skilled in recognizing the form of the response that is being called up in themselves.

Only from a fully differentiated, symbolically grounded stance that integrates auditory, perceptual and emotional stimuli, and signifies them linguistically, can one become aware of the range of unconscious meanings that are interpreted in our semantic fields.

Analysts have to become adept at moving between modalities, quickening the rate of registration of an expanded range of differentially organized facets of multidetermined communications simultaneously signaling, signifying and symbolizing, often ambiguous and ambivalent feelings and ideas. In accordance with a principle of multiple function (Waelder, 1936) our interpretive semantic necessarily activates a type of listening that, likewise, is multi-tiered, multi-vectored, with a multidimensional referential spread hovering evenly over an array of informative stimuli and significant forms. It is a type of listening that must be guided by the forms and functional organizations of the communications themselves and hence necessitates attunement to the full spectrum of human meanings, thereby firmly anchoring our investigation and interpretation of psychological phenomena in their enduring biological roots.

TOWARD AN UNDERSTANDING OF PSYCHOANALYTIC KNOWLEDGE AND OF LEARNING HOW TO ANALYZE

> It is true that psycho-analysis cannot easily be learnt and there are not many people who have learnt it properly...One learns psycho-analysis on oneself, by studying ones own personality. S.Freud, 1917,p 19

> There is nothing more disheartening to a student-analyst as the notion that analytic skill is derived not from what you do but from who you are. P. Bromberg, 1984, p 33

Anyone seriously interested in the progress of psychoanalysis today cannot have failed to notice that it is now over fifty years since Rapaport (1960) chided the field for having failed to come up with a learning theory of its own. Studies of the psychoanalytic learning process (Eckstein and Wallerstein, 1972; Tyler, 1961; Fleming, 1961; Fleming and Benedeck, 1966), and models of learning (Piers and Piers, 1965; Greenspan, 1975, 1982) have emerged, but none integrates the complex nature of psychoanalytic learning into broader conceptual foundations encompassing psychoanalytic knowledge, practice, and theory of change.

There are obvious reasons for this. A truly comprehensive psychoanalytic learning theory would have necessitated a clear picture of what sort of learning is taking place; how the various threads of experiential knowledge and information converge and how progress in their integration can be charted; it would have had to identify and name the specific referential processes of our dialogues and at least partially understand various modes of apprehension, or "levels" of learning (Greenspan, 1982), clearly articulating the central role of language in leading to conscious awareness; and this would have had to correlate with a general theory of mind(Aragno, 1997) linking psychoanalytic semantic and discourse referentiality – the practice of our method – to the acquisition of *psychoanalytic* forms of awareness. Finally, the development of a psychoanalytic learning theory would have required prior dismantling of the "instrument" metaphor replacing it with a set of functional processes and interactivities. Prolonged clinging to this metaphor has forestalled the establishment of a viable vocabulary through which to talk about and teach the technique of how this "instrument" is to be played.

Consider a comparable situation in another profession where technical acumen and interpretive artistry must join in an interpretive act. Competency in playing a musical instrument only begins by learning how to name and play the notes. Accomplished musicians must, at the very least, acquire broad knowledge of musical theory, achieve technical precision and dexterity, master sight reading, learn to transpose, embellish, phrase, etc. and, more generally, become familiar with an extensive, stylistically varied repertoire. Few achieve the technical competency required of professional musicianship and fewer still reach heights of artistry in consummate virtuoso playing. Yet it is certain that without a comprehensive notational system, technique and vocabulary, all handed down, taught and learned, music, as we know it, would not have evolved.

The comparison is obvious and only serves to highlight the problems: Psychoanalysis is the *science* of human meanings; its method is practiced in a dialogue. Yet so far no operationally integrative framework for its dialogical phenomena is handed down to help us relate communicative processes to a viable model of "mental" functioning. Lacking a conceptual framework that ties phenomenological organization (levels of experience and awareness) to communicative modes, we are offered no experience-near referents that distinguish between different kinds of unconscious meanings or that identify the formal transpositions that take place as we interpret and work-through an array of psychical manifestations all referred to broadly as "the unconscious."

"Experiential" learning or "intuition" are called on as substitutes where clearly defined terms for functional processes are lacking. Without a unifying vocabulary correlating theory, practice and technique there is little correspondence between the notes we play and the laws of sound-combination that make our music, hence, we have no clear teaching model, or cognitive map, to foster psychoanalytic learning.

This entire work is an attempt to fill these lacunae and the remaining sections are dedicated to a summation and application of its theoretical contributions. With the help of a developmental map, representing the anatomy of human interactions, in place, we can now study how psychoanalysis reengages all non-verbal and linguistic interactive modalities, and how psychoanalysts must learn to be tuned-in to different levels of meaning and different kinds of communication all transmitting different threads of information simultaneously. The component elements of the architecture of this model are complex and functionally highly interrelated. But the hierarchical theory of mind underlying it, conceptualized along a continuum from pre-semiotic to semiotically-mediated modes of communication, is relatively simple. It provides conceptual anchorage in basic transformative principles of symbolization that can serve as a foundation for a multidimensional learning theory that correlates with all other aspects of psychoanalytic training, knowledge and technique. How, then, can we define psychoanalytic knowledge? What are its unique qualities and attributes?

Descriptively, psychoanalytic knowledge is highly complex, multidimensional, polyperspectival, dense and deep. Theoretically, it is concerned with everything that is "unconscious." Practically, it is arrived at by an investigative method that employs a special attentional stance that by its unification of feeling, intellect, and observation, mends the Descartean split between emotion and reason. Everything stems from this special observational/interpretive stance, which, as we know, was essentially an extension of Freud's own investigative/analytic attitude. This new emotional/cognition, adopted in a specialized way, as a methodological necessity, is, in my opinion, the single most important scientific contribution to universal knowledge that psychoanalysis has made. Because it was tailored to register and decipher what is *unconscious*, it revolutionized the traditional split between observer and observed, placing the interpretive/investigator embedded in the semantic field.

At the center of this new consciousness is the means by which it is obtained. Psychoanalytic knowledge is contingent on an opening up of channels of human interaction that are usually defensively sealed over or diverted by language and habits of semiotic mediation during the course of development. The requirement for analysts to have themselves undergone a thorough personal analysis in addition to ensuring a measure of equilibrium and competence also ensures that bi-directional channels of introspection and empathy have been effectively opened and are accessible for interpretive use. Psychoanalytic knowledge is founded on a profound *understanding* of "another" through having investigated oneself. The capacity to tune-in to deep nonverbal levels of resonance originates in working-through and acquiring insight but is also related to having in some important way been *deeply understood* in the training analysis. To the extent that the personal analysis has reached into and worked-through tenacious defenses and the deepest, most primitive recesses of affective experience, will it have succeeded in exerting profound cognitive amplification and lasting intrapsychic re-organization. One of the unique characteristics of this type of profound personal witnessing is that it has been achieved through the integration of affect, word, and idea, by having processed emotionally-laden experiences and talked *about* and *around* associated memories reaching into the most primitive regions of the psyche. Mentation and communication, language, emotion and thought, mold each other. "Working-through," as a paradigm of verbal symbolization, leads to a specifically *psychoanalytic* way of knowing, of understanding oneself and another's psyche along many unconscious dimensions This new way of coming-to-*understand* breaks down longstanding divisions between observer and observed, conscious and unconscious, feelings and thought, operationalizing their fusion as a *methodological goal* and technical necessity.

The consequence of this participatory, interpenetrative epistemology is that it does not support divisions or divisiveness of an unconscious kind; walls are not its structures. To "understand" is not to judge or carry in preconceptions but to *enter into* the subject or object of inquiry. Such an investigative/analytic stance departs completely from interactive modes that are strictly constrained or constructed by linguistic mediation plunging to a *depth* of interpenetrative investigation that taps into modes of communication that are transmitted without words. It is not difficult to see the potentially enormous moral, ethical and political ramifications of such a stance were its value to be recognized, particularly since its domain of human exchange is firmly *dialogical.*

Personal insight is the prototype of psychoanalytic knowledge, and working-through—reflexive, expansive, integrative, laborious—its unique and far-reaching referential process. But the deepening and broadening of personal awareness through analysis is not just information tacked on to an otherwise unaltered personality or unmodified cognition. It radically alters, expands, and integrates, the *means* by which we register and understand a vast new range of unconscious meanings. Introspective efforts in analysis result in the expansion of experiential referents that feeds back, in training, to yield a new repertoire of interpretive skills (Gedo 1995). What originates and is set in motion in the personal analysis not only joins past with present and affect with intellect; it connects different functional areas of the brain, quite literally, forging new neuronal interconnections that free the intellect and reinforce capacities for resonance, reflection, attunement, and understanding. This is why psychoanalytic knowledge is tied to *emotional cognizance.* It has been forged in the process of deep personal investigation. Perhaps it is the impact of this profoundly engaging experience that endows analysts uniformly with the unshakable conviction of the efficacy of the method, a quality of belief that has rendered us vulnerable to criticisms that psychoanalysts display fervor more akin to religious fanatics than scientists.

Be that as it may, working-through produces the capacity to register and filter subjective experiences through a new emotional-cognition that produces a broad linguistic/intellectual spread. There is, however, a shadow side to this gain and one pays a price for having left the garden of undifferentiatedness: working–through works in tandem with the splitting of the ego between an experiencing and an observing self. This therapeutic dissociative process, applicable to analysands and analysts alike, has its drawbacks, the most singular being that when effectively implanted it is irreversible. More awareness carries its burdens even as it offers a subtle new "interiority." Sterba (1934) considered the development of the 'observing ego,' which gives the ability to be *in* ones experience while simultaneously *observing* it, "like an outsider," to be "*a new point of view of intellectual contemplation*," a "principle of intellectual cognition" (p.121) possibly the "extension into new fields, of the self-contemplation which from all time has been regarded as the most essential trait of man in distinction to other living beings" (Sterba, 1934, p.125). From this perspective psychoanalysis merely harnesses and exercises a new form of reflexive introspection extending it to "unconscious" referential dimensions.

The aspirant analyst will enter a profession of uncommon personal demand, a field where time, psychical elasticity, endurance and communicative skills (the bare tools of the trade) will be tried, tested and stretched in uncommon ways. Psychoanalytic candidates must learn how to come to know another person *psychoanalytically* at levels and in ways that are inaccessible by any other means and they must become adept at steering a dialogical process in such a way that it will promote profound self-awareness and personal growth. For the task, they are prepared by tripartite training programs combining didactic coursework, the personal analysis, and supervised cases. The voluminous amounts of information and knowledge to be acquired comes from different sources and is of different kinds, and each setting provides its own learning experience: candidates listen, read, experience, observe and practice analyzing under supervision, *all* while trying to metabolize the stirring impact of the personal analysis and become conversant with mountains of historical and contemporary literature in an institutional environment where hierarchies are strong and boundaries weak.

It is supposed that this vast body of new knowledge — historical, theoretical, personal, clinical, technical — can be absorbed quickly enough to justify the habitual practice of throwing candidates in cold, as it were, to begin analyzing cases at a stage in their own development when neither the benefits of the personal analysis nor their general understanding of the psychoanalytic process would warrant it, a practical necessity which, as Gedo (1990) remarked, "has compelled the American Psychoanalytic Association to recommend to its Institutes 'that they make the best of a bad situation'" (p.127). This situation is quite unique, however, unparalleled in any other profession of comparable demand and responsibility. It would be unthinkable, for instance, for a beginner pianist or violinist to play a concerto, an immature ballerina to perform a demanding leading role; or consider the potential peril in placing the novice surgeon in charge of an operation. Yet beginner analysts are routinely invited to conduct a process they have yet to complete themselves, and before their aptitude, personal maturity, or intellectual capabilities, have been sufficiently measured. [And while this is not a place to polemicize, no discussion of psychoanalytic learning can avoid noting that despite Freud's recommendations regarding the ideal education for psychoanalysts not a single institute today offers courses on the subjects he lists. Yet it is undoubtedly true that the study of philology, myth, religion, story, sociology, folklore, biology, child development, and rudiments of neuro-biology, provide the body of knowledge, the foundations of culture, and way of thinking, that is conducive to the kind of understanding espoused by a genuinely *psychoanalytic* attitude.]

Once matriculated, candidates find themselves dipping in to the divergent orientations of many "schools" in order to make sense of clinical phenomena, often adopting more than one theoretical orientation, a situation which has promulgated today's rampant eclecticism. Ideally, the enduring strength of a few common-core psychoanalytic tenets will help shape and define the basic skills and attitude required of analytic work, and optimal integration will occur. But this is an ideal: actually, given the politicized and intimidating dynamics of psychoanalytic training, institutes graduate timid analysts, ready to take their place in a profession assailed by incursions that threaten to annihilate the very premises of personal responsibility and autonomous thought upon which the entire ethical and philosophical sway of psychoanalysis as a therapy and as a movement are founded. It will take several years to sift out, sort out, and process, the entire educative experience; and it will be many more before the practice of analyzing will cultivate and yield the maturation of ones personal professional style. It is insufficiently recognized that due to the admixture of levels and types of learning that have to take place during psychoanalytic education, the full benefits and depths of its achievement only flower when their assimilation and synthesis have been integrated independently. Analytic insight and clinical skills are intimately entwined with personal maturation: the end of formal training and supervised work marks only the beginning of professional individuation.

By virtue of its tripartite structure and diverse experiential and didactic branches of study, psychoanalytic training offers an ideal panorama of different modes and "levels" of learning. A developmental model of learning in line with principles of symbolization would imply an epigenetic continuum of increasingly mediated modes but also of different kinds of information each of which contributes to psychoanalytic education. During the course of training candidates will "learn" by, i) conditioning; ii) imitation; iii) the assimilation of verbal information, and iv)by introspective analysis and personal transformation. Each of these well exercised modes of learning yield different forms of knowledge and levels of awareness, with 'conditioning' and 'identification', at the lower, more primitive end of the continuum. In addition to contributing to a growing pool of referents for the unconscious, simultaneously, a new range of interactive modalities are being opened up and brought within the spheres of consciousness through the personal analysis.

And here we meet with the most striking paradox of psychoanalytic education: what is most important for analysts to learn cannot be taught; it cannot be read or passed on as mere information, it is not dry data, or "inert knowledge" (Whitehead, 1927), but a form of emotional-cognition and understanding that is acquired in and through an experiential process that has to be lived. The particular integration of feelings and words together with the unique depth of reference that an analysis affords gradually generate closer connections between the experiencing-self and the linguistic ego. And these multiple channels of connection and communication that are opened and made accessible to verbal referencing become instrumental in attaining an analytic stance that is in tune with the many levels of meaning-transmission to which analysts must learn to resonate. "Morphic-matching," a resonance to the form in which the primary significance of a communication is made, may be likened to an empathic tuning-in to the frequency of an unconscious meaning, exactly as in Freud's "receiver" analogy. Empathic attunement is inherent in the analytic attitude and stance as a *quality* of attention, the norm rather than the exception, with its own developmental line and specialized application.

Psychoanalytic teaching and learning, then, is less pedagogical than dialogical, the educative process more *trans*formative than *in*formative: as Freud wrote, "To have heard something and to have experienced something are in their psychological nature two quite different things, even if the content of both is the same" (S. Freud, 1915, p. 176). In this sense the obligatory passage through the training analysis is not unlike a rite of passage that condenses psychological maturation with identity change (see Aragno, 1998). Actually there are more subtle similarities and differences between the two having to do with forms of internalization; the kind of learning or re-conditioning that takes place in the ritual passage occurs subliminally through the pedagogics of symbolic actions and ordeals, whereas the semanticity and investigative nature of the analytic process moves in the opposite direction — toward conscious awareness. Yet candidates, like novitiates, have to enter a liminal phase of deconstruction and personal re-construction that engages all three of Greenspan's (1982) levels of learning (somatic, consequence and representational-structural (p.661)) involving an entire hierarchy of levels of awareness (p.667). In order to learn how to analyze one must oneself have passed through this psychologically rigorous experience by which the very structures of cognition and consciousness are altered. To this is added a vast reservoir of historical, theoretical, clinical and technical information. Optimal results include optimal integration.

But by far the most difficult, practical challenge that analytic candidates face is learning how to *think* analytically, how to adopt, as second nature, the attitude and discipline that characterizes a genuine analytic stance. It is an irony of this profession that analytic skill is derived less from accumulating vast reservoirs of clinical knowledge than from a profound understanding of the analytic dialogue itself, how it proceeds, its processes and phases; that analysts benefit less from making assumptions from the general than from an investigative attitude toward the particular; and that analytic technique — which includes generating and sustaining a progressive analytic process — is developed out of a disciplined adherence to the correct analytic stance and basic interpretive strategies: the analysis of transference and resistance. In this sense, "It begins to become evident how much in each case the psychoanalytic process is a study of itself as it is created in and through the analytic dialogues" writes Shafer (1983, p. 21).

Psychoanalytic thinking is pliant, multitiered, specific, encompassing, multi-perspectival, differentiated, synthetic; it comes from a reflective, investigative attitude that allows for ambiguity, contradiction, confusion, incomprehensibility, tension, suspension, doubt and delay; and it promotes a dialogue that likewise becomes reflexive, collaborative, exploratory, formulative, integrative, open-ended.... To think psychoanalytically means to be attuned to sensory-emotional cues and being able to use these subtle private registrations as indices of meaning in the here and now; it means being able to identify, reflect upon and redefine emergent material and experiences from within a semantic space that returns insistently to an exploration of how and in what ways the current moment is an expression of the analysand's inner reality.

Familiarity with the rhythms, cycles and vicissitudes of the process comes slowly: candidates must learn to engender and enter into a semantic field in which the most salient interpretive aspects are submerged in ambiguous, polyvalent, and deeply submerged modes of communication. Since it is these very dynamisms and the tensions surrounding their unconscious levels that have to be identified and brought into the lexical sway of the dialogue, it is important in analytic training that the fusion of personal and professional result in a newly balanced hybrid combining personal sensibilities with professional responsibility. The training analysis broadens and deepens personal consciousness, however, what is most important for candidates to grasp is how to process analytic material; how to investigate, refer to, negotiate, formulate, clarify, and interpret, unconscious meanings from multiple angles and in highly individualized ways from within a dynamic core that tends, over and over again, to pull all contextual events into its enactive vortex.

Analytic thinking develops out of immersion in, and consistent exposure to, analytic discourse situations. As Vygotsky (1978) noted, learning takes place when a set of particular capabilities are exercised in relation to certain material in specific ways, "...because each activity depends on the material with which it operates, the development of consciousness is the development of a set of particular, independent capabilities, or of a set of habits" (p. 83). From this perspective, Vygotsky (1978) continues, "...special training affects overall development only when its elements, material, and processes are similar across specific domains;" (p. 83). The reflexive referentiality that began with self-observation in the personal analysis will become further faceted and amplified to include listening to the analysand and observing the process from multiple referential and interpretive perspectives. As training advances these simultaneously held experiential and interpretive viewpoints will be integrated and honed into those well-timed, intentionally focused, carefully worded communications we call "interventions." Establishing the "autonomous functioning" of the "analytic instrument"—its "calibration" (Ornstein, 1967) and "refinement" (Fleming and Benedeck, 1966)—as well as the integrative work of pulling together and synthesizing different aspects of training, is realized in supervision. In this context the candidate's main objective is learning how to "articulate the behavioral data of an analysis with explanatory concepts and theories" (Fleming and Benedeck, 1966, p. 26), while the supervisors' is to illustrate "how to apply theoretical knowledge to the treatment of patients" while teaching the "art of therapeutic communication" (p.1).

The successful use of supervision as an educative tool rests in great part on the supervisor's ability to harness and exercise the whole spectrum of modes of attunement and levels of awareness that pertain to clinical discourse, and to use the current process as a point of departure for technical or theoretical discussion. Supervision moves between the verbal, the experiential, and current process, to theory and technique: observation and abstraction of both the clinical and current process are the new dimensions this discourse articulates. Supervisors model their thinking via what they say; how and what they point to; when they inquire; how they pursue an exploration; what they draw attention to and how they reflect on it; how they negotiate the dialogue; and, ultimately, how things are understood. Supervisees learn how to listen, what to do. However, because they learn at the experiential hub of a dialogue, they learn their analyst's and supervisor's ways. Early stages of analytic learning are heavily dosed with mimicry and identification (see also Schlessinger, 1990, and Siegler, 1990).

In order to train independent analytic thinkers the supervisory process ought to encourage the supervisees' personal working-through and articulation of the material, adding to this or refining it via an enabling dialogue that, in terms of complexity of understanding, stays one step ahead of the candidate's current level of understanding. Educative exchanges take place in the gap between what the supervisee is able to grasp and formulate independently and what he/she requires supervisory guidance with. The distance between these two levels is the supervisory "zone of proximal development," that region of verbal interchange that advances the supervisee's learning. For those who understand that the discourse purpose and the supervisor's educative intent engender their own particular referential focus and communicative forms, the old dichotomy 'teach or treat,' is a moot point: supervisors identify, point to, question, indicate, explore, propose, suggest, respond, and comment on, in *active* feedback; "interpretation," in the full psychoanalytic sense, is not offered except, perhaps, for illustrative purposes, in an *educative* not a transformative dialogue.

It ought to be stressed that supervision benefits from the kind of close-process-monitoring favored by interpersonalists; they do more than pay lip service to using the contextual interchange as the source of data and attending to the current process as a vehicle of understanding. "It is our strong impression that good psychoanalytic supervision encourages the supervisee to attend to the *process of analysis*," write Caligor, Bromberg and Meltzer (1984), which they consider to be the hallmark of psychoanalysis. While its particular content and course cannot be predicted, optimally its outcome "is marked by the emergence in both participants of an increasingly reflective, non obsessive sensitivity to the multiple levels of interpersonal communication. The analyst-in-training must become an expert in this process, and be highly attuned to its nuances" (p.xv).

Candidates are leaning to resonate with and distinguish between a full range of transmissive and communicative forms; to recognize and be aware of their differences according to the nature of responses that are induced in them; to hear and interpret unconscious meanings; and to relate all of this to complex theoretical, technical and diagnostic considerations. An important aspect of the supervisor's skill lies in being able to relate what is being spoken about (or omitted) to how it is known. Bromberg (1984) illustrates this supervisory activity well:

> I am interested in what the supervisee hears, and primarily in that context, what he does. What he does, informs me of what he is hearing. What he is hearing informs me of a number of different things that can be addressed individually depending upon the relevance for a given student; how he is listening, how he thinks; his ability to conceptualize as he

> hears, his depth of knowledge, his values, and his possible blind spots due to unresolved personality conflicts of his own. (p. 38).

Papers addressing phases of learning (Dewald, 1981), teaching styles and approaches (DeBell, 1981), derailments of the process (Allpin, 1987), narcissistic issues (Brightman, 1984, 1985), questions of management (Baudry, 1993), research (Kubie, 1958), the different approaches of different schools toward the process (Caligor, Bromberg and Meltzer, eds., 1984), general principles of the process (Schlessinger, 1981), and possible teaching problems due to the supervisor's "Supertransference" (Teitelbaum, 1990), have all advanced our knowledge and understanding of the complex vicissitudes of this situation. From them have emerged such concepts as the "learning alliance," supervision as an "enabling process," awareness of the roles of modeling and identification in psychoanalytic learning, the importance of adjusting teaching style and method to fit the candidate's learning readiness, and of maintaining a "diagnostic point of view toward the candidate's learning process" (Schlessinger, 1981, p. 32).

Learning how to analyze takes place in a highly reflexive semantic field, through a dialogue that teaches how to observe itself (and oneself in it) via its own internal referential and speech activities. Here the teacher does what the student must learn to do. Yet so much of the personal dimension is employed in this discourse that the dialogue will be heavily conditioned by the theoretical penchant and personal style of the supervisor. Understandably, Hill (1958) comments "A therapist is what he does" (p 2); and what he does is an expression of what he knows. And while most self-respecting analysts try to practice what they preach, as Siegler (1990) wryly remarks, analytic supervisors face another challenge, "they must learn to *preach* what they practice" (p.145).

Despite the burgeoning interest in the supervisory process and dawning awareness of its potentially immense value as a research venue, the deeper, theoretical lacunae it sheds light on have been subtly ignored. Consider the consequences in teaching of the absence of a viable conceptual schema relating what we do to how dialogues work; or the absence of functional terms identifying the multiple referential perspectives synthesized in analytic thinking. With only dimly defined listening instructions, contrasting etiological theories and clinical models, no metatheory of mind and virtually no integrative metatheoretical map, the teaching and learning of how to analyze remains founded on hazy metaphors and foggy principles far removed from the raw phenomenology of the human encounter. Analysts are offered no tangible experience-near referents to understand their activities in process or clearly defined operative terms identifying the mental and speech processes involved in guiding the analytic dialogue through its predictable phases. Inevitably candidates learn analytic skills through imitation, "identifying" with the style and approach of their analyst and supervisors. Yet mimicry and identification lie at the least mediated, most primitive end of a continuum of learning modes, at unconscious levels far removed from the kinds of insight and deep understanding that are representative of analytic inquiry. They remain crude, unmetabolized modes of internalization, premised on neither the necessary personal integration nor full symbolic articulation that are the marks of analytic insight. I am skeptical of an educative system satisfied with such meager results.

Lastly, for a field using human communication as its prime medium, it is surprising that we have no language to talk about what we do with language. Our vocabulary stops short of providing functional concepts, dialogical terms and a theoretical framework tying together what we do, how we do it, and how it works. This study is an attempt to help fill this void yet the interrelatedness of all these problems, I believe, illustrates how impossible it is to construct a theory of learning without first establishing a psychoanalytic *epistemology*; and subsequently gaining some clarity as to the operative factors involved in what has to be learned. This analytic study of the semiotic and referential features of psychoanalytic dialogues, and the model of human communication it has generated, may, particularly in this sense, be of help.

Psychoanalytic candidates have to learn to integrate disparately acquired kinds of knowledge and to fuse and use this in making sense of what is going on, and how best to intervene, in psychoanalytically informed ways. This requires a heightened ability to register unconscious contextual experience; to refer *to* it as well as to refer *it* back to theoretical knowledge and understanding of process. Paradoxically this thinking has to become increasingly fluid and engaged as well as increasingly differentiated, objectifying, and integrative. By providing experience-near referents for interactive forms and dialogical activities the study grounds our knowledge in a comprehensive, unifying model, integrating many functional processes and phenomena. For supervisors it can serve as a tangible teaching tool, a lens through which to observe while participating in the field of an analysis: candidates may be helped by the guidance of an orienting framework that provides them, from the outset, with experience-near terms to identify what they do. In supervision, the model provides a shared conceptual schema with a new vocabulary to identify, conceptualize and discuss process-material as it emerges, enabling analysts to teach process *in* process, while talking about it in dialogical terms. Ideally, writes Siegler (1990):

> A complete psychoanalytic education should enable candidates to learn a way of *seeing*, (the development of acute powers of observation) a way of *hearing*, (listening *for* the unconscious and listening *to* it) a way of *understanding*, (familiarity with theory and strategy) and finally, a way of *speaking*. (p. 146)

Not everything, however, can be taught or learned, and there are some intangibles that depend on talent. Analytic skills engage sensory, emotional, intellectual, symbolic, and verbal formulative abilities that are not given to all in equal ways. Not everyone will achieve that rare amalgam of patience and persistence, engagement and opaqueness, restraint and spontaneity, and the acceptant optimism that underlies the psychoanalytic spirit of inquiry.

In the end there has to be some special "psychological-mindedness," akin to musicality in music, or natural giftedness, as in any other field. If this is the case then there may be, as Siegler (1990) suggests, another model of training better suited to the development of fine analysts — say that of a concert pianist: "One would begin, of course, with a passion for music, (or in our case, a passion for the mind), then one must have technical mastery over one's instrument (oneself), third, one must have musical knowledge of the entire standard repertoire (one's theory), and last, one must have interpretive skills which bring something new to the material (one's own voice)"(p.146). Ultimately, the goal is to encourage an ample interdisciplinary foundation, to provide an enriching and enabling educative process geared toward shaping independent practitioners and inspired thinkers who, to paraphrase Siegler again (1990, p. 145), will not only go by the book but will contribute new chapters of their own.

ARTISTRY IN PSYCHOANALYTIC DIALOGUES

> Nothing takes place in a psycho-analytic treatment but an interchange of words between the patient and the analyst
>
> S. Freud, 1917, p. 17

> In the mutual interaction of the good analytic hour, patient and analyst — each in his own way and on his own mental level — become both artist and medium for each other. For the analyst as artist his medium is the patient in his psychic life; for the patient as artist the analyst becomes his medium. But as living human media they have their own creative capabilities, so that they are both creators themselves.
>
> H. Loewald, 1975/1980, p.369

We think of art as consummate skill in the creative or interpretive use of a medium; of science as an acknowledged body of systematized knowledge. Psychoanalytic methodology, most analysts would agree, combines both. Yet the field has been notoriously at pains to pinpoint the locus or characteristics of either.

In the practical application of our investigative method, psychoanalysts refer to a foundation of metatheoretical knowledge and clinical principles to understand a process and to inform their interpretation of a broad range of unconscious meanings.[9]

As a therapeutic modality, however, and in the teaching of its practice, the "method" takes place in live, dynamic human interchanges, in contexts created by speech — quite simply, in dialogues. And dialogues are shaped by what we do with words. Language is our medium, words our tools; both are neutral instruments, value free, until we endow them with meanings that are context specific, bound by the semantic, referential perspectives and situational purposes that orient their use. What we know (the breadth of our knowledge), how we understand (the depth of our personal awareness), and what we say (the quality of our communications), which together constitute analytic skills, combine to create an epistemology of psychoanalytic practice. Artistry in psychoanalytic dialogues is exemplified in how skillfully and effectively we realize the dialogues purpose, or, how well we are able to use language in this particular sphere of human exchange.

Scientific knowledge, personal understanding, and aesthetic formulation are here indivisible, actualized in the pragmatics of a therapeutic dialogue. Trying to apply the usual criteria of art — truth, beauty, perfection of form, etc. — to it, however, falls short of grasping the full aesthetic merit of its goals as a *whole*, an aim that represents a quintessential post-modernist venture, the deconstruction and reconstruction of oneself, through a quintessentially humanistic venue, a dialectical "conversation." For here, as in all human endeavors, artistic value is realized through the relationship of each of the features and elements of the process to a whole, through their fit, coherence, cohesion, their expressive resolution in the overall design. Conceptualized from this deeply humanistic perspective — or Bakhtinian sensibility — "conversational" art is preoccupied with stance, understanding, responsiveness, quality of communication, cross-fertilization, inquiry, and hence, where the primal sharing that takes place between observer and observed can become "the site of another, more essential task — knowledge of the self through communicative exchange" (Emerson, 1997, p. 206).

The analyst's role and function, — ideally, I submit, a distillate of sublimated love — is to offer him/herself up as a reflective agent is to experience, contain, identify, reformulate, negotiate and give back interpretively, to use Schön's (1986) concept, what of the other they have been able to understand through themselves. The enhanced insight or new consciousness thus engendered — by this creative act but also by the aesthetic task that is its aim — resembles the participatory understanding that takes place between the viewer and the viewed through a work of art, and therefore, if properly understood, as an interpenetrative "feeling into" like empathy, might point to a paradigm for all human creativity (Emerson, 1997). Knowledge and artistry are here interwoven through the dialogues' interpretive speech activities, "their aesthetic and pragmatic value...inseparable from the activity of their formulation and delivery," (Schön, 1986, p. 308), so that, in Goodman's (1978) words, "the distinction between convention and content — between what is said and how it is said — wilts" (p.125 in Schön, 1986, p. 308).

I have found Bakhtin's (1986) articulation of the notion of speech genres, with its focal emphasis on "utterance" as the principal semantic unit of exchange, its examination of the interrelatedness of style, compositional structure and other formal and functional aspects of language in use, to be of immense value to psychoanalysis, particularly in relation to the topic of this essay. The current Bakhtinian revival is drawing accolades of appreciation from numerous academic quarters, however, many of his central ideas — the preeminence of form, creative outsideness, polyphony, the aesthetic moment, inherent responsiveness — seem to speak directly to psychoanalysts. A soviet literary intellectual, philologist, philosopher-aesthetician, he was culturally and geographically, a world apart from psychoanalytic thought. Yet his penetrating study and illuminating understanding of the nouminous power of words, of dialogue, to transform and advance human consciousness, evoked in me a gasp of recognition.

But Bakhtin's ideas are more than inspirational: they provide a bedrock of dialogical concepts yielding a set of formal attributes and characteristics of speech genres that may point to the missing conceptual links between form, content and context in our practice, suggesting that many factors championed by interpersonalists as "relational" may, in fact, be more fundamentally "dialogical" in nature. This new sensibility to our medium introduces the idea that conversational arts contain their own science, and it would behoove those of us using them to become more familiar with their operative principles.

Bakhtin (1986) begins from the premise that language is realized in various contexts of human exchange through concrete individual utterances that reflect their specific conditions and situational goals not only through thematic content and linguistic style, "— the lexical, phraseological, and grammatical resources of the language—," but primarily through their "compositional structure" (p.60). These three, "thematic content, style and compositional structure," Bakhtin writes, are organically and inseparably "linked to the *whole* of the utterance, and are equally determined by the specific nature of the particular sphere of communication" (p.60). Every linguistic context develops its own speech forms; when these have become relatively stable, identifiable types of utterance we are in the presence of a speech genre. During its formative process, a genre will absorb and subsume various other simpler or more primary genres that materialize out of less mediated forms of speech interaction. And these primary genres are altered, assuming their new more complex characteristics, as they simultaneously "lose their immediate relation to actual reality and to the real utterances of others" (Bakhtin, 1986, p. 62). [One thinks immediately of Freud's early modification of the hypnotic suggestion in the development of his method, and of the highly specialized speech forms — free-association punctuated sporadically by interpretive interventions — that derived thereof, and of his creative willingness to continue shifting and expanding his referential focus to accommodate new observations, from linking repressed affect and content, at the beginning, to the contextual interpretation of transference, resistance and the dynamically repressed, a movement from content toward form *in* process, that continues today.]

A genre, then, evolves out of specific speech conditions serving particular functions that engender its thematic contents and coherence (in our case also its particular interpretive perspectives), compositional structure and stylistic qualities. These characteristic attributes are recognized by types of sentence construction in relation to a whole utterance; in the duration of an utterance and its forms of completion; in particular phrase-cadence and expressive tonal inflections; and in particular types of exchanges prescribed by the relationship between speakers (Bakhtin, 1986, p. 64). According to these criteria, ours is a highly creative and malleable genre, characterized by extreme variability of form and individualized, particularized, spontaneous structuring: an interpretive sequence may be constituted by various utterances going on for many sentences, even over time, or it may be said in a single word.

Basically, Bakhtin (1986) asserts, we "assimilate forms of language only in forms of utterances and in conjunction with these forms" and, hence, these linguistic types (or genres) and their typical forms of utterance "enter our experience and our consciousness together, and in close connection with one another" (p.78). Given this inseparability of genre and style (and in view of what we know of unconscious internalization) we ought to be alert to the possible stultifying effects, in our field, of intergenerational transmissions of communicative style, as porous candidates assimilate their analyst's mannerisms and technique (ways of thinking and speaking) passing them down, in turn, analyst after analyst. . . . On the upside, the more fully we have mastered a genre the more freely and creatively can we manipulate it; "The better our command of genres," Bakhtin (1986) writes, "the more freely we employ them, the more fully and clearly we reveal our own individuality in them, (where this is possible and necessary), the more flexibly and precisely we reflect the unrepeatable situation of communication — in a word, the more perfectly we implement our free speech plan" (p.80).

Once we are able to cast our speech naturally and nimbly within the genres' generic forms, and have become adept at fulfilling our particular speech goals or "purposes" through its prescribed exchanges, fluidly, precisely, seamlessly, *masterfully*, then, and *only* then, do we encounter *artistry* in the use of a dialogue. For now, the dialogues ultimate aim — to increase conscious awareness — speaks through us, as does a medium achieve expressiveness *through* the artist's use of it. And, as Bakhtin divined, the proper understanding of this (essentially psychoanalytic) "aesthetic task" reveals it to be "a paradigm for all other (even the most humdrum) human tasks" (Emerson, 1997, p. 216): for here dialogue, in our methodological sense of the word, with its amalgam of scientific and artistic sources of formulation, and its mandate for contextual understanding through self-reflection and linguistically negotiated insight, becomes itself an expression and a model of the creative process. Only in art (as in love) do task and goal coincide: the interpretation of human meanings — in a dialectical, contextual exchange — will find no force, no vital process more fundamental to human experience, no regenerative power stronger, than itself. It is based on the assumption that the florid development of human consciousness, whether personal or collective, that began in a tender dialectic with at least one other person, will flourish and grow when in constant contact and through cross-fertilizing commerce with other voices.

Rudimentary practice, in our purposive contexts, begins with this basic capacity to establish a genuine subject-subject encounter; is concerned with maintaining "aesthetic" or symbolic distance, the essential "I-Thou" distinction that is requisite for "seeing" another; with not being degraded into collusive musings or actualizing communions, the loss of contour, or frame; and with assiduously avoiding the "management" of another through suggestion and condescending word or tone. More advanced skills exercise judgment and selection — of material, type of communication, etc. — of timing, phrasing, tone, style of intervention.

Since we cannot appeal to traditional aesthetic markers we must look for artistry in the formulative principles and interactive dynamisms of the dialogue itself: it is here that Bakhtin offers real, compelling ethical and aesthetic yardsticks of dialogical practice — as in any other *instrumental* art — that can be used to evaluate levels of skill and qualities of merit that may be assessed by standards of artistic excellence. As Emerson (1997) writes, dialogue is measurable by many criteria "— precision of expression, proper timing, impact on the listener, subsequent modification of behavior — and makes use of various instruments, of which words are only one" (p. 144). In Bakhtin's hands, dialogical fluency, even (or particularly) in a genre with specialized procedures and goals such as ours, includes many skills with which instrumentalists and interpretive artists are quite familiar since they are skills that apply to all arts where technique and artistry fuse in practice. "Technical" proficiency, in a dialogical sense, presupposes and subsumes a profound understanding of the genres' forms and contextual purpose, deep familiarity with ones medium, and knowledge of principles of theory and practice, the expressions of which are woven thread by thread through the whole fabric of the conversation's speech activities. The *artistic* merit of these skills can be assessed in terms of a number of attributes: clarity and precision of expression; quality of wording and tone; timing, sensitive phrasing, smooth transitions; awareness of underlying mood and thematic repetitions; attention to detail and dissonance, the placing and progression of elements in relation to the whole; ease with increasing complexity, density, intensity; prospective vision — propelling the momentum forward; endurance; artistic rendition and *understanding* of the material; imaginative use of language; interpretive depth and fullness.

As psychoanalysts we resonate with the Bakhtinian landscape; we recognize its contours, vistas and signposts of reference as resembling things we experience daily. Despite differences in terminology there is conceptual convergence in the correspondence between his ideas regarding the transmutative power of dialogues carried on over time, accretively bring about new consciousness, and the pragmatics of what we do. It stands to reason that a dialogical genre skillfully manipulated has the capacity to draw us into a whole new world view.

A fundamental skill in the art of conducting psychoanalytic dialogues is the ability to create, maintain and *use* an interpsychical semantic field for its specific therapeutic or educative purpose. The principal goals and subject matter of these situations differ but the semantic direction, referential spread and interpretive activities that inform our inquiry are the same. The nature of encounters thus engendered, within these interpsychical fields, is intricately tied to, and determined by, their specific functions and the special roles of the interlocutors in each. In fact, it is this functional indivisibility of psychoanalytic dyads (or triads) that produces the tensional dynamisms — progressive, regressive, collusive, or obstructive — and generates the uniquely interpenetrative forms of these dialogues' exchanges. There is a formal, functional and contextual unity in the epistemology of psychoanalytic practice that enables our dialogues to unfold synergistically, realizing their overall semantic orientation through their internal speech activities and specific situational goals.

In order for the inner landscape of the psychical world to come into sharp view there has to be someone present who is able to identify its manifestations, to look at them, name them, seek out their origins, co-explore and formulate an understanding of their meanings, in a psychoanalytic way. The task necessitates a willingness to enter-into yet stay outside the encounter, while generating a liminal space, or frame, which must remain loose and free to the speaker. Originally, the self came into being at the boundaries of encounter with another self; now, a new consciousness is shaped at the verbal edge, or the dialogical interface, with another voice. Clearly, the crafting of this psychical space and frame, and the requisite *symbolic* distance to be maintained within it, are as central to the task—if it is to be "aesthetic"—as the amplitude of knowledge or accuracy of interpretations.

Bakhtin refers to this aesthetic distance as "creative outsideness," a benevolent form of attention, fully differentiated yet highly engaged, which constitutes the healthy stance for any consciousness-structuring activity. For Bakhtin, a situation or an event becomes "aesthetic" when there is an outside consciousness looking in, or a second perceiving-self, capable of bestowing upon it a form-giving sense of the whole. The "aesthetic task" necessitates the presence of "someone exercising a surplus vision" (Emerson, 1997, p. 217) and certainly, in our dialogues, this external viewing or interpretive mode applies to the verbal shaping of micro-sequences (in sessions or days) as well as to macro-phases unfolding over time (months and years). To have a sense of a "whole," from this aesthetic perspective, means to give something a form: and form, in human affairs, *is* meaning. We cannot "see" something unless we stand "outside" it: any interpretive utterance in our semantic fields that may qualify as having aesthetic merit will, in its transposition of form, express and contribute some new signifying version of a heretofore indistinct or unfinalized event. Art sets forth the "idea" of a thing through the shaping of its elements: its meaning is symbolized through an interpretive act, in whatever the medium.

I must confess it is disturbing to witness the growing tendency in our field, and in our journals, to adopt an attitude that seems to condone, even encourage, an excessive blurring of psychical boundaries, whereby the aesthetic distance of a *symbolic* space, in which analysts can effectively interpret the unconscious, has necessarily collapsed. In one journal article, presumably with some pride, the author described how in deeply empathizing with his silently crying patient he, similarly, sat behind him crying silently in emotional communion. Others write freely of interventions in which they spill out their feelings, hunches, twinges and twitches, even their immediate personal reactions — as though these were legitimate responses — apparently satisfied in justifying these hasty disclosures as a way of instrumentalizing the "countertransference." But if 'psychical distance,' in the sense discussed above, is a touchstone of artistic aesthetics, in psychoanalytic contexts, it is also a touchstone of professional ethics. We are neither encharged to "manage" our clients or supervisees, nor to parade our own psyches before them, but only to use ourselves in the service of *understanding* them. From this interpretive di-stance, the counter-reactivity of countertransference proper (a mèconnaissance of the other), blurted out, is unthinkable. Artistry in our dialogues is crafting utterances that induce to *thinking,* not to wallow in like-feelings or indulge in psychical tête-à-têtes. In order to safeguard the symbolic nature of the frame and, ideally, to preserve the requisite outsideness vis-à-vis our material and interpretive tasks, we have to articulate communications that invite insight, not emotional discharge. [10]

Mastery of **frame** and **stance** then are basic in the crafting of our dialogues; but an effective guide must also know the route and be at ease in its terrain, even if the itinerary is never certain. Analysts have to be thoroughly familiar and comfortable with a multiperspectival spectrum of referential perspectives that, as we have seen, in order to be fully accessed engage us at multiple levels of listening, feeling and thought. Our dialogues wander through avenues and scenarios with unforeseeable obstacles, venturing into highly incendiary turf where staying the course means being able to avoid precipices and moving carefully through potential pitfalls. The analyst-as-guide is aware of everything that has been shown, said, done, expressed, projected into or hidden from view, recognizing the trails laid by the verbal line while tirelessly tracing the repetitive patterns traced by a shadow, counter-voice beneath.

We dwell in a domain of reference straddling at least two (probably many more) discrepant modes of making meaning, where dynamic tensions, complexity, ambiguity, ambivalence and contradiction are the norm. This makes for uncommonly paradoxical conditions: a highly artificial situation that, nonetheless, achieves extraordinary authenticity of exchange; we manage to combine intense separateness with unparalleled intimacy — a communion of rigorous differentiation. Although language is our medium, we are not limited by it; the deep tissue of our exchanges is not, in its essence, linguistic. We are less interested in what has already been wrought by words than what is still raw and visceral, unformed; in knowing about than in becoming profoundly acquainted with. More than in any others, our dialogues rely on an "interactive logic that strains words to the limit — encouraging them to take on intonation, flesh, the contours of an entire worldview" (Emerson, 1997, p.161).

To thus use language as an aesthetic, transmutative deed, requires that we constantly reconcile a number of seemingly contradictory aims: on the one hand, in order to "see" and understand, we are to contour and delineate, to identify, highlight, demarcate, denote; we have to draw boundaries with words that give shape to this organic, dynamic, transaction, fixing one-sidedly its multiple forms. On the other hand we are to remain innocent listeners, sustaining attention that is loose and free, each day fresh 'without memory or desire.' This means that we are to be fluid and bound at the same time, able to linearize what is simultaneous and freeze what is continuously moving.

This makes sense if we consider that our analysis is never textual but *con*textual: ours is not a hermeneutics of hearsay but of organic, dynamic, live interchange. The polyphony of the spontaneous account is essential to our interpretive enterprise for within its free-flowing speech it carries the hidden voices of the enacted, experiential sub tale. Moreover the "word" in our domain, heard for its wealth of condensations, is recognized as gathering unto itself all of the tributaries of meaning that originate and engender its current use, containing both the history of itself in the life of the speaker (along the vertical dimension) as well as its contextual sense in this narrative utterance at this moment in time (along the horizontal line). Words *themselves,* then, also subsume the voice of internalized interactions, in addition to how they were initially experienced and are now used. The supervisee's meticulously transcribed 'verbatim' report transports a text devitalized without its qualifying context: this blanched account carries naked words stripped of the stimulating moments that begot them. On the other hand, if we select only themes and patterns of emotion or inductions and ignore the words with which they are spun, we lose the unique fabric in which experience is woven. Balance is the key: in the confluence of content, form, subject and style; the dialectic between what is told and what is hidden, between word and action *in* interaction—unconscious meanings appear at the hub of these three. The phenomenology of spontaneous, fluid speech is fundamental to the psychoanalytic interpretive approach; it keeps us anchored in the present moment, for what is going on provides a commentary for what is being said.

Our semantic fields bear no relationship to the linear space/time dimensions of ordinary life but operate within a meta-temporal frame of psychical form and reality. For us the past is in the present until it has been worded into the dialogue to be processed, worked through, understood.

With words as our aesthetic markers we simultaneously construct and reconstruct, the dialogues progression co-authoring the story of itself superimposed on the recapitulated history it has expanded upon, completed and re-versioned. Those singularly mutative moments of the 'good analytic hour' appear at times of dyadic congruence "when re-enactment is drawn into and yields to the force field of objectifying narrative and reflection" (Loewald, 1975/1980, p. 368). They show "something of the analysts art," wrote Loewald (1975/1980), illustrating how "a piece of good analytic work is an artistic creation fashioned by the patient and analyst in collaboration….The progression in such an hour is quite similar to the progression of a work of art…at a propitious moment or period during the artists work," when the momentum of the creative process is "propelled by the directional tensions of the previous steps…and the inherent force of his medium" (Loewald, 1975/1980, p. 369). The soil from which such moments grow, as Loewald (1975/1980) pointed out, are "likely to have been prepared and cultivated…for a long time" (p.369) but when they happen, it is as though our ethical and aesthetic tasks join in the pragmatic acts of a dialogue in which, as Bakhtin (1986) counseled, we have succeeded in integrating "the real life deed with the aesthetically shaped word" (Emerson, 1997, p.240).

From this dialogical perspective, in the assessment of clinical skills, we would look, first and foremost, for qualities of craftsmanship in the shaping of the dialogue: have we created a dialectic that is maximally free? Does it lead, on its own momentum, to both understanding and apprehending potential? Is its overall movement dynamically progressive, prospective? Does the dyad, over time, come to see what is, what was, what can be? In the assessment of the novice we would look for qualities of resonance, responsiveness, wording that engenders recursiveness in the chain of communicative utterances and interactive sequences built up over time that constitute the formative, compositional elements of our purposive situations. For it is true, as Bakhtin (1986) says, that "language enters life through concrete utterances (which manifest language) and life enters language through concrete utterances as well" (p.63). But in our semantic fields it is the *psychical* that enters language through concrete utterances (which manifest the unconscious) and *dialogue* enters psyche, as well. It is all the more pressing, therefore, when assessing the novice that we consider how well he/she has been able to engender an atmosphere encouraging of inquiry, self-observation and reflection, capacities for delay, working-through and new formulation; and if he/she has imparted the value of continuous slow process, of letting speech arise and wander freely where it will, of implementing insight gained; we would observe how well the dialogues' forms have taken over its content, so that our *psychoanalytic* ways of knowing have become *the* ways of knowing in this context.

In addition to mastery of **stance, frame** and **semantic domain,** we now add **mastery of referential forms and perspectives** as requisite skills; for in a field of immense complexity and multiplicity of meanings, informed and knowledgeable *selection*, not 'intuition,' is the key. Type of communication, timing, phrasing and tone — *what* to say, *when* and *how* — which constitute the compositional elements of our interpretive chains are also the *non plus ultra* of the dialogues artistic expression. The choice of when to speak and how to couch an intervention that runs seamlessly through the moment while having its intended impact, is the essence of the *art* of psychoanalytic communication. In our work, artistry is marked by clear verbal articulation of consummate psychoanalytic understanding, at any given singular, contextual moment in time, which in turn is based on having learned how to *feel* and *think* analytically.

A psychoanalyst's understanding of the phases, stages and dynamisms of our discourse rests, ideally, on additional foundations drawn from a broad base of relevant interdisciplinary scholarship. All of this expertise, as well as personal sensibilities and maturation, come into play and converge at the moment of formulating a communication that is *intentionally* crafted as an intervention. I emphasize intent because I believe it to be an extremely powerful and transmissible force in human communication, the bearer of expression, sense, emphasis and, in great part, of the potential impact on the listener. But also, perhaps more importantly, because purposeful dialogues demand careful, judiciously worded communications condensing knowledge and understanding, pronounced from that "aesthetic distance" that is the safeguard of professional intent.

In our non linear, multistratal, semantic fields, awash in simultaneity, where condensation, displacement, enactment, and projection are commonplace, most analysts orient interpretively to no less than eight unconscious referential perspectives each with its own particular form of resistance[11] embedded in five broader *meta*psychological dimensions. Meaning, for us, is everywhere, and nothing is taken at face value. We operate from an integrated yet pliant center, moving fluidly between different levels of experience, from less-differentiated to highly- differentiated communications, equidistant between two poles along a continuum that oscillates between primary and secondary processes, from past to present, present to past, but always with an overriding prospective vision toward advancing the dialogue's purpose and new consciousness through it. In order to do this well, ideally, analysts ought to be knowledgeable of principles of progression along logical (semiotic) and *psycho*logical lines, the former related to metatheoretical principles of formal transformation, the latter to working-through of highly individual psychical issues. The interrelationships between the dialogues purpose and its internal subjects and the referential processes leading *toward* the goal—i.e., working-through of transference/resistance—*together,* lead to increased personal integration and emotional maturation.

These progressive transpositions in form result from continuously negotiated processes of increasing symbolization. The steps leading up to a "psychoanalytic" interpretation—which may be defined by its condensed, multiperspectival inclusiveness and symbolic character—however, are not all "symbolic" or "interpretive" in the same way. In the unfolding of our dialogues we would expect there to be many different types of communication paving the way, as it were, or leading up to a maximally full, genuinely symbolic, *psychoanalytic* interpretation. "Art" in such therapeutic (or educative) dialogues depends on how well one is "seeing" or understanding the current moment, and how skillfully one uses the mediational tools of the medium. The overall design of such dialogues would be progressively spiraling, phasic, dynamically taught between regression, stasis and movement, as in all *art*, and characterized by temporarily finalized elements giving shape to a whole. From this perspective we are swayed away from looking for isolated "correct" interpretations toward the idea of creating optimal *psychoanalytic* semantic fields, contexts where space/time, action, and critical judgment, are suspended in order to bring unconscious and conscious aspects into correspondence through participatory exploration and verbalization.

Understanding the primary thrust of our dialogues as being an integration of multiple facets of experience through increased symbolization was a view eloquently expressed also by Loewald (1971/1980, 1975/1980):

> It is as though what counts in mental life takes place on a kind of middle ground between two poles, and the two poles are being interpreted in terms of each other....The overall direction of a psychoanalytic investigation seems to be not so much toward consciousness per se, but toward an optimal communication, and interpenetration and balance of the two forms of mental processes and of the psychic structures their activities bring about. (1971/1980, p. 108)

And again, here encapsulating the idea of the dialogue as creating conditions for the reactivation of psychic integration through an integrative dialectic...

> Psychoanalytic interpretations establish or make explicit bridges between two minds, and within the patient bridges between different areas and layers of the mind that lack or have lost connections with each other, that are not encompassed within an overall contextual organization of personality. Interpretations establish or re-establish links between islands of conscious mentation and between the unconscious and consciousness....What is therapeutic, I believe, is the mutual linking itself by which each of the linked elements gains or regains meaning or becomes richer in meaning—meaning being our word for the resultant of that reciprocal activity. In the re-initiation and promotion of this process the interpretive activity of the analyst and the specific contents of interpretations are the enabling factor; he envisages and holds for the patient that context which makes linking possible. (Loewald, 1975/1980, p. 382)

Skill in engendering these linkages and integrative activities is enhanced when grounded in a familiarity with the principles of a mediational continuum of semiotic progression. A typology of forms through which different kinds of unconscious meanings are expressed adds an important dimension to clinical and supervisory acumen, providing a conceptual template through which to breakdown condensations and a set of principles for a parallel, multilayered model of listening.

Mastery of referential perspectives and forms, in multileveled communicative fields, results in being able to formulate interventions that include several dimensions of meaning simultaneously. Analysts in training have to learn to attune to and distinguish between a full range of transmissive and communicative forms and become aware of the qualities of their differences through the *kinds* of responses they induce in them. The hallmark of undifferentiated modes is their ability to get under ones skin, so to speak, whereas increasingly mediated interactions are more "interpersonal" and symbolic, in the full sense of the word. We may have the beginnings of a metatheoretical framework in which unmediated, semiotic and referential forms, observable in the transmutative phenomenology of psychoanalytic dialogues, reveal the complex architecture of human interactions. Through this multidimensional approach to human communication, we have arrived at the possibility of formulating a general dynamic model of human responsiveness in which interpretive principles can be singled out along multiple lines.

At different times and in different ways, analysts may be called on to filter, contain, identify, modulate, reflect, tolerate, recognize, link, differentiate, clarify, reframe, transpose, linearize, question, confront, integrate, and finally *interpret,* unconscious meanings in an atmosphere of joint inquiry and negotiated understanding. Out of this list we know that the more primitive or basic the type of function we are serving the more urgently is it needed to quell anxiety or bolster an enfeebled self, and hence the more entrenched the defenses. The analysis of disorders of very early etiology, or of the more primitive layers of the human psyche, *necessitates* attunement to these pre-semiotic, almost bio-psychical levels. Psychoanalysts have to remain open to the persistent *basso continuo*[12] of psychical life; only by resonating with its emanations can the full depths of meanings that lie beneath the spoken word be grasped.

Three broad categories of meaning-organization can be carved out of our semiotic continuum each of which benefits from an optimally matched listening mode for maximum attunement; 1) *unreferenced meanings,* functioning at signal-levels, require *participatory inference* or empathic attunement and, primarily, reflective or mirroring responses; 2) *presentational or enacted reproductions*, operating at sign-levels and through projection or evocation, once identified, have to be explored for their specific origins and nature; and 3) *verbally* referenced communications operating at symbolic levels, containing highly condensed, complex and repressed meanings, can be interpreted in a classic, psychoanalytic sense.

The art of psychoanalytic communication engages compositional skills in formulating utterances and interactive sequences that are timed, dosed, phrased, and tailored to match the functional/formal level that can best be heard, while simultaneously always pushing awareness forward with an implicit understanding that the full impact of any communication is heavily influenced by tone. This is what Gedo (1981) meant when in his epilogue, the "Art of Psychoanalysis," while commenting on technique, he stressed that one area in which analytic skills are left to clinical intuition concerns the "optimal manner in which interpretations should be articulated. Cogent ideas," he writes, "are necessary but not sufficient: *c'est le ton qui fait la musique*" (p.375). Precisely. The dynamic impact of any communication is qualified by its expressive features in which tone, inflection and volume, are central.

Conditions of timing, tone, type of communication, duration of utterance and, above all, unconscious *attitude* and *intent*, rise to the forefront and are quite as important in the analyst's communications as anything that is spoken in words. The right admixture of deliberateness and spontaneity is achieved only through lengthy practice. Unconscious transmissions and their dynamic impact go both ways, and while this subtle but pervasive bi-directionality demands rigorous personal monitoring and heightened referential acuity on the part of analysts this does not preclude the characteristic time-lapse that often divides a clinical response from an understanding of its unconscious meaning. This is why it would not do to promote a psychoanalysis oblivious to the voice of the patronizing physician, the authoritarian analyst, the overly enmeshed "empathicist" or the overly democratic "interpersonalists" planted in the equality of a contextual 'reality' that is too 'real' to be the *psychical* reality of the other. *Unconscious* attitude toward the task, the context and the client, are all important, since it is primarily the *unconscious attitude* that seeps through the dialogue saturating it with implicit messages through quality of attention, posture, tone, rhythms of response or non-responsiveness — non-responsiveness being, I believe, universally, at all stages and phases of the life cycle and in all situations, the most crippling of psychical wounds, for Thomas Mann, the very image of hell (Emerson, 1997, p. 284).

To mastery of **stance**, **frame**, **domain**, **referential forms** and **perspectives** must now be added selection of **type** and **duration of utterance** and **manner of delivery**, to complete our list of artistic criteria, with an awareness of the fluid bi-directionality and polyvalence that is ever present, at unconscious levels of human transactions. Whereas for the speaker the polyphony of voices and multiple levels of meaning must be left to emerge as freely as possible, the analysts carefully crafted communications are filtered through three voices underlying the analytic function and role: that of healer/therapist (or teacher/guide in supervision); that of the interpretive co-author; and that of the poet. These three commingled voices — the analyst as healer (or teacher) co-author and poet — always present, cross-referencing each other, alternately rising to ascendance and receding according to the requirements of the present moment and phase in the process, together, generate the dialogical therapeutics, narrative constructions and poetics, of a humanistic, aesthetic approach to the interpretive activities of psychoanalytic discourse.

From the perspective of the "healer," the analyst's therapeutic skills naturally subsume diagnostic assessments. But for this kind of knowledge not to disrupt the delicate dynamic conditions that make for an authentic encounter and in order to preserve the subject-subject equality of the dialectic, diagnostic categorizing ought not to intrude on the slow developing, progressively penetrating and increasingly particularized, open process valued by psychoanalysts. Freud cautioned against premature diagnostication. Given the slow unfolding, highly individualized, plastic quality of understanding in each analytic process, he recommended waiting until the analysis was over before finalizing its findings along diagnostic lines. In addition to the potentially contaminating effect of imposing categories that are extraneous to the complex texture of contextual exchange, and possibly clouding the unconscious dynamisms, in general, it is only later — much later — and *retrospectively* when all thematic and transferential dimensions have fully coalesced and can be grouped into component elements, that a new *psychoanalytically* full 'version' can be finalized along the lines of a "diagnosis."

If it is the voice of the **healer** who speaks directly through the analyst's therapeutic intent and interventions, it is the interpretive, co-authoring voice of the analyst as **psycho-novelist** that underlies the dyads' constructions and reconstructive activities. To become author of ones life, or to become authoring in it, one has to be able to stand back and observe oneself living and give to this fluid experience a form, or a sensible shape. In order to engender such an authoring scenario the analyst models this observing, form-finding attitude and actualizes the novelist's creative understanding by bestowing upon the emergent events, and those recounted, a new psychically inclusive *meaning*. The co-authoring, novelistic analyst serves a catalytic and participatory role, helping to complete an incomplete account by 'seeing', by taking on and giving back, worded, those aspects that are partly enacted, partly projected, partly shown and partly told, of the psychical tale. Formless experiences, lost parts of selves, undigested events and people, disavowed affects long throttled, arise from the underbelly of this shadow tale and only slowly, laboriously, will the dyad unravel new versions of mini- and meta-themes and principal life-motifs now filled out and fully narratized through a psychoanalytic interpretative lens.

But these newly authored accounts are neither story nor history; analysts are not story makers and analytic constructions are neither truth nor fiction. They are simply newly ordered, psychoanalytically crafted, particularized versions of a life, versions that are inclusive of the analyst's interpretive translation of vital messages that are transmitted coded, incompletely formed, subjectively felt and recapitulated unbidden, initially only dimly known. For there to be consciousness there has to be a "surplus vision" — a third eye — an outside perspective looking on, bestowing on the parts a sense of significance that becomes a new whole. Whether we call it "creative outsideness" (Bakhtin), "psychical distance" or analytic neutrality, aesthetic distance is *the* ethical stance, the only stance from which to fully "see" another and, hence, also to author our interpretive formulations insightfully.

The co-authoring analytic dyad, provisionally synchronized, will return again and again to a site where a dawning consciousness is being formed and, regardless of the laborious, entangling, consuming nature of the work, will continue to reach toward the unmediated contact—that which has yet to be seen, yet to be said. But where the novelistic activities piece together different narrative modes, linking and concatenating their newly interpreted elements, only a poetic mission toils to transform the raw tissue of an exchange and render it in words; it is the poet that has "commerce with a person's soul" (Emerson, 1997, p. 263). From time immemorial the poet's inner call is to become a "seer," a *voyant* (Rimbaud), an introspective "listener" (Whitman), to develop the contemplative "inner eye" (Wordsworth) that registers and duly records its private vision. The poetic analyst's deeper vision, then, is an expression of a willingness to enter into—to interpenetrate—things organically, creatively, to bore beyond, beneath and around the crust of surface presentations and touch a primary, ineffable, unmediated eidetic core and give it verbal shape; as Whyte (1960) describes this primal pollination "the primary process in everything is the coming into existence of form" (p.127).

The implicit paradox in these simultaneous tasks is that while interpreting and co-constructing necessitates standing back and 'outside' in order to identify, demarcate, delineate, and linearize, as participants we place ourselves at the disposal of the process and, like poets, become one with our material, one with our medium, wording, wording everything. The analyst endowed with poetic sensibilities is at an advantage in this verbal art and will bring to this polychromatic semantic field innate formulative tendencies habituated to distilling meanings from multiple levels of responsiveness. The poetic analyst is primed toward *seeing a felt moment worded*, is preoccupied with what Bakhtin (1984) refers to as the "architectonics" or compositional aesthetics of a purposeful discourse in which form must become part, no, *is* an essential part of content.

Unlike literati, who are experts at twisting language this way and that, analysts are experts at noting what is left out: the omitted, disavowed, minimized, the unbidden or hidden catches our eye, providing seeds out of which the kinds of meanings that we are interested in slowly surface and unfold. We become adept at dismantling camouflage, reading and decoding qualifiers that appear spread throughout the organism including the whole paraphernalia of transient sighs, sobs, jolts, and twitches, grunts, yawns, lulls, and lilting intonations that give sense and meaning to otherwise barren communications. Meaning is our milieu: and the interpretation of many types of meaning spanning presemiotic to symbolic forms exercises polychromatic sensibilities necessitating *nonlinear* erudition that is nevertheless cognizant of the proper semiotic progression that will advance the dialogical process toward conscious awareness.

Therapeutic artistry in the interpretation of so broad a spectrum of meanings, then, rests as much on a sensitivity to the primary functional organization to which any given communication is tied as on the selection of the most appropriate type of intervention that will 1) mediate the current material toward a higher plain of semiotic organization and, hence, increasingly exact verbalization and understanding, and 2) can be heard and assimilated at this particular phase in the treatment, this moment in the hour, by this particular individual, in this particular way. To the staggering complexity of these semantic fields must be added the fact that each of the analysts' three voices orients interpretively toward a different temporal dimension and all three operate simultaneously: the voice of the healer is prospective, therapeutic, always looking forward to some potential; the constructing voice of the co-author is retrospective, investigative, summative, organizing meanings into narrative completeness; and the voice of the poet "in the service of the process," is the organic voice of the present moment, feeling, understanding, wording the unworded, transcending the unwordable, transforming isolation into dialogue.

Viewed in this way, our dialogical artistry is founded on a refinement of human responsiveness that hinges as much on *quality* of attunement as on selective, interpretive and compositional skills that come together intermittently to punctuate a discourse that is inherently consciousness-enhancing, particularly at those times when understanding and communication, insight and interpretation, converge. At these moments of "surplus vision," one sees what *is* in terms of what *was* and what could be; the aesthetic responsiveness thereby engendered is expressed in fulfilling our ethical task through the formulation of an interpretive communication that will be maximally full, highly symbolic, optimally timed and focused, the chosen utterance, inclusionary, encompassing, polyvalent, integrative.

The dynamics of such aesthetic responsiveness imply complete differentiation and participation, separateness and interpenetration, thought and feeling fused and filtered through knowledge as *psycho-logical* understanding that has been honed and particularized through the analytic labor of inquiry and insight. This molding of human responsiveness toward "seeing" and forwarding another's personal consciousness can be understood as the outcome of a creative dialogue, in the maieutic tradition, in which form and function fuse in a perfect fit; a dialogue in which the analyst, who is also an artist, will be able to bring to bear on the dialogues purpose and verbal activities *qualities* of artistry whereby the dialogical therapeutics, constructions and poetics, come together.

> *Everything* is gestation and birthing. To let each impression and each embryo of a feeling come to completion, entirely in itself, in the dark, in the unsayable, the unconscious, beyond the reach of ones own understanding, and with deep humility and patience to wait for the hour when a new clarity is born: this alone is what it means to live as an artist: in understanding as in creating. (R.M.Rilke,1986, p.23-4)

FINALE

During the course of this study I believe a number of goals have been accomplished, a summary of which follows:

1) The study effectively utilizes psychoanalytic methodology and our dialogical processes as research vehicles, culling from allied disciplines information that is relevant, even essential, to stimulate new observations while weaving the yields of their synthesis into theoretical propositions that encompass all metapsychological dimensions.

2) By making interactions and communicative processes *themselves* the focus of scrutiny and analysis, the study shifts the locus of theory onto process-phenomena that *can* be systematized along a mediational continuum, advancing our understanding of the complex functioning of pre-verbal and linguistic interactions while obviating the epistemologically flawed one- or two-person psychology arguments.

3) Because it is based on participant-observation of communicative processes from an interpenetrative-epistemological viewpoint, it continues to implement the paradigm shift begun in my 1997 developmental study of Symbolization. The situational analyses of two psychoanalytic dialogues tracing the internalization of referential activities and tri-phasic design of predictable stages in these dialogues, point to actual operative factors impacting on intrapsychic structure as the unconscious is made conscious through a psychoanalytic, interpretive prism.

4) The model's hierarchic design effectively accommodates the baffling problem of simultaneity or heterogeneity of form, along the vertical axis, as

well as the trans-formational mediations occurring in dialogical sequences over time, along the horizontal line. It provides a visual image and conceptual underpinnings for principles of attunement—or morphic matching—that lead to a bio-psychological model of psychoanalytic listening that embodies the meaning of 'meeting' analysands at their functional levels of communication. This developmental orientation toward communication is crucial in other ways: by tracing the morphological transpositions that constitute functional progressions and differentiation in ontogenesis it enables us to recognize the ways in which similar semiotic and referential progressions are recapitulated in dialogues, as well as providing insight into the phenomenological experience and degree of awareness of the speaker. This knowledge informs with respect to the kind of intervention he/she would more likely be able to hear.

5) The 'process' orientation of this study generated dialogical concepts and terms that unify principles of metatheory and practice, yielding a conceptual vocabulary of experience-near referents that can be put to use in the contextual particulars of each situation.

6) The semiotic grounding of this study introduces morphological principles of form that replace the spatial connotations of topography forcing us to examine and reexamine the mediational transformations inherent in communication and dialogues themselves, looking for answers to the important question "what *kinds* of talking cure." This study represents a first attempt to generate a typology of transmissive and communicative forms and to break down the inter- and intra-referential processes involved in working-through and psychoanalytic insight. I would emphasize again that a semiotic approach to mind is anything but capricious, seeking "the high gloss of science…" (Goldstein 1995, p.513), and I fear that it is only those who fail to grasp its importance who choose to devalue it. Rather, it is, the bedrock of our science, the only explanatory framework through which can be systematized the complexities of human meanings, interactions, responsiveness and the extraordinary dialogical activities that enable psychoanalysis to *function* as well as *classify* as a science of mind.

7) With the help of this model it may be possible to integrate phenomena of the paranormal and telepathic variety that are common occurrences in psychoanalytic practice but that have remained, for the most part, shrouded in secrecy. What has thus far received tacit acknowledgement by the field now has a contemporary scientific paradigm and an explanatory framework to legitimize it.

8) Approaching our situations as special kinds of dialogues brought me to the gateway of avenues opened up by the great vision of Mikhail Bakhtin whose formidable understanding of the power of dialogue led from the possibility of articulating the unique ethical and aesthetic dimensions of our discourse to an appreciation of how, in them, the singular fit between function, form, subject and purpose — outer speech and inner transformation — is mutually adaptive. The world of Bakhtin introduced me to the concept of *prosaics*, or "prosaic harmony" (Emerson, 1997, p. 36) described as a worded order that is "accretive and temporary," valuing "slow, open processes" and rewarding those "who are successful at developing, over time, flexible, particularized, nonrepeating relations among differentiated parts" (p.36) relations, that according to Bakhtin, are among the most fundamental to human experience.

But it is in supervision where the intricate medley of surface exchanges and rippling inter-transmissive undercurrents complicate the dynamics within these triadic fields that knowledge of communicative forms is most edifying. A primary supervisory task is to distill from an array of swiftly-passing, unevenly-organized, partly enacted and partly narrated reportorial modes, those hybrid parallel patterns that thread dynamically through both situations, while steering the dialogical process in such a way as to become a catalyst for its understanding. The task is not unlike that of the conductor who, similarly, shapes the orchestral sound so as to bring out and render the music's inherent expressiveness. Both the conductor and psychoanalytic supervisor function as guides as well as conduits in their interpretive roles; doing this well requires profound knowledge and understanding of the material and consummate skills in manipulating the medium.

One might say that music exists *in potentia* in the notes and staffs of a musical score and that it is up to the conductor's musical insight and artistry to find its vital pulse by selecting the richest, most full and fitting play of tempi, volume, color and phrasing to draw out what is inherent in the music's compositional form. To do this masterfully requires deep familiarity with all aspects of the piece and beyond that with orchestration and music in general: the conductor is aware of the tonal qualities and capabilities of each instrument and of each instrument group in relation to the others at any point in the score and knows how to titrate and balance each orchestral part in relation to the whole. The great conductor can be singled out by a capacity, through exquisite sensitivity and attention to detail, to fulfill the deepest expressive nuances seemingly emanating from within the music itself.

For the analytic supervisor, although certainly with lest rapture, the job is similar. And those familiar with an orchestral score will have recognized the visual and conceptual parallels I have been drawing between the layered instrumentation of the one, the layered communicative modes of the other, and the hierarchic design representing condensations they both share. One of the prime functions of the conductor is to balance the orchestral sound by highlighting certain instruments while subduing others. This interpretive sensibility is in part inspired by a talent we refer to as *musicality* but it also has to be supported by technical proficiency in performance as well. Similarly, the supervising analyst focuses on different aspects and facets of the clinical report responding to different levels of communication, weighing considerations of timing and relevance, tone and form. Supervisory skills have to encompass sensitivity and a capacity to assess what, at any given time, is the most immediately relevant learning issue for the supervisee and how to address it so as to advance the process. For both conductors and supervisors, their artistry is realized through the skill with which they implement their understanding of their medium and material *in process* and how effectively their interpretive activities actualize, or realize, the music's or dialogue's purpose.

Armed with a taxonomy of communicative organizations—a grammar of form — the analytic supervisor is better equipped to recognize the salient features and configurations in the report, the nature of his/her induced responses, and to weave the complex, multi-leveled web of unconscious meanings into a coherent whole. By proposing an attentional stance resonant to form and a technique attuned to the informative value of reciprocally matched modes of responsiveness, the model can become a useful instrument to appraise the functional organization and degree of awareness of the speaker. Distinguishing clearly between resonance to *form* and counter-reactivity to dynamics, the model clarifies a long standing misuse of the term "countertransference" as an umbrella for what are actually different and discrete responses to interpsychical phenomena. It seems to me that increased understanding of pre-semiotic and mediated communicative modes is essential for psychoanalysis if systematizing different forms of unconscious manifestations is to be translated into technical skill.

The theoretical and practical purpose of the model here presented is to serve as a unifying template integrating principles of semiotic progression with functional shifts in the phenomenology of experience and of how things are known through symbolization, discourse, and semantic referentiality. Implicitly it has pointed toward a psychoanalytic theory of learning providing new referents for teaching. Because principles of form are logical and observable it provides a conceptual framework that can generate research hypotheses, and for the same reasons it lends itself to future microanalysis of microgenetic progressions of interactional sequences. It offers a comprehensive, unified system of ideas to organize the interpretation of unconscious meanings through the manifest forms in which they appear. Finally, I believe it is a model that would warm Freud's heart, empiricist that he was, since he believed that the foundations of science "upon which everything rests;…is observation alone" (Freud, 1914, p. 77).

This study emerged out of my observations of the supervisory process and serves primarily as a conceptual guide to identify and name communicative configurations that replay the history and nature of unconscious internalizations. It has yielded a conceptual model that traces microgenetic shifts in communicative forms as unconscious experience and knowledge is processed consciously, a model that reveals how the voices of psyche can be seen.

CODA

It may interest the reader to know that this work has been written three times over — from start to finish. And this third writing is not merely another revision but an entirely new *version*, reformulated, reconceptualized, rearticulated — thoroughly worked through — as though the material had to be filtered by my brain many times over, sifted like sand through a sieve or the steady slow steaming of a pungent sauce, until the resulting distillate was sufficiently clear to be presented, worded, on the written page. This may not be all that remarkable to seasoned editors for whom multiple 'drafts' are commonplace, but for those of us studying our own processes in relation to subject matter, this says much about revisions and the painfully slow pace of paradigm change. In many ways I frequently felt less that I was writing this book than that the book was writing me — often I bemoaned the inadequacy of one mind to do the job. It could not have materialized had I not submitted my thinking to constant questioning by means of a dialectic within an inner dialogue, much like early philosophical and scientific writings that were written in dialogical form.

The complexity and multidimensionality of the topic, as it unfolded before me, swallowed me up daily sending me back, wordless, again and again to think, rethink and generate keener, clearer formulations for aspects of phenomena that have been largely ignored by the field, searching for a new language conceptually encompassing enough to integrate and articulate the noumena of our phenomena. Discussions begun enthusiastically, albeit naively — the questions and ideas with which I started — appeared daunting up close and the only reward for persevering was that somehow the material swept me along, seemingly by its own momentum: inch by inch formulations appeared, passages cleared. The end result is a work that does more than present a study of communication; potentially it reorients our metatheoretical purview toward phenomena that can be systematized and that are relevant for the integration of metatheory, clinical theory and practice.

Like an explorer, I have wandered uncharted territories, finding and forging pathways while examining the landscape. The lonely hike was marked by sobering setbacks and halting hurdles: rapid advances led to dead ends turning me back to go it the slow way. And, of course, at the end, the journey is not over. My writing process, I have reasoned, must itself embody some essential aspects of the material. To ease the strain, I entered more deeply into a conversation with myself coming face to face with the immense power of dialogue, even when solitary, as an instrument of reference, definition, cogitation, increased awareness and clarification. I learned that recursivity, openness and unfinalizability, three inherent qualities of dialogue, promote their own progressive processes, that dialogues garner their own semantic kinesis, impacting accretively; by their very momentum new forms of consciousness are stirred and set free. The condition is one of coming to know — by diverse means and through different channels of formulation and understanding.

It is perhaps a testament to the paradoxes of evolution and the unpredictable consequences of human pursuits that we live at a time in which far more is known about the technology for transmitting information than about the complex architecture of meanings and human communication itself. At no other time in the course of civilization has communication between people been more instantaneous, direct or continuous, or have communicative means so radically altered the multi-paletted tissue of human experience and interchange, transforming codes of discourse and relationship, transcending time and space, altering the quality of life, even the nature of reality. The entire globe is now wrapped in an "internet" which, while defying temporal and geographical boundaries and providing a mind-boggling supply of information, severely constricts the plane of interaction to a single flat verbal screen. The E-mail contact, similarly, reduces communication to a highly abbreviated linguistic code. We need no longer have contact to make contact; even intimate conversations occur between people who will never meet.

Paradoxically, the faster we can press a button or flick a switch the less effectively do we seem to be able to reach each other, to forge relationships that are likely to hold, to moderate impulse, or mediate difference by discussion rather than aggression. The interpolation of so much machinery between each other and the natural world has bred its own strains of disease. Modern "isolation" (and dissociation), the most prevalent ailments of our age, make it increasingly difficult to bridge the far more alienating distance created by the dry impersonality and sloganistic conditioning of the modern world and its symptomatic sequelae spread through our daily lives. Again, paradoxically, the more accessible communication has become the less do we seem able to do it meaningfully. Attempting to reach a person has become frustrating; an institution, futile; but try having an indepth conversation! The art of conversing *about* anything has been all but extinguished by the preponderant use of the time-pressured three millisecond utterance overwhelmingly favored by the impatient interlocutor who, were one to attempt a slightly more developed sentence, might cut you off or, worse still, put you on hold! Signals or coded signs, rather than symbols, are the median currency of exchange — heaven knows what complex consequences for the human brain this primitivization of interchange, and degradation of form, will have.

We grow accustomed to listening through clipped messages recited by sterile voices listing "menus" from which we obediently pinch our select morsels of information, raging silently at an inanimate machine for having wasted all the time it was supposed to save. Lost within these sterile techno-labyrinths, we fail to find a vital human response at the other end that could lead us out. We have become a species of information mongers, knowing more and more about less and less, oblivious to the difference between information and knowledge, digitalized data and human intelligence. The new humans are rapidly briefed into becoming the breathless button-pushing, screen-scanning, channel-switching, icon-gazing techno-puppets most fitted adaptively to our great, giant dazzling technocracy. But the loss of slow process, careful formulation, reflection, and frequent, diversely phrased and paced, face to face interchange, only reinforces a rampant collective narcissism nourished by the omnipotent control of the almighty switch that can, at will, turn you on or flick you off. We ought to be vigilant to the potentially disjunctive effects of technology on human relationships; seemingly simple habits may have deep seated and widespread impact on the human mind.

Clearly there is more to human communication than the mere transmission of information: in fact, within the woof and warp of all exchanges are embedded a blend of moral and ethical codes of conduct, national and individual personality traits, the entire lattice work of values, beliefs and principles for living that tie us to a family, a culture, and to the traditions of a particular society of which, as animals of kinship, we must feel a part. If it is to be truly human then communication must continue to encompass all of those codified, affiliative signs and gestures, subliminal cues and expressive symbols that are essential to the making of meaning and the use of communication as a means of bonding. For myself, I have grown appreciative of the privilege inherent in the daily practice of an intimate, purposeful dialogue, where unconscious meanings are of the essence. This engagement has convinced me that, more than ever, we must hold dear those venerable forms of discourse — poesis, narrative, ritual, drama, story, debate, conversation, exegesis — that continue to preserve our needs to participate and represent, to transmit, articulate, listen and respond, via personal communication.

This has been an effort in synthesis and integration and as with all such efforts the results are partial and provisional. My hope is that by continuing to use psychoanalytic methodology and psychoanalytic dialogues for research purposes it will have paved a way for others to build upon.

BIBLIOGRAPHY

I have included in this bibliography not only works cited from but also all papers and books read that I consider to be pertinent and important readings subsumed and woven through this text.

Adler, E. and Bachant, J. L., (1996), "Free Association and Analytic Neutrality: The Basic Structure of the Psychoanalytic Situation," *Journal of the American Psychoanalytic Association*, 44:1021-1046.

Allphin, C., (1987), "Perplexing or Distressing Episodes in Supervision: How they can Help in the Teaching and Learning of Psychotherapy," *Clinical Social Work Journal*, 15:236-245.

Aragno, A., (1997), "Symbolization: Proposing a Developmental Model for a New Psychoanalytic Theory of Mind," Madison, Connecticut: International Universities Press.

_______, (1998), "Die So that I May Live: A Psychoanalytic Essay on the Adolescent Girls Struggle to Delimit Her Identity," in *The Mother Daughter Relationship: Echoes Through Time*, ed. G. I. Fenchel, Northvale, NJ: Jason Aronson, pp. 85-133.

————, and Schlachet, P., (1996), "The Accessibility of Early Experience through the Language of Origin: A Theoretical Integration," *Psychoanalytic Psychology*, 13(1):23-34.

Arlow, J. (1961), "Silence and the Theory of Technique," *Journal of the American Psychoanalytic Association*, 9:44-55

_______, (1963), "The Supervisory Situation," *Journal of the American Psychoanalytic Association*, 11(3):576-594.

_______, (1969), "Fantasy, Memory and Reality Testing," *Psychoanalytic Quarterly*, 38:28-51.

_______, (1979), "The Genesis of Interpretation," *Journal of thAmerican Psychoanalytic Association*, 24 (suppl.):192-206.

_______, (1993),"Two Discussions of 'The Mind of the Analyst,'" *International Journal of Psycho-Analysis*, 74:1147-1155.

Atwood, G., and Stolorow, R., (1984), *Structures of Subjectivity*, Hillsdale, New Jersey: The Analytic Press.

Augustine, (1973), *An Augustine Reader*, Edited, with an introduction by J. J. O'Meara, Garden City, NY: Doubleday.

Austin, J., (1962), *How to do Things with Words*, Oxford: Oxford University Press.

Bachrach, H. M., (1976), "Empathy," *Archives of General Psychiatry*, 33:35-38.

Bakhtin, M. M., (1981), *The Dialogic Imagination*, Ed. M. Holquist, Austin: University of Texas Press.

_______, (1984), *Problems of Dostoyevsky's Poetics*, Ed. and Trans. C. Emerson, Minneapolis: University of Minnesota Press, Orig. Pub. in Russia, 1929.

_______, (1986), *Speech Genres and Other Late Essays*, ed. Caryl Emerson and Michael Holquist, trans. V. W. McGee, Austin: University of Texas Press.

Balter, L., Lothane, Z. and Spencer, J., (1980), "On the Analyzing Instrument," *Psychoanalytic Quarterly*, 49:474-504.

Barabasi, A.L., (2003), *Linked,* London, England: Penguin Books Ltd.,

Barratt, B. B., (1994), "Critical Notes on the Psychoanalyst's Theorizing," *Journal of the and American Psychoanalytic Association*, 42(3):697-725.

Barroso, F., Freedman, N., (1992), "The Nonverbal Manifestations of Cognitive Processes in Clinical Listening," *Journal of Psycholinguistic Research*, Vol. 21: pp. 87-110.

Barroso, F., & Freedman, N., Grand, S., & van Meel, J., (1978), "Evocation of Two Types of Hand Movements in Information Processing," *Journal of Experimental Psychology: Human Perception and Performance*, 4:2, May 1978, pp. 321-329.

Basch, M. F., (1973), "Psychoanalysis and Theory Formation," *The Annual of Psychoanalysis*, 3:3-20, New York: International Universities Press.

_______, (1976a), "The Concept of Affect: A Re-examination," *International Journal of Psychoanalysis* 24:759-777.

_______, (1976b),"Psychoanalysis and Communication Science," *Annual of Psychoanalysis*, 4:385-422.

_______, (1976c), "Theory Formation in Chapter VII," *Journal of the American Psychoanalytic Association*, 24:61-100.

_______, (1981) "Psychoanalytic Interpretation and Cognitive Transformation," *International Journal of Psychoanalysis*, 62:151-175.

_______, (1983), "Empathic Understanding: A Review of the Concept of Some Theoretical Considerations, *Journal of the American Psychoanalytic Association*, 31:101-126.

Bateson, G., (1972), *Steps to an Ecology of Mind*, New York: Balantine Books.

_______, (1979), *Mind in Nature: A Necessary Unity*, New York: E. P. Dutton.

Baudry, F., (1993), "The Personal Dimension and Management of the Supervisory Situation with a Special Note on the Parallel Process," *Psychoanalytic Quarterly*, LXII, pp. 588-614.

Beres, D., (1957), "Communication in Psychoanalysis and the Creative Process: A Paralle." *Journal of the American Psychoanalytic Association*, Vol. 5: pp. 408-423.

_______, (1968),"The Role of Empathy in Psychotherapy and Psychoanalysis," J. Hillsdale Hospital, 17:362-369.

Beres, D.,and Arlow, J. A., (1974), "Fantasy and Identification in Empathy," *Psychoanalytic Quarterly*, 43:26-50.

Bermann, L.,(1949), "Countertransference and Attitudes of the Analyst in the Therapeutic Process," *Psychiatry*, 12:159-166.

Birdwhistell, R. L., (1952), *Introduction to Kinesics*, Louisville, Kentucky: University of Louisville Press.

_______, (1970), *Kinesics and Context: Essays on Body Motion Communication*, Philadelphia: University of Pennsylvania Press.

Black, M., (1962), *Models and Metaphors: Studies in Language and Philosophy*, Ithaca: Cornell University Press.

Blakeslee, S., (1991), "Brain Yields New Clues on Its Organization for Language," *The New York Times*, Science Section, September 10, 1991, pp. 1 and 10.

Bowlby, J., (1969), "Attachment and Loss—Vol. 1," *Attachment*, New York: Basic Books.

_______, (1973), "Attachment and Loss—Vol. 2," *Separation*, New York: Basic Books.

_______, (1980), "Attachment and Loss—Vol. 3," *Loss*, New York: Basic Books.
Breuer, J. and Freud, S., (1893-1895), *Studies on Hysteria*, Standard Edition Vol. 2, pp. 1-305, London: Hogarth Press, 1955.
Brightman, B. K., (1984-85), "Narcissistic Issues in the Training Experience of the Psychotherapist," *International Journal of Psychoanalytic Psychotherapy*, 10:293-317.
Bromberg, P.,(1982), "The Supervisory Process and Parallel Process in Psychoanalysis," *Contemporary Psychoanalysis*, 18:92-111.
________, (1984), "The Third Ear," in L. Caligor, P. Bromberg and J. Meltzer (Eds.), *Clinical Perspectives on the Supervision of Psychoanalysis and Psychotherapy*, New York: Plenum Press, pp. 29-44.
Bruner, J., (1969), "Eye, Hand and Mind." In: *Studies in Cognitive Development*, ed. D. Elkind and J. H. Flavelle, New York: Oxford University Press, pp. 223-235.
________ (1983), *Child's Talk: Learning to Use Language*, New York, London: W. W. Norton & Co.
Buck, R., (1993), "What is this Thing Called Subjective Experience? Reflections on the Neuropsychology of Qualia," *Neuropsychology*, 7(4):490-499.
Buie, D. H.,(1981), "Empathy. It's Nature and Limitations," *Journal of the American Psychoanalytic Association*, 29:281-307.
Bull, P., (1983), *Body Movements and Interpersonal Communication*, New York: John Wiley & Sons.
Bullough, E., (1912), "'Psychical Distance' as a Factor in Art and as an Aesthetic Principle" in *British Journal of Psychology*, V, part II, pp. 87-118.
Burlingham, D., (1967), "Empathy Between Infant and Mother," *Journal of the American Psychoanalytic Association*, 15:764-780.
Caligor, L., (1984), "Parallel and Reciprocal Processes in Psychoanalytic Supervision," in L. Caligor, P. Bromberg and J. Meltzer (Eds.), *Clinical Perspectives on the Supervision of Psychoanalysis and Psychotherapy*, New York: Plenum Press, pp. 1-28.
Caligor, L., Bromberg, P., and Meltzer, J., eds., (1984), *Clinical*

Perspectives on the Supervision of Psychoanalysis and Psychotherapy, New York; London: Plenum Press.
Carpenter, W. B., (1874), *Principles of Mental Physiology*, 1st ed., London: H. S. King.
Cassirer, E., (1874-1945), Philosophy of Symbolic Forms, trans. W. Hendel, New Haven: Yale University Press, 1953-1957.
The Concise Oxford Dictionary, (1951), 4th Ed., Oxford: The Clarendon Press.
Creighton, J. E., (1921), "Reason and Feeling," *Philosophical Review*, XXX, 5:465-481.
Crowley, R., (1984), "Being and Doing in Continuous Consultation," in *Clinical Perspectives on the Supervision of Psychoanalysis and Psychotherapy*, Caligor, L., Bromberg, P., and Meltzer, J., eds., pp. 75-87, New York; London: Plenum Press.
Damasio, A. R., (1994), *Descartes' Error. Emotion, Reason, and the Human Brain*, New York: Grosset/G. P. Putnam & Sons.
Darwin, C., (1872), *The Expression of the Emotions in Man and Animals*, New York: D. Appleton & Co., 1899 ed.
Davies, P. C. W., (1984), *Superforce*, London: Heinemann.
DeBell, D. F., (1963), "A Critical Digest of the Literature on Psychoanalytic Supervision," *Journal of the American Psychoanalytic Association*, 11:546-575.
DeBel, D., (1981), "Supervisory Styles and Positions," in *Becoming a Psychoanalyst*, Wallerstein, R. S., ed., Madison, Connecticut: International Universities Press.
Derrida, J., (1980), "The Law of Genre," in *On Narrative*, W. S. T. Mitchell, ed., Chicago, London: University of Chicago Press 1980, pp. 51-77.
Descartes, R., (1955), *The Philosophical Works of Descartes—Vol. 1*, Trans. L. S. Haldane and G. R. T. Ross, New York: Dover.
Deutsch, F.,(1947), "Analysis of Postural Behavior,"*Psychoanalytic Quarterly*, 16:195-213.
________,(1952), "Analytic Posturology," *Psychoanalytic Quarterly*, 21:196-214.
Deutsch, F., & Madler, R. A., (1975), "Empathy: Historic and Current

Conceptualizations, Measurement and a Cognitive Theoretical Perspective," *Human Development*, 18:267-287.
Deutsch, H., (1926), "Occult Processes Occurring During Psychoanalysis," in *Psychoanalysis and the Occult*, ed. G. Devereux, New York: International Universities Press, 1970, pp. 133-146.
Dewald, P. A., (1981), "Aspects of the Supervisory Process," *The Annual of Psychoanalysis*, IX:75-89.
Dilthey, W., (1976), *Selected Writings*, Ed. and Introduced by H. P. Rickman, London: Cambridge University Press, first published 1883-1911.
Doerhman, M., (1976), "Parallel Processes in Supervision and Psychotherapy," *Bulletin of the Menninger Clinic*, 40:9-83.
Dorpat, T., (1992), "The Primary Process Revisited" in Dorpat, T., and Miller, M., (1992), *Clinical Interaction and the Analysis of Meaning: A New Psychoanalytic Theory*, pp. 29-58, Hillsdale, New Jersey, London: The Analytic Press.
Easser, B.R. (1974) "Empathic Inhibition and Psychoanalytic Technique," *Psychoanalytic Quarterly*, 43:557-580.
Eckstein, R., and Wallerstein, R. (1972), *The Teaching and Learning of Psychotherapy*, Second Edition, New York: International Universities Press.
Edelson, M., (1975), *Language and Interpretation in Psychoanalysis*, Chicago, London: The University of Chicago Press.
Eichle, S., (1995), "Freud in America," *Journal of the American Psychoanalytic Association*, 43(3):835-851.
Ekman, P., (1973), "Cross Cultural Studies of Facial Expression," in P. Ekman (ed.), *Darwin and Facial Expression*, pp. 169-223, New York: Academic Press.
________, (1977), "Biological and Cultural Contributions to Body and Facial Movement," in J. Blacking (ed.), *Anthropology of the Body*, pp. 39-84, London: Academic Press.
Ekman, P. and Freisen, W. V., (1969), "The Repertoire of Non-Verbal Behavior: Categories, Origins, Usage and Coding," *Semiotica*: 1:49-98.
________, (1974) "Detecting Deception from the Body or Face," *Journal of Personality and Social Psychology*, 29:288-298.
Ekman, P. and Oster, H. (1979) "Facial Expression of Emotion," *Annual Review of Psychology*, 30:527-555.

Emde, R. N., (1990), "Mobilizing Fundamental Modes of Development: Empathic Availability and Therapeutic Action," *Journal of the American Psychoanalytic Association*, 38(4):881-913.

Emerson, C., (1997), *The First Hundred Years of Mikhail Bakhtin*, Princeton, NJ: Princeton Universities Press.

Epstein, L., and Feiner, A. H., (1979),"Countertransference: The Therapist's Contribution to Treatment," *Contemporary Psychoanalysis*, 13:1-15.

_______, (1979), *Countertransference: The Therapists Contribution to Treatment*, New York: Jason Aronson, Inc.

Escalona, S., (1953), "Emotional Development in the First Year of Life," in *Problems of Infancy and Childhood*, ed. Milton J. E. Senn. Transactions of the Sixth Conference, March 17-18, 1952. New York. Sponsored by J. Macy, Jr. Foundation. 16 West 46th Street, New York 10036, pp. 11-92.

Feiner, K., and Kiersky, S., (1994), "Empathy. A Common Ground," *Psychoanalytic Dialogues*, 4(3):425-440.

Fenichel, O., (1934), "Defense Against Anxiety, Particularly by Libidinization," in *Collected Papers*, 1:303-317, New York: Norton, 1953.

_______, (1945), *The Psychoanalytic Theory of Neuroses*, New York: Norton.Ferenczi, S., (1914), "On Embarrassed Hands," in *Further Contributions to the Technique and Theory of Psychoanalysis*, London: Hogarth Press 1926, pp. 315-316.

________, (1919), "Thinking and Muscle Innervation," in *The Theory and Technique of Psychoanalysis II*, New York: Basic Books 1953.

Fliess, R., (1942), "The Metapsychology of the Analyst," *Psychoanalytic Quarterly*, 11:211-227.

Fleming, J. and Benedeck, T. F., (1966), *Psychoanalytic Supervision. A Method of Clinical Teaching*, New York: Grune and Stratton, Inc.

Fosshage, J., (1995), "Countertransference as the Analyst's Experience of the Analysand: Influence of Listening Perspectives," *Psychoanalytic Psychology*, 12(3):375-391.

Frank, G., (1998), "The Psychoanalytic Process: The Search for Common Ground" *Psychoanalytic Psychology*, 15(2):296-304.

_______, (2000), "The Status of Psychoanalytic Theory Today, There is an

Elephant," *Psychoanalytic Psychology*, 17(1):174-179.
Freedman, N., (1971), "The Analysis of Movement Behavior During the Clinical Interview," in *Studies in Dyadic Communication*, ed. A. Siegman and B. Pope, New York: Pergamon Press, pp. 153-175.
Freedman, N., Barroso, F., Bucci, W., and Grand, S., (1978), "The Bodily Manifestations of Listening," *Psychoanalysis and Contemporary Thought*, 1:157-194.
Freedman, N., and Hoffman, S. P., (1967), "Kinetic Behavior in Altered Clinical States: An Approach to the Objective Analysis of Motor Behavior During Clinical Interviews," *Perceptual and Motor Skills*, 24:525-539.
Freedman, N. & Lavender, J., (1997), "On Receiving the Patient's Transference: The Symbolizing and Desymbolizing Countertransference" in *Journal of the American Psychoanalytic Association*, 45(1):79-103.
Freedman, N., O'Hanlon, J., Oltman, P. & Witkin, H. A.,(1972), "The Imprint of Psychological Differentiation on Kinetic Behavior in Varying Communicative Contexts," *Journal of Abnormal Psychology*, 79:239-258.
Freedman, N., Blass, T., Rifkin, A. & Quitkin, F., (1973) "Body Movements and the Verbal Encoding of Aggressive Affect," *J. Pers. Soc. Psch.*, 26:72-85.
Freedman, N., and Steingart, I., (1975) "Kinesic Internalization and Language Construction," *Psychoanalysis. Contemporary Science*, 4:355-404.
Freedman, N., & Grand, S., (1984), "Shielding: An Associative Organizer," in G. Stricker & R. H. Keisner (Eds.), *From Research to Clinical Practice*, pp. 353-374, New York: Plenum Press.
Freedman, N. and Berzofsky, M., (1995), "Shape of the Communicated Transference in Difficult and Not So Difficult Patients. Symbolized and Desymbolized Transference," *Psychoanalytic Psychology*, 112:363-374.
Freud, A., (1936), *The Ego and the Mechanisms of Defense*, New York: International Universities Press (1946).
Freud, S., (1900), *The Interpretation of Dreams*, Standard Edition Vol. 4-5, London: Hogarth Press, 1953.
_______, (1904), *Freud's Psychoanalytic Procedure*, Standard Edition, Vol. VII, London: Hogarth Press, 1953, pp. 247-254,

_______, (1905), *Jokes and Their Relation to the Unconscious*, Standard Edition, Vol. 8, pp. 1-236, London: Hogarth Press, 1960.
_______, (1906), *Delusions and Dreams in Jensen's Gradiva*, Standard Edition, Vol. 9, pp. 1-96, London: Hogarth Press, 1959.
_______, (1911), *Formulations Regarding the Two Principles of Mental Functioning*, Standard Edition, Vol. 12, London: Hogarth Press, 1958, pp. 215-226.
_______, (1912), *Recommendations to Physicians Practicing Psycho Analysis*, Standard Edition Vol. 12, London: Hogarth Press 1958, pp. 111-120.
_______, (1913a), *On Beginning the Treatment: Further Recommendations in the Technique of Psychoanalysis*, Standard Edition, Vol. 12, London: Hogarth Press 1958, pp. 121-144.
_______, (1913b), *On Psycho-Analysis*, Standard Edition, Vol. 12, London: Hogarth Press, 1958, pp. 207-211.
_______, (1913c), *The Claims of Psychoanalysis to Scientific Interest*, Standard Edition Vol. 13, pp. 163-190, London: Hogarth Press, 1955.
_______, (1914a), *Remembering, Repeating and Working Through*, Standard Edition, Vol. 12, London: Hogarth Press 1958, pp. 147-156.
_______, (1914b), *Observations on Transference Love (Further Recommendations on the Technique of Psychoanalysis) III*, Standard Edition Vol. 13, pp. 159-171, London: Hogarth Press 1958.
________, (1914c), "On Narcissism," Standard Edition Vol. 14, pp. 77-, London: Hogarth Press, 1957.
_______, (1914d), *History of the Psychoanalytic Movement*, Standard Edition Vol. 14, pp. 7-66, London: Hogarth Press, 1957.
_______, (1915), *The Unconscious*, Standard Edition Vol. 14, pp. 161-215, London: Hogarth Press, 1957.
_______, (1916), "Parapraxes," Standard Edition Vol. 15, pp. 60-79, London: Hogarth Press, 1963.
_______, (1917), *Introductory Lectures on Psychoanalysis*, Standard Edition Vol. 15-16, London: Hogarth Press, 1963.
_______, (1918), *From the History of an Infantile Neurosis*, Standard Edition Vol. 17, pp. 1-122, London: Hogarth Press, 1955.
_______, (1921), "Group Psychology and the Analysis of the Ego,"

Standard Edition Vol. 18, pp. 69-143, London: Hogarth Press, 1955.
_______, (1923), "The Ego and the Id," Standard Edition Vol. 9, pp. 19-27, London: Hogarth Press 1961.
_______, (1925), "Joseph Breuer," G. S., 11, 281; G. W., 14, 562 (XXVIII).
[Trans. *International Journal of Psychoanalysis*; 6,459: Standard Ed. 19] London: Hogarth Press 1955.
_______, (1926), "The Question of Lay Analysis," Standard Edition Vol. 20:177-250, London: Hogarth Press, 1959.
_______, (1932), "New Introductory Lectures on Psychoanalysis," editors and translated by James Strachey, New York: Norton, 1965.
_______, (1933), *Dreams and Occultism*, "New Introductory Lectures on Psycho-Analysis," Standard Edition Vol. 22, London: Hogarth Press 1964, pp. 31-56.
________, (1937), *Analysis Terminable and Interminable*, Standard Edition Vol. 23, pp. 209-253, London: Hogarth Press, 1964.
_______, (1940), *An Outline of Psycho Analysis*, Standard Edition Vol. 23, pp. 141-207, London: Hogarth Press, 1964.
Freud, S. and Breuer, J., (1893-1895), *Studies on Hysteria*, Standard Edition, Vol. II, London: Hogarth Press 1955, pp. 1-305.
Fromm, G., (1995), "What Does *Borderline* Mean?" *Psychoanalytic Psychology*, 12(2):233-245.
Furer, M., (1967) "Some Developmental Aspects of the Superego," *International Journal of Psychoanalysis*, 48:277-280.
Furth, H. G., (1970), "On Language and Knowing in Piaget's Developmental Theory," *Human Development*, 13:241-257.
Gal'perin, P. Ya, (1969), "Stages in the Development of Mental Acts" in M. Cole and I. Maltzman, eds., *A Handbook of Contemporary Soviet Psychology*, New York: Basic Books.
Gardner, H., (1982), *Art, Mind and Brain*, New York: Basic Books.
_______, (1983), *Frames of Mind*, New York: Basic Books.
Gediman, H., and Wolkenfeld, F., (1980), "The Parallelism Phenomenon in Psychoanalysis and Supervision: Its Reconsideration as a Triadic System," *Psychoanalytic Quarterly*, 49:234-254.
Gedo, J., (1979), *Beyond Interpretation: Toward a Revised Theory for Psychoanalysis*, New York: International Universities Press.

_______, (1988), *The Mind in Disorder*, Hillsdale, NJ: Analytic Press.

_______, (1990), "Position Statement on the Training Analysis Question," in *Tradition & Innovation in Psychoanalytic Education*, Hillsdale, New Jersey: Clark Conference on Psychoanalytic Training for Psychologists, Hove and London Lawrence Erlbaum Associates Publishers, pp. 125-129.

_______, (1993), "On Fastball Pitching, Astronomical Clocks, and Self-Cognition," in *Self-Analysis*, ed. J. Barron, Hillsdale, New Jersey: Analytic Press, pp. 133-146.

_______, (1995), "Working Through as a Metaphor and as a Modality of Treatment," *Journal of the American Psychoanalytic Association*, 43(2) pp. 339-356.

_______, (1997), "Reflections on Metapsychology, Theoretical Coherence, Hermeneutics, and Biology," *Journal of the American Psychoanalytic Association*, 45(3):779-806.

Gedo, P., & Pollock, G., (Eds.), (1976), *Freud: The Fusion of Science and Humanism*, New York: International Universities Press.

Gedo, J. and Goldberg, A., (1979), *Models of the Mind: A Psychoanalytic Theory*, Chicago and London: The University of Chicago Press.

Gibson, J. J., (1966), *The Senses Considered as Perceptual Systems*, Boston: Houghton-Mifflin.

_______, (1979), *The Ecological Approach to Visual Perception*, Boston: Houghton-Mifflin.

Gill, M., (1994), *Psychoanalysis in Transition. A Personal View.*, Hillsdale, NJ, London: The Analytic Press.

Goldstien, R. G., (1995), "The Higher and Lower in Mental Life: An Essay on J. Hughlings Jackson and Freud," *Journal of the Psychoanalytic Association*, 43(2) pp. 495-515.

Gombrich, E. H., (1961), *Art and Illusion: A Study in the Psychology of Pictorial Representation*, 2nd ed., rev. Princeton: Princeton University Press.

Goodman, N., (1978), *Ways of World Making*, Indianapolis: Hackett Publishing Co.

_______, (1980), "Twisted Tales; Or Story, Study and Symphony," in *On Narrative,* ed. W. J. T. Mitchell (1980), London, Chicago: The University of Chicago Press, pp. 99-115.

_______, (1984), *Of Mind and Other Matters*, Cambridge, MA ,
London, England: Harvard University Press.
Gostynski, E., (1951), "A Clinical Contribution to the Analysis of Gestures," *International Journal of Psychoanalysis*, 32:310-318.
Greenacre, P., (1954), "The Role of Transference," *Journal of the American Psychoanalytic Association*, 2:671-684.
Greenson, R., (1960), "Empathy and Its Vicissitudes," *International Journal of Psychoanalysis*, 41:418-424.
_______, (1961), "On the Silence and Sounds of the Analytic Hour," *Journal of the American Psychoanalytic Association*, 9:79-84.
_______, (1965), "The Working Alliance and the Transference Neurosis," *Psychoanalytic Quarterly*, 343:155-181.
_______, (1967), *The Technique and Practice of Psychoanalysis*, Vol. I, New York: International Universities Press.
_______, (1971), "The Real Relationship Between the Patient and the Psychoanalyst," in *The Unconscious Today*, ed. M. Kanzer, New York: International Universities Press, pp. 213-232.
Greenspan, S. I., (1975), "A Consideration of Some Learning Variables in the Context of Psychoanalytic Theory: Toward a Psychoanalytic Learning Perspective," (Psychological Issues Monogram 33), New York: International Universities Press.
________, (1982), "Three Levels of Learning: A Developmental Approach to 'Awareness' and Mind-Body Relations," *Psychoanalytic Inquiry*, 1(4):659-694.
_______, (1989), *The Development of the Ego Implications for Personality Theory, Psychopathology, and the Psychotherapeutic Process*, Madison, Connecticut: International Universities Press.
_______, (1996), *Developmentally Based Psychotherapy*, Madison, Connecticut: International Universities Press.
Greimas, A. J., (1976), "The Cognitive Dimension of Narrative Discourse," in *New Literary History*, Vol. VII, No. 3, Spring 1976.
Grinberg, L., (1990), "Theory of Identification," in *The Goals of Psychoanalysis*, London, New York: Karnac, pp. 83-97.
_______, (1991), "Countertransference and Projective Counteridentification in Nonverbal Communications," in *Psychoanalysis in Europe*, European Psychological Federation Bulletin: 36, pp. 11-23.

_______, (1995), "Nonverbal Communication in the Clinic with Borderline Patients," *Contemporary Psychoanalysis*: 31, 1, January 1995, pp. 92-105.

Guthrie, W. K. C., (1960), *The Greek Philosophers from Thales to Aristotle*, New York: Harper and Rowe.

Hall, E. T., (1959), *The Silent Language*, New York: Fawcett World Library 1965.

_______, (1966), *The Hidden Dimension*, New York: Anchor Book Edition 1969.

Hanson, N. R., (1958), *Patterns of Discovery: An Inquiry into the Conceptual Foundations of Science*, Cambridge: Cambridge University Press.

Hanson, J. H., (1977), "René Descartes and the Dream of Reason," in *The Narcissistic Condition*, ed. Marie Coleman Nelson, New York: Human Sciences Press.

Hartmann, H., (1964), "Understanding and Explanation," in *Essays on Ego Psychology*, New York: International Universities Press, pp. 369-403.

Hayes, G. E., (1994), "Empathy. A Conceptual and Clinical Deconstruction," *Psychoanalytic Dialogues*, 4(3):409-424.

Heimann, P., (1950) "On Countertransference," *International Journal of Psychoanalysis*, 31:81-84.

Hill, L., (1958) "On Being Rather Than Doing in Psychotherapy," *International Journal of Group Psychotherapy*, 8:1-9.

Hoffman, M. L., (1978), "Toward a Theory of Empathic Arousal and Development," in *The Development of Affect: Genesis of Behavior*, Vol. 1, ed. M. Lewis and L. E. Rosenblum, New York: Plenum Press.

Holquist, M., and Emerson, C., (1981), Glossary. In Bakhtin (1981).

Holzkamp, K., (1956) "Ausdrucksverstehen als Phänomen, Funktion und Leistung," in *Yahrbuch für Psychologie und Psychotherapie*, IV (1956) pp. 297-323.

Horowitz, M. J., (1972) "Modes of Representation of Thought," *Journal of the American Psychoanalytic Association*, 20:793-819.

Hutten, F., (1981), "Meaning and Information in Group Process," in *The Evolution of Group Analysis*, ed. M. Pines, London: Routledge, Kegan Paul.

Il'enkov, E. V., (1977), *Dialectical Logic: Essays on its History and Theory*, Moscow: Progress Publications.

Izard, C. E. and Tomkins, S. S., (1966), "Affect and Behavior: Anxiety as a Negative Affect," in C. D. Spielberger (ed.), *Anxiety and Behavior*, pp. 81-125, New York: Academic Press.

Izard, C. E., (1971), *The Face of Emotion*, New York: Appleton Century-Croft.

_______, (1977), *Human Emotions*, New York: Plenum Press.

Jacobs, A., (1958), *A New Dictionary of Music*, Harmondsworth: Middlesex, Penguin Books Ltd.

Jacobs, T., (1993), "The Inner Experiences of the Analyst: Their Contributions to the Analytic Process," *International Journal of Psychoanalysis*, 74:7-14.

Jacobson, J. G., (1994), "Signal Affects and Our Psychoanalytic Confusion of Tongues," *Journal of the American Psychoanalytic Association*, 42(1):15-42.

Jameson, F., (1981), *The Political Unconscious: Narrative as a Socially Symbolic Act*, Ithaca: New York, 1981.

Jung, C. G., (1971), *The Portable Jung*, trans. R. F. C. Hull, New York: The Viking Press Inc.

Kagan, J., (1984), *The Nature of the Child*, New York: Basic Books.

Kaplan, B., and Wapner, S., (1981), Foreword to Schafer's 1981 "Narrative Actions in Psychoanalysis," Heinz Werner Lecture Series, Vol. XIV, Worcester, Mass.: Clark University Press.

Katz, A. G., (1998), "Where the Action Is: The Enacted Dimension of Analytic Process," *Journal of the American Psychoanalytic Association*, 46(4):1129-1167.

Keeney, B., (1982), "What is an Epistemology of Family Therapy?" *Family Process*, 21(2):153-168.

Kermode, F., (1980), "Secrets and Narrative Sequence," in *On Narrative*, ed. W. J. T. Mitchell (1980), London, Chicago: The University of Chicago Press, pp. 79-97.

Kern, J. W., (1995), "On Focused Association and the Analytic Surface: Clinical Opportunities in Resolving Analytic Stalemate," *Journal of the American Psychoanalytic Association*, 43(2) pp. 393-422.

Kernberg, O., (1975), *Borderline Conditions and Pathological Narcissism*, New York: Jason Aronson, Inc.
_______, (1984), *Severe Personality Disorders*, New Haven: Yale University Press.
Kestenberg, J., (1975), *Children and Parents: Pscyhoanalytic Studies in Development*, New York: Jason Aronson.
Kohut, H. (1959) "Introspection, Empathy and Psychoanalysis," *Journal of the American Psychoanalytic Association*, 7:459-483.
_______ (1966) "Forms and Transformations of Narcissism," *Journal of the American Psychoanalytic Association*, 14:243-272.
_______ (1971) *The Analysis of the Self*, New York: International Universities Press.
_______ (1977) *The Restoration of the Self*, New York: International Universities Press.
Knoblauch, S. H., (1996), "The Role of the Analysts Questions," *Psychologist Psychoanalyst*, Vol. 16(3):14.
Krause, R., (1995), Book Review: *Affect, Imagery, Consciousness: Vol. 3. The Negative Affects: Fear and Anger*, Tomkins, S. S., (1991) in *Journal of the American Psychoanalytic Association*, 43(3):929-938.
Kris, E., (1952), *Psychoanalytic Explorations in Art*, New York: International Universities Press.
Kubie, L. S., (1953), "The Distortion of the Symbolic Process in Neurosis and Psychosis," in *Symbols and Neurons*, Monogram 36, Psychological Issues 19, New York: New York University Press 1978.
_______, (1958), "Research Into the Process of Supervision in Psychoanalysis."
Psychoanalytic Quarterly, 27:226-236.
Kuhn, T. S., (1962), *The Structure of Scientific Revolutions*, London, Chicago: The University of Chicago Press.
Landauder, K., (1938), "Affects, Passions and Temperament," in *International Journal of Psychoanalysis*, 19:388-415.
Langer, S. K., (1942), *Philosophy in a New Key*, Cambridge, MA: Harvard University Press.
_______, (1953), *Feeling and Form*, New York: Scribner.
_______, (1957), *Problems of Art*, New York: Scribner.

_______, (1962), *Philosophical Sketches*, Baltimore: John Hopkins Universities Press.
_______, (1967), *Mind: An Essay on Human Feeling*, Vol. 1, Baltimore and London: Johns Hopkins University Press.
_______, (1972), *Mind: An Essay on Human Feeling*, Vol. II, Baltimore, MD: John Hopkins Universities Press.
_______, (1982), *Mind: An Essay on Human Feeling*, Vol. III, Baltimore, MD: John Hopkins Universities Press.
Langs, R., (1976), *The Bipersonal Field*, New York: Jason Aranson.
_______, (1994), "Combining Supervision with Empowered Psychotherapy," *Contemporary Psychoanalysis*, Vol. 30(1):25-47.
Lashley, E., (1938), "Cerebral Organization and Behavior," in *The Brain and Human Behavior*, ed. H. C. Solomon, et al, Baltimore: William & Wilkins, pp. 1-18.
Levenson, E. A., (1994), "The Uses of Disorder: Chaos Theory and Psychoanalysis," *Contemporary Psychoanalysis*, Vol. 30(1):5-24.
Levi-Strauss, C., (1964), *The Raw and Cooked*, New York: Harper Torchbook, 1970.
Lichtenberg, J., Lachmann, F., and Fosshage, J., (1992), *Self and Motivational Systems: Toward a Theory of Technique*, Hillsdale, New Jersey: The Analytic Press.
Little, M. I. (1951), "Countertransference and the Patient's Response to It,' *International Journal of Psychoanalysis*, 32:32-40.
Loewald, H., (1960), "On the Therapeutic Action of Psychoanalysis," in *Papers on Psycho-Analysis*, New Haven, London: Yale University Press, 1980, pp. 221-256.
_______, (1962), "Internalization, Separation, Mourning and the Superego, in *Papers on Psycho-Analysis*, New Haven, London: Yale University Press, 1980, pp. 257-276.
_______, (1970), "Psychoanalytic Theory and the Psychoanalytic Process," *The Psychoanalytic Study of the Child*, Vol. XXV, pp. 45-68.
_______, (1970), "Psychoanalytic Theory and the Psychoanalytic Process," in *Papers on Psycho-Analysis*, New Haven, London: Yale University Press, 1980, pp. 277-301.
_______, (1971), "On Motivation and Instinct Theory," in *Papers on*

Psycho-Analysis, New Haven, London: Yale University Press, 1980, pp. 102-137.

_______, (1973), "Some Considerations on Repetition and Repetition Compulsion," in *Papers on Psycho-Analysis*, New Haven, London: Yale University Press, 1980, pp. 87-101.

_______, (1973), "On Internalization," in *Papers on Psycho-Analysis*, New Haven, London: Yale University Press, 1980, pp. 69-86.

_______, (1975), "Psychoanalysis as an Art and the Fantasy Character of the Psychoanalytic Situation," in *Papers on Psycho-analysis*, New Haven, London: Yale University Press 1980, pp. 352-371.

_______, (1978a), "Primary Process, Secondary Process and Language," in *Papers on Psycho-Analysis*, New Haven, London: Yale University Press, 1980, pp. 178-193.

_______, (1978b), "Instinct Theory, Object Relation and Psychic Structure Formation," in *Papers on Psycho-Analysis*, New Haven, London: Yale University Press, 1980, pp. 207-218.

_______, (1979), "Reflections on the Psychoanalytic Process and Its Therapeutic Potential," in *Papers on Psycho-Analysis*, New Haven, London: Yale University Press, 1980, pp. 372-383.

_______, (1988), *Sublimation: Inquiries into Theoretical Psychoanalysis*, New Haven, London: Yale University Press.

Lorenz, M., (1953), "Language as Expressive Behavior," *A.M.A. Archive Neurol and Psychiatry*, 70.

Luber, P., (1991), "A Patient's Transference to the Analyst Supervisor: Effect of the Setting on the Analytic Process," *Journal of the American Psychoanalytic Association*, 39(3), pp. 705-725.

Mackay, D. M., (1969), *Information, Mechanism and Meaning*, Cambridge, MA: M.I.T. Press.

Mahl, C., (1977), "Body Movement, Ideation and Verbalization during Psychoanalysis," in *Communication Structures and Psychic Structures*, ed. N. Freedman, S. Grand, New York: Plenum, pp. 291-310.

Mahler, M., Pine, F., & Bergman, A., (1975), *The Psychological Birth of the Human Infant: Symbiosis and Individuation*, New York: Basic Books.

Major, M. and Miller, P., (1984), "Empathy, Antipathy and Telepathy in the

Analytic Hour" in *Empathy*, Vol. II, ed. J. Lichtenberg, et al. Hillsdale, New Jersey: Analytic Press, pp. 227-249.
Makari, G. and Shapiro, T., (1993), "On Psychoanalytic Listening: Language and Unconscious Communication," *Journal of the American Psychoanalytic Association*, 41(4):991-1021.
Malcove, L., (1975), "The Analytic Situation: Toward a View of the Supervisory Experience," *Journal of the Philadelphia Association of Psychoanalysis*, II:1-19.
Marshack, A., (1972), *The Roots of Civilization*, New York: McGraw-Hill.
_______, (1989), "Evolution of Human Capacity: The Symbolic Evidence," *Yearbook of Physical Anthropology*, Yearbook Series Vol. 32, pp. 1-34.
Masson, S. M., Trans. & Ed., (1985), *The Complete Letters of Sigmund Freud to Wilhelm Fliess 1887-1904*, Cambridge, Massachusetts; London, England: The Belknap of Harvard University Press.
Maturana, H., and Varela, F., (1980), *Autopoesis and Cognition: The Realization of the Living*, Dordrecht, Holland, D. Reidl.
McCullogh, W., (1965), *Embodiments of Mind*, Cambridge, Mass., M.I.T. Press.
Meisels, M. & Shapiro, E.R., Eds., (1990), *Tradition & Innovation in Psychoanalytic Education*, Hillsdale, NJ: Clark Conference on Psychoanalytic Training for Psychologists, Hove and London Lawrence Erlbaum Associates Publishers.
Meissner, W. W. S., (1996), *The Therapeutic Alliance*, New Haven: Yale University Press.
_______, (1998), "Neutrality, Abstinance and the Therapeutic Alliance," *Journal of the American Psychoanalytic Association*, 46(4):1089-1128.
Mink, L.O., (1972), "Interpretation and Narrative Understanding," in *The Journal of Philosophy*, 1969, pp. 735-737.
_______, (1978), "Narrative Form as a Cognitive Instrument in the Writing of History," *Literary Form and Historical Understanding*, ed. Robert H. Canary and Henry Kozicki, Madison, Wisconsin, 1978.
_______, (1980), "Every Man His or Her Own Annalist," in *On Narrative,* ed. W. J. T. Mitchell (1980), London, Chicago: The University of Chicago Press, pp. 233-239.

Moore, B. E., and Fine, B. D., Eds., (1968), *A Glossary of Psychoanalytic Terms and Concepts*, Second Edition, New York: American Psychoanalytic Association.

Morris, D., (1967), *The Naked Ape*, New York: Dell Publishing Company.

_______ (1978), *Manwatching*, Triad/Grenada.

New York Psychoanalytic Institute, (1963), *Minutes of the Faculty Meeting*, October 14, 1963. Unpublished.

New York Psychoanalytic Institute, (1957), *Minutes of the Curriculum Committee Meeting on "Problems of Supervision,"* November 6, 1957. Unpublished.

New York Psychoanalytic Institute (1963), *Minutes of the Faculty Meeting*, November 20, 1963. Unpublished.

Ogden, T. H. (1979) "On Projective Identification," *International Journal of Psychoanalysis*, 60:357-373.

Olden, C., (1953), "On Adult Empathy with Children," *The Psychoanalytic Study of the Child*, Vol. 8:111-126, New York: International Universities Press.

_______, (1958), "Notes on the Development of Empathy," *The Psychoanalytic Study of the Child*, Vol. XIII, pp. 505-518.

Olds, D. D(2000) "A Semiotic Model of Mind." *Journal of the American Psychoanalytic Association*, vol. 48,(2); 497 -529.

Ornstein, P. H., (1967), "Selected Problems in Learning How to Analyze," *International Journal of Psychoanalysis*, 48:448-461.

_______, (1979), "Remarks on the Central Position of Empathy in Psychoanalysis," *Bulletin of the Association of Psychoanalytic Medicine*, 18:95-108.

Person, Ethel Spector, (1989), "Plagiarism and Parallel Process: Two Maladaptive Forms of Cultural (or Interpersonal) Transmission," in *Psychoanalysis: Toward the Second Century*, Eds. A. M. Cooper, O. F. Kernberg, Ethel Spector Person, New Haven, London: Yale University Press 1989, pp. 52-69.

Peterfreund, E., (1971) *Information, Systems and Psychoanalysis*, New York: International Universities Press.

_______ (1973) "On Information Processing Models for Mental Phenomena," in *International Journal of Psychoanalysis*, 54:351-357.

_______ (1975) "The Need for a New General Theoretical Frame of Reference for Psychoanalysis," *Psychoanalytic Quarterly* 44:534-549.

_______ (1975) "How Does the Analyst Listen? On Models and Strategies in the Psychoanalytic Process," *Psychoanalysis and Contemporary Science*, 4:459-101, New York: International Universities Press.

_______ (1980) "On Information and Systems Models for Psychoanalysis," *International Review of Psychoanalysis*, 7:327 345.

Philips, D. C., (1987), *Philosophy, Science and Social Inquiry*, Oxford, NY: Pergammon Press.

Piaget, J., (1923), *Language and Thought of the Child*, New York: Meridian, 1955.

_______, (1936), *The Origins of Intelligence in Children*, New York: International Universities Press (1952).

_______, (1937), *The Construction of Reality in the Child*, London: Rutledge, Kegan, Paul.

_______, (1962), *Play, Dreams and Imitation in Childhood*, trans. C. Gattegno and F. M. Hodgson, New York, London: W. W. Norton & Company.

_______, (1970), *Genetic Epistemology*, New York: Columbia University Press.

Piaget, J. and Inhelder, B., (1969), *The Psychology of the Child*, New York: Basic Books.

Pierce, C. S., (1893-1910), *Philosophical Writings of Pierce*, ed. J. Buchler, New York: Dover 1955.

_______, (1931-1935), *Collected Papers of Charles Sanders Pierce*, Ed. C. Hortshorne and P. Weiss, Cambridge, Mass.: Harvard University Press.

Piers, G. and Piers, M. W., (1964), "Modes of Learning and the Analytic Process," *Sixth International Congress of Psychotherapy*, London, 1964, Selected Lectures, pp. 104-110, S. Karger Basel, New York, 1965.

_______, (1965),"Modes of Learning and the Analytic Process," in *Proceeds of the Sixth International Congress of Psychotherapy*, London; Basel: Kayer.

Plutchick, R., (1980), *Emotions: A Psychoevolutionary Synthesis*, New York: Harper & Row.

_______, (1984), "Emotions: A General Psychoevolutionary Theory," in *Approaches to Emotions*, eds. K. R. Scherer, P. Ekman, Hillsdale, NJ: Lawrence Erlbaum Associates, Inc.

Plutchick, R. and Kellerman, H. eds., (1980), *Emotions: Theory, Research and Experience*, New York: Academic Press.

Polanyi, M., (1964), *Personal Knowledge*, New York: Harper & Row.

Post, S. L., (1980) "Origins, Elements and Functions of Therapeutic Empathy," *International Journal of Psychoanalysis*, 61:277-293.

Pribram, K. H., (1971), *Languages of the Brain*, Englewood Cliffs, NJ: Prentice-Hall.

Propp, V., (1968), *Morphology of the Folk Tale*, Austin, Texas: University of Texas Press.

Quine, W. V. O., (1973), *The Roots of Reference*, LaSalle, IL: Open Court Publishing.

Racker, H., (1957) "The Meaning and Uses of Countertransference," *Psychoanalytic Quarterly*, 26:303-357.

_______, (1968) *Transference and Countertransference*, London: Maresfield Library.

Rangell, Leo, (2000) "Psychoanalysis at the Millenium: A Unitary Theory," *Psychoanalytic Psychology*, 17(3):451-466.

Rapaport, D., (1940) *Emotions and Memory*, 3rd ed., NY: International Universities Press, 1950.

_______, (1941) Book Review: Heinz Werner, *Comparative Psychology of Mental Development (1941)* in *The Collected Papers of David Rapaport,* ed. M. M. Gill, New York, London: Basic Books, Inc., (1967), pp. 74-79.

_______, (1942) "The History of the Awakening of Insight" in *The Collected Papers of David Rapaport,* ed. M. M. Gill, New York, London: Basic Books, Inc., (1967), pp. 100-112.

_______, (1944), "The Scientific Methodology of Psychoanalysis" in *The Collected Papers of David Rapaport*, ed. M. M. Gill, New York, London: Basic Books, Inc., (1967), pp. 165-220.

_______, (1951a), "The Conceptual Model of Psychoanalysis" in *The Collected Papers of David Rapaport,* ed. M. M. Gill, New York, London: Basic Books, Inc., (1967), pp. 405-431.

_______, (1951b), "Interpersonal Relationships, Communication and Psychodynamics" in *The Collected Papers of David Rapaport,* ed. M. M. Gill, New York, London: Basic Books, Inc., (1967), pp. 440-449.
_______, (1953), "On the Psychoanalytic Theory of Affects" in *The Collected Papers of David Rapaport,* ed. M. M. Gill, New York, London: Basic Books, Inc., (1967), pp. 476-512.
_______, (1959), "The Theory of Attention Cathexis: An Economic and Structural Attempt at the Explanation of Cognitive Processes" in *The Collected Papers of David Rapaport,* ed. M. M. Gill, New York, London: Basic Books, Inc., (1967), pp. 778-794.
_______, (1960a), "Psychoanalysis as a Developmental Psychology" in *The Collected Papers of David Rapaport,* ed. M. M. Gill, New York, London: Basic Books, Inc., (1967), pp. 820-852.
_______, (1960b), *The Structure of Psychoanalytic Theory — A Systematizing Attempt*, New York:International Universities Press.
Rapaport, D. and Gill, M., (1959/1996), "Points of View and Assumptions of Metapsychology," in *The Collected Papers of David Rapaport*, Northvale, NJ, London: Jason Aronson Inc., pp. 795-811.
Reed, G., (1995), "Relativism and Clinical Truth" *Journal of the American Psychoanalytic Association*, 43(3):713-739.
Reich, A., (1951), *On Countertransference. Psychoanalytic Contributions*, New York: International Universities Press, 1973, pp. 136-154.
_______, (1973), "Empathy and Countertransference (1966)," *Psycho-Analytic Contributions*, New York: International Universities Press, 1973, pp. 344-360.
Reich, W., (1933), *Character Analysis*, New York: Orgone Institute Press, 1945.
Reik, T., (1948), *Listening with the Third Ear. The Inner Experience of the Psychoanalyst.* New York: Farrar, Strauss & Company.
Rilke, R. R., (1986), *Letters to a Young Poet*, translated by Stephen Mitchell, Vintage Books Edition, Div. of Random House: New York.
Ricoeur, P., (1984), "Narrative Time," in *On Narrative*, ed. W. J. T. Mitchell (1980), London, Chicago: The University of Chicago Press, pp. 165-186.
Rommetveit, R., (1974), *On Message Structure: A Framework for the Study of Language and Communication*, New York: Wiley.

_______, (1979a), *On Meanings of Situations and Social Control of Such Meaning in Human Communication*, Paper presented at the Symposium on The Situation in Psychological Theory and Research: Stockholm (in Wertsch).

_______, (1979b) *The Role of Language in the Creation and Transmission of Social Representations*, University of Oslo, Typescript (in Wertsch).

Russell, B., (1910/1953) "Knowledge by Acquaintance and Knowledge by Description," in *Mysticism and Logic and Other Essays*: Melbourne, London, Baltimore: Penguin Books, pp. 197-218.

_______ (1912), *Problems of Philosophy*, New York: Oxford University Press.

_______ (1914b/1953), "On Scientific Method in Philosophy," in *Mysticism and Logic and Other Essays*: Melbourne, London, Baltimore: Penguin Books, pp. 95-119.

_______, (1914c/1953), "The Relation of Sense-Data to Physics," in *Mysticism and Logic and Other Essays*: Melbourne, London, Baltimore: Penguin Books, pp. 139-170.

_______, (1915/1953), "The Ultimate Constituents of Matter," in *Mysticism and Logic and Other Essays*: Melbourne, London, Baltimore: Penguin Books, pp. 120-138.

Rycroft, C., (1956), "Symbolism and its Relationship to the Primary and Secondary Processes," *International Journal of Psychoanalysis*, 37:137-146.

_______ 1958) "An Enquiry into the Function of Words in the Psychoanalytic Situation," *International Journal of Psychoanalysis*, 39:408-415.

Sachs, D.M., and Shapiro, S. H., (1976), "On Parallel Process in Therapy and Teaching," *Psychoanalytic Quarterly*, 45:394-415.

Sandler, J. (1976)"Countertransference and Role-responsiveness," *International Journal of Psychoanalysis*, 3:4-47.

_______, (1992) "Reflections on Developments in the Theory of Psychoanalytic Technique," *International Journal of Psychoanalysis*, 73:189-198.

_______ (1993), "On Communication from Patient to Analyst: Not

Everything is Projective Identification," *International Journal of Psychoanalysis*, 74:1097-1107.
Sawyier, F. H. (1975) "A Conceptual Analysis of Empathy," *Annual of Psychoanalysis*, No. 3:37-47.
Schafer, R.(1959), "Generative Empathy in the Treatment Situation," *Psychoanalytic Quarterly*, 28:342-373.
_______ (1968), *Aspects of Internalization*, New York: International Universities Press.
_______ (1976), *A New Language for Psycho-analysis*, New Haven, London: Yale University Press.
_______ (1980) "Narration in the Psychoanalytic Dialogue," in *On Narrative,* ed. W. J. T. Mitchell (1980), London, Chicago: The University of Chicago Press, pp. 25-49.
_______ (1981) "Narrative Actions in Psychoanalysis," Vol. XIV, 1980, Heinz Werner Lecture Series, Worcester: Mass.: Clark University Press, pp. 1-58.
_______, (1983), *The Analytic Attitude*, New York: Basic Books, Inc.
Schaughnessy, P. (1995), "Empathy and the Working Alliance: The Mistranslation of Freud's *Einfühlung*," *Psychoanalytic Psychology*, 12(2):221-231.
Scheflin, A. E.,(1963), "Communication and Regulation in Psychotherapy," *Psychiatry*, 26:126-136.
_______ (1968), "Quasi-Courtship Behavior in Psychotherapy," *Psychiatry*, 28:245-257.
Schilder, P. (1924), *Medical Psychology*, ed. tr. D. Rapaport, New York: International Universities Press, 1953.
Schlessinger, H. J. (1981), "General Principles of Supervision," in *Becoming a Psychoanalyst*, Wallerstein, R. S., ed., Madison, Connecticut: International Universities Press.
_______ (1990), "Supervision and the Training Analysis: Repetition or Collaboration?" in *Tradition and Innovation in Psychoanalytic Education*, ed. M. Meisels and E. E. Shapiro, pp. 135-140.
_______ (1995), "The Process of Interpretation and the Moment of Change," *Journal of the American Psychoanalytic Association*, 43(3):663-688.

Scholes, R., (1980), 'Language, Narrative, and Anti-Narrative," in *On Narrative,* ed. W. J. T. Mitchell (1980), London, Chicago: The University of Chicago Press, pp. 200-208.

Schön, D. A., (1986), "Making Meaning. An Exploration of Artistry in Psychoanalysis," *Annual of Psychoanalysis*, Vol. 14, pp. 301-316.

Schore, A. N., (1996), "The Experience-Dependant Maturation of a Regulatory System in the Orbital Prefrontal Cortex and the Origin of Developmental Psychopathology," *Development and Psychopathology*, 8:59-87.

_______ (1997a), "Interdisciplinary Developmental Research as a Source of Clinical Models," in *The Neurobiological and Developmental Basis for Psychotherapeutic Intervention*, ed. M. Moskowitz, C. Monk, C. Kaye, S. J. Ellman, New Jersey & London: Jason Aronson, pp. 2-71.

_______ (1997b), "A Century After Freud's Project: Is a Rapprochement Between Psychoanalysis and Neurobiology at Hand?" *Journal of the American Psychoanalytic Association*, 45(3):807-840.

Schwaber, E. A., (1984), "Empathy: A Mode of Psychoanalytic Listening," in *Empathy*, Vol. II, ed. J. Lichtenberg, et al. Hillsdale, New Jersey: Analytic Press, pp. 143-185.

_______ (1986), "Reconstruction and Perceptual Experience: Further Thoughts on Psychoanalytic Listening," *Journal of the American Psychoanalytic Association*, 34:911-932.

Searles, H. (1955) "The Informational Value of the Supervisor's Emotional Experiences," in *Collected Papers on Schizophrenia and Related Subjects*, 1965, New York: International Universities Press, pp. 157-176.

_______ (1962), "The Differentiation Between Concrete and Metaphorical Thinking in the Recovering Schizophrenic Patient,' *Journal of the American Psychoanalytic Association*, 10 pp. 22-42.

_______ (1965) *Collected Papers on Schizophrenia and Related Subjects*, New York: International Universities Press.

_______ (1979), "The Countertransference With the Borderline Patient," in *Advances in Psychotherapy of the Borderline Patient*, ed. J. LeBoit and A. Capponi, New York: Jason Aronson, pp. 309-346.

Shapiro, T.(1974) "The Development and Distortion of Empathy," *Psychoanalytic Quarterly*, 43:4-25.

_______ (1970) "Interpretation and Naming," *Journal of the American Psychoanalytic Association*, 18:399-421.
_______ (1979), *Clinical Psycholinguistics*, New York: Plenum Press.
_______ (1981), "Empathy: A Critical Reevaluation," *Psychoanalytic Inquiry*, 1:423-448.
_______, (1986), "Sign, Symbol and Structural Theory," *Psychoanalysis: The Science of Mental Conflict*, Hillsdale, NJ: Analytic Press.
_______, (1988), *Language, Structure and Psychoanalysis*, Madison, CT: International Universities Press.
_______, (1991), "Words and Feelings in the Psychoanalytic Dialogue," *Journal of the American Psychoanalytic Association*, 39(supplement):321-348.
Sharpe, E. F., (1940), "Psycho-Physical Problems Revealed in Language: An Examination of Metaphor," in *Collected Papers on Psycho-Analysis*: London: Hogarth Press 1950, pp. 155-169.
Sheldrake, R., (1981), *A New Science of Life: The Hypothesis of Formative Causation*, New Edition London: Blond and Briggs, 1985.
_______, (1988) *The Presence of the Past: Morphic Resonance and the Habits of Nature*, London: Collins.
_______, (1991) *The Rebirth of Nature*, Rochester, VT: Park Street Press.
Shevrin, H., (1978) "Semblance of Feeling in the Imagery of Affect in Empathy, Dreams and Unconscious Processes — A Revision of Freud's Several Affect Theories," in *The Human Mind Revisited*, ed. S. Smith, New York: International Universities Press, pp. 263-294.
Siegler, A., (1990), "Finding Ones Voice in the Analytic Chorus: Some Thoughts About Psychoanalytic Education," in *Tradition & Innovation in Psychoanalytic Education*, Hillsdale, NJ: Clark Conference on Psychoanalytic Training for Psychologists, Hove and London Lawrence Erlbaum Associates Publishers, pp. 141-146.
Smith Herrnstein, B., (1980), "Narrative Versions, Narrative Theories," in *On Narrative,* ed. W.
J. T. Mitchell (1980), London, Chicago: The University of Chicago Press, pp. 209-232.
Spence, D., (1982), *Narrative Truth and Historical Truth*, New York, London: W. W. Norton & Company.

Spence, D. P., Mayes, L. C., Dahl, M., (1994), "Monitoring the Analytic Surface," *Journal of the American Psychoanalytic Association*, 42(1):43-64.

Spotnitz, H., (1979), "Narcissistic Countertransference," in *Countertransference: The Therapist's Contribution to Treatment*, Eds. L. Epstein and A. H. Feiner, New York: Jason Aranson.

_______, (1985), *Modern Psychoanalysis of the Schizophrenic Patient—Theory of a Technique*, Human Science Press Inc., 72 Fifth Avenue, New York, NY 10011.

Springman, R.R. (1986) "Countertransference: Clarifications in Supervision," *Contemporary Psychoanalysis*, Vol. 22, 2:252-277.

Sterba, R. (1934), "The Fate of the Ego in Analytic Therapy," *International Journal of Psychoanalysis*, 15:117-126.

Stern, D. (1985), *The Interpersonal World of the Infant*, New York: Basic Books.

Stolorow. R. and Atwood G.E. (1992), *Contexts of Being. The Intersubjective Foundations of Psychological Life*, Hillsdale, NJ, London: The Analytic Press.

Stone, L., (1954), "The Widening Scope of Indications for Psychoanalysis," *Journal of the American Psychoanalytic Association*, 2:565-620.

_______, (1961), *The Psychoanalytic Situation*, New York International Universities Press.

Tarnas, R (1991), *The Passion of the Western Mind, Understanding the Ideas that have Shaped Our World View*, New York; Ballantine Books.

Thompson, D'Arcy, (1942), *On Growth and Form*, 2nd Ed.: 2 Vols., 1st Ed., 1917, Cambridge: University Press, 1942.

Teitelbaum, S., (1990), "Supertransference: The Role of the Supervisor's Blind Spots," *Psychoanalytic Psychology*, 7(2):243-258.

Tomkins, S. S., (1962), *Affects, Imagery, Consciousness Vol. 1—The Positive Affects*, New York: Springer.

_______, (1963), *Affects, Imagery, Consciousness Vol. 2—The Negative Affects*, New York: Springer.

_______, (1970), "Affects as the Primary Motivational System," in *Feelings and Emotions*, ed. M. B. Arnold, New York: Academic Press, pp. 101-110.

_______, (1992), *Affect Imagery, Consciousness Vol. 4*, New York, Springer.
Tower, L. E., (1956), "Countertransference," *Journal of the American Psychoanalytic Association*, 4:224-255.
Turner, V., (1974), *Dramas, Fields and Metaphors: Symbolic Action in Human Society*, Ithaca; London: Cornell University Press.
_______, (1980), "Social Dramas and Stories About Them," in *On Narrative,* ed. W. J. T. Mitchell (1980), London, Chicago: The University of Chicago Press, pp. 137-164.
_______, (1982), *From Ritual to Theatre: The Human Seriousness of Play*, New York: PAJ Publications.
Tyler, R., (1974), "Coper Commission 1," *The Tripartite System of Psychoanalytic Education*, New York: American Psychoanalytic Association.
Van Gennep, A., (1909/1960), *The Rite of Passage*, trans. M. Vizedom and G. Caffee, London: Routledge, Kegan Paul.
Viderman, S., (1979), "The Analytic Space: Meaning and Problems," *Psychoanalytic Quarterly*, 48:257-291.
Volkelt, J., (1920), *Das Aesthetische Bewusstsein; Prinzipienfragen der Aesthetik*, Munich: Beck.
Von Bertalanffy, L., (1968), *General Systems Theory*, New York: Balantine.
Vygotsky, L., (1934), *Thinking and Speech: Psychological Investigations*, Moscow and Leningrad: Gosudarstvennoe Sotial'no. Ekonomicheskoe Isdalatel'stvo.
_______, (1960), *Razvitic vysshykh psikhicheskikh funktsii (The Development of Higher Mental Functions)*, Moscow: Izdatel'stvo Academi Pedagogicheskikh Nauk.
_______, (1977), *From the Notebooks of L. S. Vygotsky*, Moscow University Record: Psychology Series 15:89-95.
_______, (1978), *Mind in Society: The Development of Higher Psychological Processes*, ed. M. Cole, V. John-Steiner, S. Scribner, and E. Souberman, Cambridge, MA: Harvard University Press.
_______, (1981a/1985), "The Instrumental Method in Psychology," in Wertsch (1995), *Vygotsky and the Social Formation of Mind*,

Cambridge, MA, London, England: Harvard University Press.
Watzlawick,P Beavin,J.and Jackson,D. (1967), *Pragmatics of Human Communication*, New York, Norton.
Webster's New World Dictionary, (1966), Cleveland and New York: The World Publishing Company.
Webster's Third New International Dictionary of the English Language, Unabridged, (1971), Vol. III, Chicago, William Burton Ed.
Werner, H. and Kaplan, B., (1963), *Symbol Formation*, New York: J. Wiley, 1967 Edition.
Wertsch, J. V. (1985), *Vygotsky and the Social Formation of Mind*, Cambridge, MA, London, England: Harvard University Press.
_______, (1991), *Voices of the Mind*, Cambridge, MA: Harvard University Press.
Westrup, J. A., and Harrison, F. W., eds. (1959), *Collins Music Encyclopedia*, London and Glasgow: William Collins & Sons, Ltd., 1959 ed.
White, H., (1980a), "The Value of Narrativity in the Representation of Reality," in *On Narrative,* ed. W. J. T. Mitchell (1980), London, Chicago: The University of Chicago Press, pp. 1-23.
_______, (1980b), "The Narratization of Real Events," in *On Narrative,* ed. W. J. T. Mitchell (1980), London, Chicago: The University of Chicago Press, pp. 249-254.
Whitehead, A. N., (1927), *Symbolism. Its Meaning and Effect*, New York: Fordham University Press.
Wilson, O. E., (1978) *On Human Nature*, Cambridge, Massachusetts. London, England: Harvard University Press
Whyte, L. L., (1960), *The Unconscious Before Freud*, New York: Basic Books.
Wilson, A., (1995), "Mapping the Mind in Relational Psychoanalysis: Some Critiques, Questions and Conjectures." In *Psychoanalytic Psychology*, 12(1):9-29.
Wilson, A. and Weinstein, L., (1992), "An Investigation into Some Implications of a Vygotskian Perspective on the Origins of Mind: Psychoanalysis and Vygotskian Psychology, Part 1," *Journal of the American Psychoanalytic Association*, 40(2):349-379.

_______, (1992), "Language and the Pscyhoanalytic Process: Psychoanalysis and Vygotskian Psychology, Part 2," *Journal of the American Psychoanalytic Association*, 40(3):725-759.
_______, (1996), "The Transference and the Zone of Proximal Development," *Journal of the American Psychoanalytic Association*, 44:167-200.
Winnicott, W. D., (1947), "Hate in the Countertransference," in *Through Paediatrics to Psycho-Analysis*, London: Hogarth Press, pp. 194-203.
_______, (1960), "Counter-transference," *British Journal of Medical Psychology*, 33:17-21.
Winson, J., (1986), *Brain and Psyche*, New York: Vintage Books.
Wittgenstein, L., (1922/1961), *Tractatus Logico-Philosophicus*, trans. D. F. Pearce and B. F. McGuiness, London: Rutledge & Kegan Paul.
_______, (1953), *Philosophical Investigations*, Oxford: Blackwell.
Yakubinskii, L. P., (1923), *On Dialogic Speech*, Petrograd: Trudy Foneticheskogo Instituta Prakticheskogo Izucheniya Yazkov.
Zeligs, M. A., (1961), "The Psychology of Silence: Its Role in Transference, Countertransference and the Psychoanalytic Process," *Journal of the American Psychoanalytic Association*, 9:7-43.
Zetzel, E. R., (1956), "The Concept of Transference," in *The Capacity for Emotional Growth*, New York: International Universities Press, 1970, pp. 168-181.
Zinchenko, V. P., and Davidov, V. V., (1985), Forward in Wertsch (1985), *Vygotsky and the Social Formation of Mind*, Cambridge, Mass.; London, England: Harvard University Press.

ENDNOTES

[1] It ought to be pointed out that Freud's topographical ideas had much to recommend them by way of unification; he himself recognized the theoretical lacunae, later to be filled by Piaget, when he wrote "Our psychical topography has *for the present* nothing to do with anatomy; it has reference not to anatomical localities but to regions in the mental apparatus, wherever they may be situated in the body." (1915, p. 175)

[2] The intrinsic value for psychological integration of 'talking out" rather than "acting out" can be logically demonstrated according to principles of symbolization that are corroborated by the functional anatomy of brain circuitry and the effects on it of symbolic mediation. In the psychoanalytic process, the translation of sense-abstractions into verbal form *transforms* the nature of meanings as well as the organic impact they have upon us.

[3] Piaget's genetic epistemology, a developmental theory of cognition, notoriously underplays this crucial *affective* dimension of sensorimotor intelligence.

[4] In my vernacular this is also a *formal* transposition; hence functional/form designates psychic *organization*, in the old topographical sense, and is observably manifest in the *form* of communication.

[5] See Loewald (1979/80) particularly p. 379 where he writes: "Unless the analyst grasps that he is, on the now pertinent level of the patients mental functioning, drawn into this undifferentiated force field, he will not be able to interpret adequately the transference meanings of the patients communications. To do so, he has to be in touch with that mental level in himself, a level on which for him, too, the distance and separateness between himself and the patient are reduced or suspended."

[6] Since the first writing of this essay (1996) it has come to my attention that J. Gedo (1996) also used this title for a section in his "Languages of Psychoanalysis." Any overlap in content is purely coincidental.

[7] Only Freud attempted such comprehensive integration — albeit with the aid of metaphors and analogies — and even he, in his great wisdom, openly declared that his was not yet a theory at all but a first stock taking of the data of observation (1940, p. 18).

8 Bromberg (1982) and others have turned to Grinberg's (1962) notion of "projective counter-identification" (p. 236) to define the reciprocal processes and multiple role switching (Caligor, 1981) that has been observed in supervisory contexts. Many others, in line with Searles (1955), Greenson (1960) and Arlow (1963), consider the same interpenetrative phenomena to be a result of oscillations in stance between transitory empathic identification and objective observation "The supervisor observes, participates, and observes once again," writes Arlow (1963, p. 587) acting like the analyst in the "psychoanalysis of a psychoanalysis" (p.587). It is my preference to view these intertransmissive phenomena, in accordance with the framework of this model, as evidence of the enduring presence in human interchange of less differentiated modes of communication and unmediated sensibilities that are identified in psychoanalytic situations and brought into the dialogue by virtue of our semantic and referential spread, particularly so in supervision, where they are part of the supervisory learning experience.

9 Loewald (1975/1980) expressed very similar ideas : "In one sense of art, psychoanalytic *technique* may be called the art of applying psychoanalytic knowledge and the psychoanalytic method to a particular clinical case. Perhaps the latter, the method of investigation and interpretation, may more specifically be called an art (a skill), whereas the body of psychoanalytic observation and theory — the science of psychoanalysis — is made use of in this art." (p. 353)

10 It is my hope that through this contribution cross-fertilized by similar ideas issuing from other quarters that Freud's much maligned and misunderstood principles of neutrality and abstinence will be reconsidered for their obvious aesthetic *and* ethical value.

11 See The Psychoanalytic Semantic (Second Movement) in which I distinguish between the following eight referential perspectives and different types of resistances tied to each; 1) the unrepresented distant past; 2) the unrepresented recent past; 3) the dynamically repressed (the dynamic unconscious); 4) the creative unconscious (dreams, slips of the tongue, etc.); 5) the archetypal unconscious; 6) internalized early interactions; 7) psychological defenses; 8) thought processes. The five metapsychological dimensions are: the topographical, the dynamic, the genetic, the economic, and the adaptive.

12 This musical term is a particularly apt analogy for this form of human sensibility: it was a type of base-line written for a keyboard instrument playing an accompaniment or

participating in an ensemble. Given a single base note, players had to work out independently the correct harmonics to play above this note. To *play the continua* then is to interpret and play the correct harmonics above this particular kind of base. (A New Dictionary of Music, 1958, p. 82)

Printed in the United States
128491LV00002B/25/P

9 781606 103555